Anxiety Disorders and Related Conditions

Christos Charis • Georgia Panayiotou
Editors

Anxiety Disorders and Related Conditions

Conceptualization and Treatment from Psychodynamic and Cognitive Behavioral Perspectives

Springer

Editors
Christos Charis
Private Practice for Psychotherapy
Dillenburg, Hessen, Germany

Georgia Panayiotou
Department of Psychology & Center
for Applied Neuroscience
University of Cyprus
Nicosia, Cyprus

ISBN 978-3-031-56797-1 ISBN 978-3-031-56798-8 (eBook)
https://doi.org/10.1007/978-3-031-56798-8

This Springer imprint is published by the registered company Springer Nature Switzerland AG
The registered company address is: Gewerbestrasse 11, 6330 Cham, Switzerland

Paper in this product is recyclable.

Introduction to the Volume

The main purpose of the volume is to instigate a dialog between the psychoanalytic and the cognitive-behavioral traditions on conceptualization and treatment of anxiety disorders and related conditions through contributions of respective experts. It presents current findings and current theories and conceptualizations with regard to the mechanisms of etiology and maintenance of anxiety and related conditions, as well as innovative, new, or experimental approaches to treatment that target core difficulties found in patients with anxiety. The book integrates basic research with conceptualization and treatment, while giving space for multiple perspectives to treatment. Both psychotherapeutic and pharmacological treatments as well as basic behavioral and neurosciene research are being described. Chapters include (a) conceptualization and treatment of anxiety and panic from psychodynamic perspectives, (b) 2nd wave CBT treatment and the use of virtual reality, (c) 3rd wave perspectives, (d) neuroendocrine factors, and (e) pharmacotherapy perspectives. Wherever possible, case studies were included. Different theoretical approaches are presented highlighting the strengths and the evidence in favor of each approach, with an effort to highlight common underlying themes like safety behaviors and avoidance, social support, and role of learning history. In this way, the book presents a combination of theory, science, and practice aiming to be an excellent resource for researchers, clinicians, and students of mental health professions.

Contents

Functional Analysis Case Conceptualization and Acceptance and Commitment Therapy for the Treatment of Anxiety-Related and Rumination Problems

Maria Karekla and Katerina Georgiou

Acceptance and Commitment Therapy (ACT) Applied to Anxiety Problems

Acceptance and commitment therapy (ACT; Hayes et al. 1999) is a process-based third-wave cognitive-behavior therapy (Hayes 2004). What differentiates ACT from other third-wave approaches is the philosophical and theoretical framework underlying it (McCracken and Vowles 2014). ACT is rooted in functional contextualism (FC; Hayes et al. 1988) and relational frame theory (RFT; Hayes et al. 2001). Functional contextualism as a philosophical framework which explains psychological events as interactions between individuals and their contexts and posits that each behavior (internal or external) however maladaptive or problematic may have at some point or in some context served a function for the person (Hayes 2004). The theoretical framework behind ACT is RFT, which presents that learning can occur verbally via rules and relations among cues including verbally constructed arbitrary cues (Hayes 2004). For example, a person may learn to fear an animal they have never encountered or had direct experience with, just because somewhere in the person's history, someone may have verbally expressed that this animal was dangerous and something to be feared.

In contrast to other therapeutic approaches, ACT acknowledges the omnipresence of hardships and does not aim to decrease pain or other emotions, symptoms, or thoughts or bring about "positive" internal experiences (Eifert and Forsyth 2005, p. 28). In other words, ACT rejects the assumption of "healthy normality" and rests on the notion that typical psychological processes may become destructive and create psychological suffering when applied inflexibly and incongruently to the specific context (Harris 2006). The focus of ACT is instead on fostering acceptance

M. Karekla (✉) · K. Georgiou
Department of Psychology, University of Cyprus, Nicosia, Cyprus
e-mail: karekla.maria@ucy.ac.cy

C. Charis, G. Panayiotou (eds.), *Anxiety Disorders and Related Conditions*,
https://doi.org/10.1007/978-3-031-56798-8_1

toward all psychological events, detangling from such events (e.g., what may be considered negative thoughts and emotions), and promotes committed action in line with one's values (Zhang et al. 2018). Subsequently, the main aim of ACT is to increase psychological flexibility (PF; Hayes et al. 2011), which refers to an array of inter-personal and intra-personal skills (Gloster and Karekla 2020) and has been conceptualized as the skill to identify and adjust to situations, adapt mindsets or behaviors to facilitate personal and social functioning, preserve balance in personally important domains of life and approach values-congruent behaviors with awareness openness and commitment (Kashdan and Rottenberg 2010). PF is comprised of six core inter-related processes which we will discuss below and include experiential acceptance, cognitive defusion, contact with the present moment, self-as-context, values clarification, and values-committed action (Hayes et al. 2012b). PF is thought to have a flip side of contextual inflexibility or rigidity considered to contribute to problems and psychopathology. Psychological inflexibility involves behaviors guided by internal experiences and avoidance of such experiences (experiential avoidance and cognitive fusion) at the cost of living in the present with self-awareness and values-based actions (Levin et al. 2014).

Experiential avoidance refers to the unwillingness to stay in contact with internal experiences such as thoughts, feelings, and bodily sensations (Hayes et al. 2004) at all cost, even when fighting to control or get rid of these experiences causes long-term problems in the persons' life (Hayes-Skelton and Eustis 2020). It is important to note that experiential avoidance has an evolutionary function which facilitates adaptation to environmental challenges (e.g., running away when faced with a life-threatening situation such as an encounter with a bear; Dinis et al. 2015). Experiential avoidance thus becomes problematic when it becomes the "go-to" coping technique irrespective of context and especially when engaging in it contributes to problems. *Experiential acceptance*, a flexible and functional responding based on the context at hand, is proposed as the antidote to experiential avoidance in ACT (Zacharia and Karekla 2021). This involves actively approaching and being open to all internal experiences, without seeking to modify their frequency or form (Hayes et al. 2006). Experiential acceptance must not be confused with passive resignation (Eifert and Forsyth 2005). Rather, through acceptance, both positive and negative aspects of internal experience are acknowledged, and the person then chooses actions to take in line with their values (Hulbert-Williams et al. 2015). Within the context of anxiety, ACT aims to help clients accept all internal experiences, especially those considered "negative or unwanted" such as fear, worry, elevated heart rate, and intrusive thoughts. The person learns that rather than attempting to avoid them at all cost, they can recognize them for what they are and instead be guided toward living the life they want (Eifert and Forsyth 2005 in Berman et al. 2010).

Cognitive fusion refers to a process where the person intertwines private events or internal experiences with behavior, whereby actions are driven by these internal experiences (Ruiz et al. 2017; Noureen and Malik 2021). For example, a person may think that when their heart beats fast, something is wrong with them and as such they avoid attending a social event so as not to have this unwanted thought and associated symptom. Cognitive fusion is targeted within ACT with *cognitive defusion*, which involves experiencing internal events as they are (i.e., a thought is just a though), rather than believing what the mind says they are (i.e., something dangerous or tragic; Eifert et al. 2009; Twohig and Levin 2017). When working with clients suffering from anxiety problems, cognitive defusion techniques aid the person to not respond to the literality of their thoughts and instead view their thoughts from a different perspective or create distance between the person and the thought through language (i.e., my fast heart beat means that I am having a heart attack vs. *I have the thought* that I am having a heart attack due to my heart beating fast).

Engaging in experiential avoidance and cognitive fusion tends to lead to the person predominantly leaving in the past or to a catastrophic future at the expense of being aware of the present and living in the moment (Zacharia and Karekla 2021). The counter or therapeutic process is *contact with the present moment or present moment awareness* and refers to experiencing and responding to both private and public events as they occur in the here-and-now (Twohig 2012). Mindfulness exercises are utilized to promote present moment awareness (Hayes et al. 2012a).

Attachment to a conceptualized self refers to the self-narrative used to describe oneself (Hayes et al. 2012a, b). This self-narrative involves fused and evaluative accounts about the self, focusing on the content of this narrative and defined by these events (Hayes et al. 2013). On the contrary, *self-as-context* within ACT refers to defining oneself as a person who notices thoughts, feelings, and experiences (Flaxman et al. 2011) and recognizes that who we are is more than a simple compilation of our thoughts, stories, and feelings. For example, the person learns to regard themselves as more than any thought or label they have been telling themselves (e.g., I am socially anxious as opposed to I am a person who experiences anxious thoughts and feelings when faced with a social encounter). In treatment, work conducted toward self-as-context involves disentangling from the evaluative accounts of the self and achieving a different perspective (Twohig and Levin 2017) while adopting a compassionate stance toward the self and lived-experiences (Karekla and Kelly 2022).

Values are viewed as one's desires in life which act as forms of positive reinforcement (Blackledge and Barnes-Holmes 2009). Within the context of ACT, values and goals are differentiated (Wilson et al. 2010). Goals are conceptualized as consequences of an action which can be achieved and has an end point, whereas values are chosen qualities of action which can never be completed, but the person can always strive toward living in accordance to them (Chase et al. 2013). For example, a person who values being a supportive friend can always strive for more actions to live with this stated value and avoiding attending a social event with their friend because of anxiety would be incongruent to living with this value. Attending one party with a friend is a goal that is in line with this value. Once attended, it is not finished however. There will continue to be subsequent opportunities for the person to engage in activities in line with the value of being a supportive friend. Often, clients with anxiety difficulties realize that their efforts to control anxiety-related experiences stand in the way of living in harmony with their values (Eifert et al. 2009). Clarifying what is of importance to the person can bring meaning into action to be taken even if anxiety shows up in the prospect of engaging in these actions

(Karekla et al. 2019a; Karekla and Kelly 2022). Thus, *values clarification* can serve to motivate individuals to engage in previously avoided situations and therapeutically lead to exposure and new learning to occur.

When *actions are inconsistent with values*, behavioral repertoires become restricted (Karekla et al. 2018) leading to inflexible behavioral patterns (Hayes et al. 2006). *Committed action* in ACT refers to behavior which leads to effective action in line with one's personal values (Hayes et al. 2012a, b; Moran 2015). Thus, following values clarification, the person comes into contact with their behavioral choices, coined as a "choice moment" (see Karekla and Kelly 2022). Individuals are encouraged at each moment to consider what is of value to them and to choose actions that lead them toward living their lives in accordance with their values. So, if going to a party serves the value of connection with others and friendship, the person chooses to go to the party even if anxious thoughts and feelings appear.

Briefly, ACT conceptualization of anxiety problems is that they arise from six processes: (1) unwillingness to experience private events (thoughts, emotions, memories) associated with anxiety; (2) normal anxiety-related experiences are viewed as health threats; (3) attempts to control such experiences; (4) escape or avoidance strategies to control anxiety-related experiences; (5) reinforcement of avoidance and control strategies as they work in the short term; and (6) patterns of psychological and behavioral inflexibility due to escape/avoidance responses (Orsillo et al. 2005). Intervention then focuses on each of these, and utilizing the tenets of ACT attempts to reverse these (considered psychological inflexibility processes) and achieve psychological flexibility and values-committed actions.

Why ACT for Anxiety?

ACT has demonstrated promising results regarding the management of several psychological conditions, including anxiety problems (Forman et al. 2007; Hancock et al. 2018; Ruiz et al. 2020; Caletti et al. 2022; Larsson et al. 2022). Specifically, evidence suggests that ACT is efficacious for the treatment of anxiety difficulties in clinical and non-clinical populations, regardless of format, individual, or group (Swain et al. 2013). Moreover, ACT is associated with decreased rates of treatment dropout or dropouts for non-treatment-related reasons (Ferreira et al. 2022; Karekla et al. 2019b) and is effective even for clients deemed to be treatment-resistant when treated with other types of therapies (Gloster et al. 2015).

ACT is a scalable approach concerning the format, number, and length of therapeutic sessions (Fashler et al. 2018). That is, it is flexible and adaptable to the needs and severity of the clients' difficulties and allows for learning and practicing its tenets through metaphors and experiential exercises (Zacharia and Karekla 2021). Additionally, since values-clarification and values-based living hold a central role within the ACT framework, values can be a motivator for change not only during therapy but also for maintaining treatment gains after therapy (Arch and Craske 2008).

Experiential avoidance, a key target within ACT, is a well-known contributor to anxiety pathology genesis (Berman et al. 2010; Panayiotou et al. 2014b) and maintenance (Panayiotou et al. 2014a). Those who suffer from anxiety difficulties, in their effort to avoid anxiety-related internal events, employ escape or avoidance strategies as part of the evolutionary process of the fight or flight response. However, when avoidance is applied inflexibly irrespective of context and long-term consequences, they are responsible for the development and maintenance of anxiety (Hayes et al. 1996; Panayiotou et al. 2014a). Excessive reliance on experiential avoidance for managing stress is also implicated in the gender differences common in anxiety problems (Panayiotou et al. 2017).

The use of ACT in treating anxiety has produced similar results to other active psychotherapy approaches (Bluett et al. 2014; Gloster et al. 2020). For example, it has shown reduction in experiential avoidance at a greater level in comparison to cognitive behavioral therapy (CBT), in individuals with social anxiety disorder (Niles et al. 2014) and panic disorder (Karekla 2004; Levitt and Karekla 2005). When comparing ACT to CBT for individuals with mixed anxiety disorders, ACT demonstrated higher improvement in psychological flexibility (Arch et al. 2012). Although evidence suggests that ACT demonstrates similar results regarding treatment effectiveness and efficacy to other active psychotherapeutic approaches, more research is needed to better understand treatment moderators when working with ACT (Landy et al. 2015). Yet, ACT is a promising intervention that specifically targets those aspects that contribute to the initiation and maintenance of anxiety problems and has demonstrated its effectiveness in numerous trials (Gloster et al. 2020; Swain et al. 2013; Sharp 2012).

Functional Analysis Case Conceptualization and Treatment Plan: The Case of a Woman Suffering from Repetitive Negative Thinking and Anxiety Problems

To demonstrate how we would apply ACT, we describe below the case of Skepsi, a woman who sought for psychological services for anxiety difficulties, complaining of repetitive negative thinking (RNT). To protect the client's identity, information including the persons' name have been disguised according to the General Data Protection Regulation (GDPR). We first present how we utilize functional analysis based on the psychological flexibility model, followed by proposing hypothesized mechanism of problem maintenance and suggesting a treatment plan based on ACT. The structure of the case conceptualization and treatment plan is partly based on the following sources: Dr. Karekla's lectures at the University of Cyprus and similar approaches presented in Eifert et al. (2009) and Eifert and Forsyth (2005).

Presenting Problem

Skepsi is a woman in her early 20 s who sought psychological support due to what she described as repetitive negative thinking (RNT) and elevated anxiety. RNT refers to worry and/or rumination which is related to emotional difficulties (Ehring et al. 2011). Specifically, she reported continuously having negative and unwanted thoughts regarding her romantic relationship, her professional future, and the ways in which others perceive her. Additionally, she noted a difficult relationship with her "absent" father. At the moment of seeking treatment, she was a full-time college student and was not employed.

List of Presenting Problems

Thoughts and Memories

Here are the thoughts she presented: "My behavior is a burden for my partner"; "If my partner is not with me at all times, that means he doesn't love me"; "If my partner is not with me at all times, that means we have a bad relationship, similar to the one between me and my father"; "I want to tell my partner that he does not give me the attention I need"; "I want to be able to voice my opinion, wants, and needs, but I am afraid others will reject me"; "I would like to be myself and be comfortable with who I am"; "I always have to portray my best possible self in front of others, because if I don't they will reject me"; "If I'm not perfect, everyone will leave me"; "I need to be perfect"; "If I show my true self to others, they will judge me"; "I will not be able to find a job because I am incompetent in certain areas"; "I won't make it"; "I will fail"; "I don't want to try to improve my skills because I will fail anyway"; "Nobody understands me and the pressure I feel"; "Is it my fault that I have a bad relationship with my father?"; and "Why isn't my father accepting of me?"

Skepsi has memories of the absence of her father while growing up and the absence of acceptance and support from him. Memories relating to the discourse between her parents cause her great discomfort.

Emotions and Physical Sensations

The client reported experiencing feelings of insecurity, anxiety, distress, embarrassment, guilt, fear of rejection, and elevated heart rate for about 3 years prior to seeking help. She explains that these feelings however increased around 6 months ago.

Behavior

Skepsi reports many avoidance behaviors including the following: voicing her opinion during social gatherings, doing daily activities and chores to avoid her thoughts, avoiding short meetings with her boyfriend to prevent sadness when they part, avoiding going to classes and exposing herself to situations where perfection may not be guaranteed, engaging in rumination and crying as a means to control her thoughts, constant mental checking of behavior and excessively using social media to distract from her thoughts and feelings.

Predisposing Factors

Predisposing factors, also known as vulnerability or risk factors, are factors proposed to predict the trajectory of psychological symptoms throughout life (Merikangas and Pine 2002). Parental psychopathology is associated with offspring psychopathology (McLaughlin et al. 2012). In this case, the client mentioned her father struggling with psychological issues, which may suggest a predisposing factor toward emotional difficulties.

Perfectionism as a general trait may constitute an additional risk factor for the development of anxiety (Limburg et al. 2017). Specifically, maladaptive perfectionism is associated with avoidant coping strategies (Montgomery et al. 2019). Moreover, perfectionism is correlated with checking and safety behaviors (Lee et al. 2011). Skepsi mentioned that she always felt the need to "be perfect." She has associated this need with mental checking of her behavior when in social settings or avoidance of social gatherings altogether. Additionally, her strive for perfectionism contributes to feelings of anxiety.

Parental exhibitions of avoidant behaviors when interacting with their children may instill fear of mistakes and failures in children (Segrin et al. 2019). Additionally, parental neglect predicts anxious symptomatology (Van Veen et al. 2013; Spinhoven et al. 2010). In this case, Skepsi mentioned an absence of a fatherly figure throughout her childhood. She remembers limited interactions with her father which always left her longing for his acceptance and affection.

Exposure to familial conflict and violence, especially between parents, is associated with anxiety in young adulthood (Schiff et al. 2014). Similarly, violence toward a woman in the household is associated with higher risk of child maltreatment (Øverlien 2010). Moreover, adopting a care-taker role for the victims (i.e., the mother) of familial violence may lead to severe emotional distress (Holt et al. 2008). Skepsi reported frequent arguing among her parents. She remembers at least one incident where her father was physically violent toward her mother, and she intervened by putting herself in the middle of her parents. All these memories and experiences possibly contribute to her ruminative thoughts and the anxiety she experiences.

Precipitating Factors

Precipitating factors are any "events or situations that actually provoke the onset of the problem…" (Westbrook et al. 2011, p. 199). Experiencing stressful life events is associated with rumination as a response to distress (Michl et al. 2013). Specifically, the occurrence of stressful life events acts as a reinforcer of worry for anxious individuals (Francis et al. 2012). In this case, Skepsi has experienced stressful life events such as witnessing domestic violence, adopting the role of a care-taker for her mother, and experiencing rejection from her father.

The most recent factor, which seems to have contributed to the exacerbation of symptoms and led to her seeking treatment, is her upcoming college graduation and subsequent entering into the workforce. The transition from being a university student to an employee is a major life event. Such transitions can be challenging for some individuals and have been associated with anxiety (McBeath et al. 2018).

Mechanisms of Maintaining the Problem According to the Psychological Flexibility/Inflexibility Model

In Fig. 1 we depict the psychological inflexibility model of an ACT case conceptualization for this client, based on Luoma et al. (2017). Ratings for the pervasiveness for each of the six components for the persons' difficulties, ranging from a scale of 1 (limited) to 5 (very extensive), are provided (see Luoma et al. 2017). Below, we describe each component of the psychological inflexibility model relating to this case.

Experiential Avoidance

Internal Emotional Control Strategies: Rumination, worry, and distraction.

Overt Emotional Control Strategies: Avoidance of social situations and conversations, stays at home, avoids visiting parents' home, excessive use of social media, and avoids seeing her partner for a limited amount of time to prevent herself from experiencing emotions of sadness when her partner leaves.

Strategies for Avoiding Emotions and Emotional Control Observed During Sessions: She focuses exclusively and with rigidity on other people's feelings and understandings of situations rather than her own. She also focuses on thoughts, facts, and logic to avoid negative emotions. In session, she is apprehensive toward any activity that may cause her to confront uncomfortable emotions.

Generally, Skepsi employs various avoidance methods to control her emotions. These control efforts are pervasive across most of her life areas, thus receiving a score of 5 on the scale mentioned above (see Fig. 1).

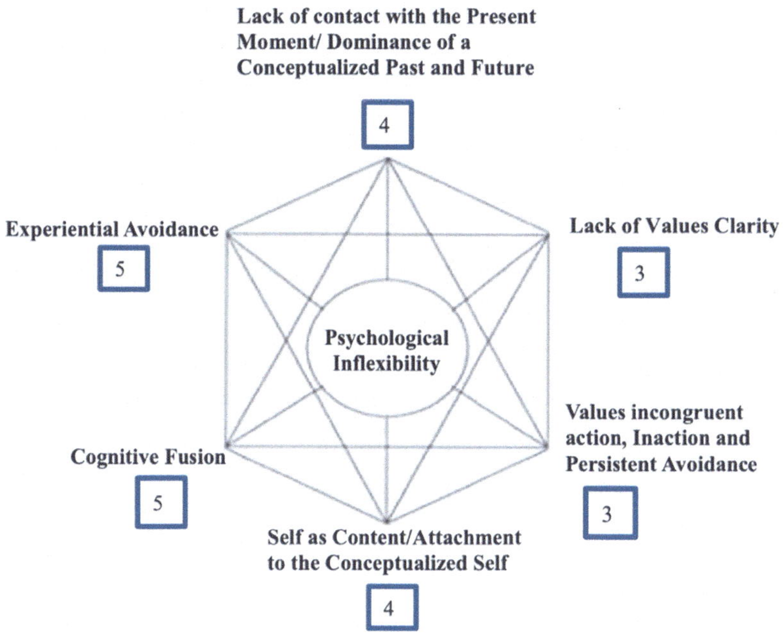

Fig. 1 Assessment of the client based on the psychological inflexibility model

Cognitive Fusion

Skepsi presents with being stuck (fusion) with continuous overthinking/rumination, efforts that serve a protective function from future challenges and problems. At times, she appears fearful of the prospect of not engaging with her thoughts. She is also attached to her self-image and repeatedly presents the thought that no one will accept her as she is and therefore needs to portray an ideal self. Additionally, she mentions several internal rules by which she regulates her overt behavior especially in social settings. She views herself as incompetent regarding professional employment, and she argues that these thoughts prevent her from improving her skills. The client received a rating of 5 regarding the extent of cognitive fusion.

Self as Content/Attachment to a Conceptualized Self

Skepsi sees herself as "just the thoughts and difficulties" she faces. The image she has of herself is of an "incompetent person." She characterizes herself as a burden to her romantic relationship because she constantly seeks attention and reassurance. When describing thoughts about herself, she uses words such as "silly" or phrases such as "I know it doesn't make sense," yet she is unwilling to let go of them. She exhibits difficulty with seeing beyond her relationship with her father and its consequences in her romantic life. Specifically, she equates the quality of her relationship with her father to the quality of her relationship with her significant other. The only area where she appears to regard herself as something more than her problems and difficulties is when it comes to her relationship with her mother and siblings. For instance, she expresses that she knows she is a good daughter and sister and is appreciated by her family. In terms of the extent of Skepsi's pervasiveness of attachment to a conceptualized self, we gave her a score of 4.

Lack of Contact with the Present Moment/Dominance of a Conceptualized Past and Future

Skepsi appears to lose herself in her thoughts about her past problems with her father and is preoccupied with possible future failures. She is mostly attached to the future since she often ruminates about possible scenarios regarding her romantic and social relationships and professional career. She also appears to hold the belief that her relationship with her father has caused her a significant amount of damage which is evident in her current romantic relationship. She only seems to focus on the present when she expresses feelings of inadequacy regarding her ability to be assertive and about her self-image. Regarding rating the level of pervasiveness of a conceptualized past and future, Skepsi received a score of 5.

Lack of Values Clarity

Skepsi is able to identify as important values her friendships, romantic relationship, health, community, education, and family. From these she expresses that the most important values are having close and trustworthy relationships with her family members (her mother and her siblings) and having a close supportive romantic relationship. According to Skepsi, she often lost contact with the value of family as she avoided visiting her mother and her siblings. Her romantic relationship is the only value where she mostly lives in line with as she does invest a lot in it, yet many times the investment is mobilized by fear rather than a connection to her values. Being a supportive friend is another value that she exhibits. Regarding the level of lack of values clarity, she received a score of 3.

Values-Incongruent Action, Inaction, and Persistent Avoidance

Skepsi acts somewhat in accordance with her values in the romantic relationship domain since she invests in this relationship and has maintained it for a long time. She also acts partly according to the value of being a good friend, as she provides emotional support to her friends. She notes that this gives her life meaning, but she feels these actions are most often one-sided, i.e., that she provides support but does not ask for support when she needs it. Skepsi avoids social gatherings and meetings with friends, and she avoids visiting her family members. Similarly, although she recognizes actions which would bring her closer to her value of education, she does not behave accordingly, i.e., she avoids attending classes or investing in her learning experiences. In her effort to live a life free of anxiety, her behavioral repertoire has become narrow. As a result, we gave her a score of 3 regarding the level of inaction and persistent avoidance behavior.

Maintenance mechanisms can also be observed by exploring the "ABCs," that is, A = antecedents, B = behavior, and C = consequences (see Table 1; for more information, see Ramnero and Torneke 2008).

Synthesis of Hypothesized Mechanism

Skepsi had been struggling with ruminative thoughts and anxiety for more than 3 years before seeking psychological services. Her symptomatology appeared to be exasperated by her approaching college graduation.

Table 1 Indicative ABCs to examine mechanisms that maintain problems

A Activating events/antecedents	B Behavior	C Consequences (behavioral mechanism/function)
Thoughts of the lack of relationship with her father and feels sad Thought: "I do not want my romantic relationship to be as bad as my relationship with my father is"	Isolates herself from her family Avoids meeting her significant other Does house chores and other activities instead Spends excessive amount of time on social media Calls best friend to vent	Immediate emotional relief (positive reinforcement) Emotional pain is not exacerbated (negative reinforcement) Distraction from thoughts (positive reinforcement)
Opportunity for socialization	Thought: "I need to be perfect, to not be rejected" Avoids voicing her opinions or wants Avoids going out Mental checking of behavior (noticing of how she replies to others, smiling, nodding, agreeing with everything)	Immediate relief (positive reinforcement) Thought: "I have not disagreed with anyone; therefore I am liked and accepted" (positive reinforcement)
Alone at home Thoughts: "I failed in the past," "I have a bad relationship with my father," "My partner is tired of me," "I will not find a job," and "I am incompetent"	Rumination ("I will sign up for extra classes, and then I will be in a better position to be hired," "I am an inadequate partner so I must do xyz to better myself") Crying	Immediate relief (positive reinforcement) Reduction of distress (negative reinforcement) Belief/rule: "Ruminating helps me find solutions to my problems and protects me from possible future threats" (positive reinforcement)

Her historical context of a problematic relationship with her absent father may have contributed to her critical attitude toward herself, the insecurities she has regarding her romantic and other relationships, and her RNT.

According to ACT, anxiety arises due to one's behavioral repertoire becoming restricted due to psychological inflexibility and continuous context-incongruent experiential avoidance. In the case of Skepsi, she uses behavioral and experiential avoidance in almost all areas of her life. She avoids social settings, visiting her family and even her partner, out of fear of rejection. This fear leads her to focus exclusively on the emotions, thoughts, and behaviors of others rather than her own. For example, when asked about her emotions, thoughts, and behaviors on a particular event, she responded with "I think/feel that my boyfriend/friends/family feels/thinks…." This further restricts her behavior as she is apprehensive toward any situation which may evoke negative feelings. Skepsi uses rumination as another avoidance tactic to regulate her emotions. Through rumination, she successfully controls her emotions in the short term. However, in the long term, these emotions become more difficult to avoid, and her rumination efforts grow larger. She focuses on the literality of her thoughts to avoid negative emotions. Her rumination efforts seem to be reinforced through loops of positive and negative reinforcement, which further maintain dysfunctional behavior and exacerbated feelings of anxiety.

While being preoccupied with her thoughts, she loses contact with the present moment. She often worries about possible future threats and failures. She frequently dwells on the experience of rejection from her father which propels her to predict future rejection from others and especially her partner. Skepsi becomes "stuck" with her thoughts about a future filled with rejection. Similarly, her fear of rejection combined with feelings of professional inadequacy lead to thoughts about a catastrophic future. Specifically, she becomes consumed by thoughts of unemployment due to lack of professional skills.

Her attachment to her thoughts and experiences prevents her from viewing herself as a whole. Specifically, she struggles regarding herself as a person with difficult thoughts, feelings, and emotions. In particular, she is self-critical ("inadequate," "incompetent" "imperfections lead to rejection") and believes herself to be the problem. She also has difficulty recognizing herself as being more than just her thoughts and emotions and is overly critical toward herself, lacking any self-compassion.

Skepsi has some clarity regarding what is important to her (e.g., in the domains of family, romantic relationship, friendships), but in most cases, she does not act in accordance with her values in these domains. She often exhibits behaviors which lead to immediate emotional relief even when these behaviors do not align with her values. Avoidance behaviors (e.g., not visiting her family, avoiding social events) and "fusion" with her thoughts interfere from living a meaningful life.

The function of her avoidance behaviors and RNT (and subsequent anxiety) is reinforced both negatively and positively. Via positive reinforcement, staying home to do house chores or other activities, engaging in excessive social media use, venting to a friend, and mental checking of behavior (e.g., smiling, nodding, and agreeing), she feels better and in control for a short while. Isolating from her family, avoiding social gatherings, avoiding meeting with her partner, not voicing her opinion, and crying reduce her distress and emotional pain and thus are reinforced negatively. In the long term, all these behaviors contribute and exacerbate her problems, anxiety, life dissatisfaction, and psychological inflexibility.

Clients' Strengths That Can Aid the Intervention

Skepsi sought psychological services of her own volition, indicating that she recognized the difficulties she was facing. Additionally, she presents as ready to participate in therapy and make changes to better her life. Her family (excluding her father), her romantic partner, and her best friend act as her support network. She is also nearing the completion of course which despite difficulties will probably be completed successfully. Skepsi's therapy prognosis is very good.

External Barriers or Obstacles to the Intervention

The difficult relationship with her father may act as an obstacle to the intervention as there does not seem to be a way to repair that relationship. The acquired patterns of interaction within the family in general may serve as a barrier and a trigger when she visits her family home.

Treatment Plan

Treatment began by targeting the processes of the psychological flexibility model. As it is hypothesized that these processes are interlinked, targeting one process may also affect other related processes. In Skepsi's case, we began by targeting the components which seem the most pervasive and contribute most to her difficulties. The first intervention targets were acceptance and cognitive defusion while incorporating components relating to self-as-context and values-guided actions. To reduce experiential avoidance, "creative hopelessness" was introduced to illustrate the ineffectiveness of efforts to control thoughts and emotional distress. Recent research suggests that individuals are more likely to open up to their thoughts and feelings (acceptance) once they experience directly the inevitability of avoidance practices for controlling internal states (Konstantinou et al. 2023). The use of metaphors and experiential exercises in ACT aims to enhance learning through direct experience. For this reason, we used metaphors such as "The Hungry Tiger Cub" (Hayes et al. 1990). At this point, we normalized and validated her experience by highlighting that she has used all logical means and strategies to cope with her thoughts and emotions. Experientially, we examined and recognized how these control efforts did not have lasting results. This led to the conclusion that she now has a choice to adopt an alternative way of coping (willingness) with negative internal experiences. To illustrate willingness as an alternative to control efforts, we used "The Chinese Finger Trap" exercise (Eifert and Forsyth 2005, adapted from Hayes et al. 1999). To emphasize active acceptance, we carried out the "Tug of War with the Anxiety Monster" exercise (Hayes et al. 1990), further highlighting the conscious choice of fighting and not fighting with internal experiences.

We simultaneously focused on cognitive defusion by firstly educating the client on the function of anxiety and fear as survival instincts. Also, we introduced the notion that all emotions serve important evolutionary purposes for humans, and as such no emotion is problematic. Emotions become problematic when we try to control them or struggle to extinguish some or expect to always experience others. To aid in creating distance between the client and her thoughts, we devised an exercise where the client wrote down all her unwanted thoughts and feelings on a white board. Then, both therapist and client stood extremely close to the whiteboard, and the client was asked to describe what she could see. The exercise continued by moving away, facing other points in the room, and asking the client what she could see. The aim of this exercise was to introduce the client to the notion that these negative internal events exist even when she is not focused on them or sees them, but the choice of getting unstuck and behaving in accordance with her values was hers to make. The "choice moment" exercise (Karekla and Kelly 2022) was frequently used to remind her that she has a choice at each moment as to where she will pivot her attention and efforts—toward or away from her values and making a committed choice with her actions. Correspondingly, the process of self-as-context was promoted. Upon creating distance between herself and her thoughts, Skepsi started to regard herself as a whole rather than defining herself on the basis of her negative experiences. To further illustrate self-as-context, we used the "Anxiety News Radio" metaphor (Eifert and Forsyth 2005, adapted from Karekla 2004).

Throughout the sessions, we fostered contact with the present moment using mindfulness techniques. Specifically, these techniques aimed to train the client to be aware of thoughts, feelings, and bodily sensations in the moment they happen without judgment. An additional aim was to bring awareness to events during the session and her daily life. We began each session with centering/mindfulness exercises. The first centering exercises were shorter, around 3 min long, and focused on bringing attention to breathing, bodily sensations, and sounds. The following exercises were longer and focused on noticing private experiences (emotions and thoughts). These exercises were also used to gradually expose the client to her difficult thoughts and emotions and achieve new learning as to how to interact with them.

Following, we focused on areas of valued living and committed action. We used exercises such as "The 80th Birthday Party" (Harris 2007) and the "Game of Life" (Karekla and Kelly 2022) to recognize first and come into contact with her values. Next we examined whether she lives her life currently, in accordance with these values, and how her struggling with her anxiety, thoughts, and emotions gets in the way of living the life she would like. To further enhance this idea experientially with an eye on moving toward committed action, we used the "Passengers on the Bus" metaphor (Hayes et al. 1999). Through our values exploration, the distinction between values and goals was made. She then identified, set, and committed to setting goals which would lead her on her valued living path. She was encouraged to set small, measurable, and attainable goals for each week. She was able to complete almost all her goals before each session; in cases where valued living goals were not met, these were discussed and barriers were identified and dealt with in an ACT manner.

Finally, skills training and practice were employed for areas which the client had identified as lacking in skills. We carried out assertiveness training regarding her difficulties and insecurity as to the most fruitful way to voice her opinion/needs/wants. During sessions scenarios and role-playing exercises were used to elicit "difficult" thoughts and feelings for the client and practice psychologically flexible ways to communicate her thoughts, feelings, and needs. The client practiced these skills in social settings between sessions. Additionally, exercises relating to self-confidence and self-compassion were adopted. All exercises included elements of self-as-context and cognitive defusion as described above and elements of exposure. Treatment termination was decided in collaboration with the client at 15 sessions.

Assessment of Progress

Evaluation of her progress was continuous utilizing the "ACT Daily Record" sheet (Eifert and Forsyth 2005; Karekla 2004) which assessed suffering, struggle, workability, and valued action for each day. Through the course of the treatment, although suffering and struggle were present, valued actions increased. Additionally, the client qualitatively assessed her progress toward the mid-point of treatment and identified further areas that needed improvement (e.g., expressed difficulties with assertiveness and self-confidence).

Toward the mid-point of therapy, she reported minimal in any RNT and rumination. In line with this, she reported being more compassionate to herself and acknowledged that although her negative experiences were a part of her story, they did not define her—so her language use regarding her thoughts and emotions was observed to change. Similarly, she used mindfulness exercises during her day which helped her foster contact with the present moment. She reported recognizing how her "stuckness" with her thoughts prevented her from living a full life and began engaging in actions in line with her values by setting and meeting her goals. She finally reported exposing herself to social activities and becoming more assertive in her interactions with others, while she aimed to engage in all previously avoided activities including her education.

Termination and Relapse Prevention

Termination was decided together with Skepsi. The therapeutic sessions with Skepsi ended once all therapeutic goals were achieved and the client was engaging in valued actions even in the face of negative internal events. Follow-up check-in sessions have at this point been scheduled for 6- and 12-weeks post-termination.

For relapse prevention, the client identified internal and external triggers which may lead to relapse. Collaboratively, Skepsi and the therapist developed a relapse prevention plan which included skills learned in therapy to help with the management of triggers, ways to monitor her own progress, and ways to enhance psychological flexibility (in line with Karekla and Kelly 2022). Additionally, her prevention plan included ways in which she can support her progress and enhance her resilience.

In summary, this chapter illustrated the ACT approach to conceptualization and treatment of a client dealing with anxiety and RNT. This approach appears effective for general anxiety experienced by outpatients (Swain et al. 2013) and managing RNT for individuals with specific anxiety disorders (Ruiz et al. 2019). ACT is a flexible and scalable approach that has been used in the treatment of various forms of psychopathology (Zacharia and Karekla 2021). Finally, the psychological flexibility model is easily adaptable in meeting the individualized needs of each client, as illustrated by the case presented in this chapter.

References

Arch, J. J., Eifert, G. H., Davies, C., Vilardaga, J. C. P., Rose, R. D., & Craske, M. G. (2012). Randomized clinical trial of cognitive behavioral therapy (CBT) versus acceptance and commitment therapy (ACT) for mixed anxiety disorders. *Journal of consulting and clinical psychology*, *80*(5), 750.

Arch, J. J., & Craske, M. G. (2008). Acceptance and commitment therapy and cognitive behavioral therapy for anxiety disorders: Different treatments, similar mechanisms?. *Clinical psychology: Science and practice*, *15*(4), 263.

Berman, N. C., Wheaton, M. G., McGrath, P., & Abramowitz, J. S. (2010). Predicting anxiety: The role of experiential avoidance and anxiety sensitivity. *Journal of anxiety disorders*, *24*(1), 109–113.

Blackledge, J. T., & Barnes-Holmes, D. (2009). Core processes in acceptance and commitment therapy. *Acceptance and commitment therapy: Contemporary theory, research, and practice*, 41–58.

Bluett, E. J., Homan, K. J., Morrison, K. L., Levin, M. E., & Twohig, M. P. (2014). Acceptance and commitment therapy for anxiety and OCD spectrum disorders: An empirical review. *Journal of anxiety disorders*, *28*(6), 612–624.

Caletti, E., Massimo, C., Magliocca, S., Moltrasio, C., Brambilla, P., & Delvecchio, G. (2022). The role of the acceptance and commitment therapy in the treatment of social anxiety: An updated scoping review. *Journal of Affective Disorders*.

Chase, J. A., Houmanfar, R., Hayes, S. C., Ward, T. A., Vilardaga, J. P., & Follette, V. (2013). Values are not just goals: Online ACT-based values training adds to goal setting in improving undergraduate college student performance. *Journal of Contextual Behavioral Science*, *2*(3–4), 79–84.

Dinis, A., Carvalho, S., Gouveia, J. P., & Estanqueiro, C. (2015). Shame memories and depression symptoms: The role of cognitive fusion and experiential avoidance. *International Journal of Psychology and Psychological Therapy, 15*(1), 63–86.
Ehring, T., Zetsche, U., Weidacker, K., Wahl, K., Schönfeld, S., & Ehlers, A. (2011). The Perseverative Thinking Questionnaire (PTQ): Validation of a content-independent measure of repetitive negative thinking. *Journal of behavior therapy and experimental psychiatry, 42*(2), 225–232.
Eifert, G. H., Forsyth, J. P., Arch, J., Espejo, E., Keller, M., & Langer, D. (2009). Acceptance and commitment therapy for anxiety disorders: Three case studies exemplifying a unified treatment protocol. *Cognitive and behavioral practice, 16*(4), 368–385.
Eifert, G. H., & Forsyth, J. P. (2005). *Acceptance and commitment therapy for anxiety disorders: A practitioner's treatment guide to using mindfulness, acceptance, and values-based behavior change*. New Harbinger Publications.
Fashler, S. R., Weinrib, A. Z., Azam, M. A., & Katz, J. (2018). The use of acceptance and commitment therapy in oncology settings: a narrative review. *Psychological reports, 121*(2), 229–252.
Ferreira, M. G., Mariano, L. I., de Rezende, J. V., Caramelli, P., & Kishita, N. (2022). Effects of group Acceptance and Commitment Therapy (ACT) on anxiety and depressive symptoms in adults: A meta-analysis. *Journal of Affective Disorders.*
Flaxman, P. E., Blackledge, J. T., & Bond F. W. (2011). Acceptance and Commitment Therapy: The CBT distinctive features series. Hove, England: Routledge.
Forman, E. M., Herbert, J. D., Moitra, E., Yeomans, P. D., & Geller, P. A. (2007). A randomized controlled effectiveness trial of acceptance and commitment therapy and cognitive therapy for anxiety and depression. *Behavior modification, 31*(6), 772–799.
Francis, J. L., Moitra, E., Dyck, I., & Keller, M. B. (2012). The impact of stressful life events on relapse of generalized anxiety disorder. *Depression and anxiety, 29*(5), 386–391.
Gloster, A. T., & Karekla, M. (2020). A multi-level, multi-method approach to testing and refining intervention targets. In S.G. Hoffman & S. Hayes (Eds.), Beyond the DSM: Toward a process-based alternative for diagnosis and mental health treatment (pp. 226–249). Oakland, CA: Context Press/New Harbinger Publications.
Gloster, A. T., Walder, N., Levin, M. E., Twohig, M. P., & Karekla, M. (2020). The empirical status of acceptance and commitment therapy: A review of meta-analyses. *Journal of Contextual Behavioral Science, 18*, 181–192.
Gloster, A. T., Sonntag, R., Hoyer, J., Meyer, A. H., Heinze, S., Ströhle, A., ... & Wittchen, H. U. (2015). Treating treatment-resistant patients with panic disorder and agoraphobia using psychotherapy: A randomized controlled switching trial. *Psychotherapy and psychosomatics, 84*(2), 100–109.
Hancock, K. M., Swain, J., Hainsworth, C. J., Dixon, A. L., Koo, S., & Munro, K. (2018). Acceptance and commitment therapy versus cognitive behavior therapy for children with anxiety: Outcomes of a randomized controlled trial. *Journal of Clinical Child & Adolescent Psychology, 47*(2), 296–311.
Harris, R. (2007). Acceptance and commitment therapy (ACT) introductory workshop handout. *Psych Med.*
Harris, R. (2006). Embracing your demons: An overview of acceptance and commitment therapy. *Psychotherapy in Australia, 12*(4), 70–6.
Hayes-Skelton, S. A., & Eustis, E. H. (2020). Experiential avoidance.
Hayes, S. C., Levin, M. E., Plumb-Vilardaga, J., Villatte, J. L., & Pistorello, J. (2013). Acceptance and commitment therapy and contextual behavioral science: Examining the progress of a distinctive model of behavioral and cognitive therapy. *Behavior therapy, 44*(2), 180–198.
Hayes, S. C., Pistorello, J., & Levin, M. E. (2012a). Acceptance and commitment therapy as a unified model of behavior change. *The Counseling Psychologist, 40*(7), 976–1002.
Hayes, S. C., Strosahl, K. D., & Wilson, K. G. (2012b). *Acceptance and commitment therapy: The process and practice of mindful change* (2nd ed.). New York, NY: Guilford Press.

Hayes, S. C., Strosahl, K. D., & Wilson, K. G. (2011). *Acceptance and commitment therapy: The process and practice of mindful change*. Guilford press.

Hayes, S. C., Luoma, J. B., Bond, F. W., Masuda, A., & Lillis, J. (2006). Acceptance and commitment therapy: Model, processes and outcomes. *Behaviour research and therapy*, *44*(1), 1–25.

Hayes, S. C. (2004). Acceptance and Commitment Therapy, Relational Frame Theory, and the third wave of behavioral and cognitive therapies. *Behavior Therapy, 35, 639–665.* https://doi.org/10.1016/S0005-7894(04)80013-3.

Hayes, S. C., Strosahl, K., Wilson, K. G., Bissett, R. T., Pistorello, J., Toarmino, D., … & McCurry, S. M. (2004). Measuring experiential avoidance: A preliminary test of a working model. *The psychological record*, *54*, 553–578.

Hayes, S. C., Barnes-Holmes, D., & Roche, B. (Eds.). (2001). *Relational frame theory: A post-Skinnerian account of human language and cognition*. Springer Science & Business Media.

Hayes, S. C., Strosahl, K. D., & Wilson, K. G. (1999). *Acceptance and commitment therapy* (p. 6). New York: Guilford press.

Hayes, S. C., Wilson, K. G., Gifford, E. V., Follette, & V. M., Strosahl, K. (1996). Experiential avoidance and behavioral disorders: A functional dimensional approach to diagnosis and treatment. *Journal of Consulting and Clinical Psychology, 64, 1152–1168.* https://doi.org/10.1037/0022-006X.64.6.1152

Hayes, S. C., Wilson, K., Afari, N., & McCurry, S. (1990, November). *The use of Acceptance and Commitment Therapy in the treatment of agoraphobia*. Paper presented at the meeting of the Association for Advancement of Behavior Therapy, San Francisco.

Hayes, S. C., Hayes, L. J., & Reese, H. W. (1988). Finding the philosophical core: A review of Stephen C. Pepper's World Hypotheses: A Study in Evidence. *Journal of the experimental analysis of behavior*, *50*(1), 97.

Holt, S., Buckley, H., & Whelan, S. (2008). The impact of exposure to domestic violence on children and young people: A review of the literature. *Child abuse & neglect*, *32*(8), 797–810.

Hulbert-Williams, N. J., Storey, L., & Wilson, K. G. (2015). Psychological interventions for patients with cancer: psychological flexibility and the potential utility of Acceptance and Commitment Therapy. *European journal of cancer care*, *24*(1), 15–27.

Karekla, M., (2004). A comparison between acceptance-enhanced panic control treatment and panic control treatment for panic disorder. *Dissertation Abstracts International, Section B: The Sciences and Engineering, 65* (9-B), 4835.

Karekla, M., & Kelly, M. M. (2022). *Cravings and Addictions: Free Yourself from the Struggle of Addictive Behavior with Acceptance and Commitment Therapy*. New Harbinger Publications.

Karekla, M., Karademas, E. C., & Gloster, A. T. (2019a). The common sense model of self-regulation and acceptance and commitment therapy: Integrating strategies to guide interventions for chronic illness. *Health psychology review*, *13*(4), 490–503.

Karekla, M., Konstantinou, P., Ioannou, M., Kareklas, I., & Gloster, A. T. (2019b). The phenomenon of treatment dropout, reasons and moderators in acceptance and commitment therapy and other active treatments. *Clinical Psychology in Europe*, *1*(3), 1–36.

Karekla, M., Zacharia, M., & Koushiou, M. (2018). Accept pain for a vital life: Acceptance and Commitment Therapy for the treatment of chronic pain. *Somatoform and Other Psychosomatic Disorders: A Dialogue Between Contemporary Psychodynamic Psychotherapy and Cognitive Behavioral Therapy Perspectives*, 163–191.

Kashdan, T. B., & Rottenberg, J. (2010). Psychological flexibility as a fundamental aspect of health. *Clinical psychology review*, *30*(7), 865–878.

Landy, L. N., Schneider, R. L., & Arch, J. J. (2015). Acceptance and commitment therapy for the treatment of anxiety disorders: a concise review. *Current Opinion in Psychology*, *2*, 70–74.

Konstantinou, P., Trigeorgi, A., Georgiou, C., Michaelides, M., Gloster, A. T., Georgiou, E., Panayiotou, G., & Karekla, M. (2023). Functional versus Dysfunctional Coping with Physical Pain: An Experimental Comparison of Acceptance vs. Avoidance Coping. *Behaviour Research and Therapy*, https://doi.org/10.1016/j.brat.2023.104339

Larsson, A., Hartley, S., & McHugh, L. (2022). A randomised controlled trial of brief web-based acceptance and commitment Therapy on the general mental health, depression, anxiety and stress of college Students. *Journal of Contextual Behavioral Science*, *24*, 10–17.

Lee, M., Roberts-Collins, C., Coughtrey, A., Phillips, L., & Shafran, R. (2011). Behavioural expressions, imagery and perfectionism. *Behavioural and Cognitive Psychotherapy*, *39*(4), 413–425.

Levin, M. E., MacLane, C., Daflos, S., Seeley, J. R., Hayes, S. C., Biglan, A., & Pistorello, J. (2014). Examining psychological inflexibility as a transdiagnostic process across psychological disorders. *Journal of contextual behavioral science*, *3*(3), 155–163.

Levitt, J. T. & Karekla, M. (2005). *Integrating Acceptance and Mindfulness with Cognitive Behavior Treatment for Panic Disorder.* In M. M. Antony (Ed.). Acceptance and Midfulness-Based Approaches to Anxiety: Conceptualization and Treatment. New York, NY, US: Klumer Academic/Plenum Publisher.

Limburg, K., Watson, H. J., Hagger, M. S., & Egan, S. J. (2017). The relationship between perfectionism and psychopathology: A meta-analysis. *Journal of clinical psychology*, *73*(10), 1301–1326.

Luoma, J. B., Hayes, S. C., & Walser, R. D. (2017). *Learning ACT: An acceptance & commitment therapy skills-training manual for therapists* (2nd ed.). Oakland, CA: New Harbinger Publications, Inc.

McBeath, M., Drysdale, M. T., & Bohn, N. (2018). Work-integrated learning and the importance of peer support and sense of belonging. *Education+ Training*, *60*(1), 39–53.

McCracken, L. M., & Vowles, K. E. (2014). Acceptance and commitment therapy and mindfulness for chronic pain: model, process, and progress. *American psychologist*, *69*(2), 178.

McLaughlin, K. A., Gadermann, A. M., Hwang, I., Sampson, N. A., Al-Hamzawi, A., Andrade, L. H., ... & Kessler, R. C. (2012). Parent psychopathology and offspring mental disorders: results from the WHO World Mental Health Surveys. *The British Journal of Psychiatry*, *200*(4), 290–299.

Merikangas, K. R., & Pine, D. (2002). Genetic and other vulnerability factors for anxiety and stress disorders. *Neuropsychopharmacology: The fifth generation of progress*, 868–82.

Michl, L. C., McLaughlin, K. A., Shepherd, K., & Nolen-Hoeksema, S. (2013). Rumination as a mechanism linking stressful life events to symptoms of depression and anxiety: longitudinal evidence in early adolescents and adults. *Journal of abnormal psychology*, *122*(2), 339.

Montgomery, S., Gregg, D. H., Somers, C. L., Pernice-Duca, F., Hoffman, A., & Beeghly, M. (2019). Intrapersonal variables associated with academic adjustment in United States college students. *Current Psychology*, *38*, 40–49.

Moran, D. J. (2015). Acceptance and commitment training in the workplace. *Current Opinion in Psychology*, *2*, 26–31.

Niles, A. N., Burklund, L. J., Arch, J. J., Lieberman, M. D., Saxbe, D., & Craske, M. G. (2014). Cognitive mediators of treatment for social anxiety disorder: Comparing acceptance and commitment therapy and cognitive-behavioral therapy. *Behavior therapy*, *45*(5), 664–677.

Noureen, S., & Malik, S. (2021). Conceptualized-self and depression symptoms among university students: Mediating role of cognitive fusion. *Current psychology*, *40*, 5106–5114.

Orsillo SM, Roemer L, Block-Lerner J, LeJeune C, & Herbert JD (2005). ACT with anxiety disorders. In SC Hayes & KD Strosahl (Eds.). *A Practical Guide to Acceptance and Commitment Therapy* (pp. 103–132). New York: Springer Science & Business Media.

Øverlien, C. (2010). Children exposed to domestic violence: Conclusions from the literature and challenges ahead. *Journal of social work*, *10*(1), 80–97.

Panayiotou, G., Karekla, M., & Leonidou, C. (2017). Coping through avoidance may explain gender disparities in anxiety. *Journal of Contextual Behavior Science*, *6*(2), 215–220.

Panayiotou, G., Karekla, M. & Mete, I. (2014a). Dispositional coping in individuals with anxiety disorder symptomatology: Avoidance predicts distress. *Journal of Contextual Behavior Science*, *3*(4), 314–321. https://doi.org/10.1016/j.jcbs.2014.07.001.

Panayiotou, G., Karekla, M. & Panayiotou, M. (2014b). Direct and indirect predictors of social anxiety: The role of anxiety sensitivity, behavioral inhibition, experiential avoidance and self-focused attention. *Comprehensive Psychiatry, 55*(8), 1875–1882.

Ramnero, J., & Törneke, N. (2008). *The ABCs of human behavior: Behavioral principles for the practicing clinician*. New Harbinger Publications.

Ruiz, F. J., Peña-Vargas, A., Ramírez, E. S., Suárez-Falcón, J. C., García-Martín, M. B., García-Beltrán, D. M., … & Sánchez, P. D. (2020). Efficacy of a two-session repetitive negative thinking-focused acceptance and commitment therapy (ACT) protocol for depression and generalized anxiety disorder: A randomized waitlist control trial. *Psychotherapy, 57*(3), 444.

Ruiz, F. J., García-Beltrán, D. M., Monroy-Cifuentes, A., & Suárez-Falcón, J. C. (2019). Single-case experimental design evaluation of RNT-focused acceptance and commitment therapy in GAD with couple-related worry. *International Journal of Psychology and Psychological Therapy, 19*(3), 261–276.

Ruiz, F. J., Suárez-Falcón, J. C., Riano-Hernández, D., & Gillanders, D. (2017). Psychometric properties of the cognitive fusion questionnaire in Colombia. *Revista Latinoamericana de Psicología, 49*(1), 80–87.

Schiff, M., Plotnikova, M., Dingle, K., Williams, G. M., Najman, J., & Clavarino, A. (2014). Does adolescent's exposure to parental intimate partner conflict and violence predict psychological distress and substance use in young adulthood? A longitudinal study. *Child abuse & neglect, 38*(12), 1945–1954.

Sharp, K. (2012). A review of acceptance and commitment therapy with anxiety disorders. *International Journal of Psychology and Psychological Therapy, 12*(3), 359–372.

Segrin, C., Kauer, T. B., & Burke, T. J. (2019). Indirect effects of family cohesion on emerging adult perfectionism through anxious rearing and social expectations. *Journal of Child and Family Studies, 28*, 2280–2285.

Spinhoven, P., Elzinga, B. M., Hovens, J. G., Roelofs, K., Zitman, F. G., van Oppen, P., & Penninx, B. W. (2010). The specificity of childhood adversities and negative life events across the life span to anxiety and depressive disorders. *Journal of affective disorders, 126*(1–2), 103–112.

Swain, J., Hancock, K., Hainsworth, C., & Bowman, J. (2013). Acceptance and commitment therapy in the treatment of anxiety: a systematic review. *Clinical psychology review, 33*(8), 965–978.

Twohig, M. P., & Levin, M. E. (2017). Acceptance and commitment therapy as a treatment for anxiety and depression: a review. *Psychiatric clinics, 40*(4), 751–770.

Twohig, M. P. (2012). Acceptance and commitment therapy: Introduction. *Cognitive and Behavioral Practice, 19*(4), 499–507.

Van Veen, T., Wardenaar, K. J., Carlier, I. V. E., Spinhoven, P., Penninx, B. W. J. H., & Zitman, F. G. (2013). Are childhood and adult life adversities differentially associated with specific symptom dimensions of depression and anxiety?

Westbrook, D., Kennerley, H., & Kirk, J. (2011). *An introduction to cognitive behaviour therapy: Skills and applications*. Sage.

Wilson, K., Sandoz, E. K., Flynn, M. K., Slater, R. M., & DuFrene, T. (2010). Understanding, assessing, and treating values processes in mindfulness-and acceptance-based therapies. *Assessing mindfulness and acceptance processes in clients: Illuminating the theory and practice of change*, 77–106.

Zacharia, M., & Karekla, M. (2021). The acceptance and commitment therapy perspective: Case conceptualization and treatment of depression in cancer. In *Depression Conceptualization and Treatment: Dialogues from Psychodynamic and Cognitive Behavioral Perspectives* (pp. 123–147). Cham: Springer International Publishing.

Zhang, C. Q., Leeming, E., Smith, P., Chung, P. K., Hagger, M. S., & Hayes, S. C. (2018). Acceptance and commitment therapy for health behavior change: a contextually-driven approach. *Frontiers in psychology*, 2350.

Fear, Anxiety and Their Meaning for Our Life from Psychodynamic Point of View. Modern Psychoanalytical Approaches to Anxiety Disorders

Christos Charis

Anxiety as an affect is experienced on a psychological level and is associated with other affects such as despair, anger, hopelessness and other negative feelings. Moreover, fear is accompanied by physical reactions: increase in heart rate and blood pressure, muscle tension, dizziness, change in voice and facial expression and shock-like paralysis. Fear is therefore a psycho-socio-somatic phenomenon (Ermann 2019). In this sense, fear is (a) a basic feeling of human existence and is attributed to the foreboding of death and the presentiment of the limitedness of human existence (b) also to the abysses of the human soul (the unconscious), which elude immediate access. Fear in certain situations (situational fear) serves to cope with or avoid concrete dangers. Freud (1926) called this signal anxiety (Rudolf and Heningsen 2017). It is an alarm signal and serves to protect against real threats by evoking appropriate reactions (see more below). Fear has shaped in a very deep way the cultures of our world over the millennia. In religion, in philosophy and in art, this fundamental affect has a lasting impact. Psychoanalysis, with its more than 100 years of tradition, has contributed significantly to research into pathological anxiety, as has behavioural therapy. It arises from the psychodynamics of conflicts or crises (see more below).

In the Greek mythology, death and sleep Hypnos and Thanatos were brothers (Askitopoulou 2015). Death is the greatest fear factor in our civilisation (Becker 1973). Becker, an American cultural anthropologist, came to the conclusion on the basis of his research that the repressed fear of death in humans plays a central role in our lives. Fear is one of the fundamental emotions in human life, i.e. it has a great influence on our life or on how we cope with life. That is why through the ages of mankind, all kinds of disciplines have dealt with this emotion. They try to express the fear, to explore it and to ultimately show a way how man can cope with fear.

C. Charis (✉)
Private Practice for Psychotherapy, Dillenburg, Hessen, Germany
e-mail: christos-charis@outlook.de

C. Charis, G. Panayiotou (eds.), *Anxiety Disorders and Related Conditions*,
https://doi.org/10.1007/978-3-031-56798-8_2

They try to mitigate the power of fear by finding descriptive terms. Parallel to the variety of personifications of the different varieties and intensities of anxiety, a broad spectrum of linguistic terms has developed to put the symptoms of anxiety into words. What is remarkable here is the concentration of terminology on an illustration of exclusively physical symptoms, which has remained almost unchanged up to the present day, when we still speak of the fact that, due to anxiety, the hair stands on end, the eyes are wide open and the pupils dilated, the ears buzz, the breath stops (often also the image of the throat being tightened), the voice fails, the pulse races, the knees go weak and so on. The word ‘anxiety’ derives from the Greek word *ἄγχω* (verb) and Latin word *ango* (verb) which means ‘to constrict’, ‘to press together’, ‘to draw off the breath’ and ‘to strangle’, related to the German word ‘Enge’ (substantive), and is not only connected to the image of the ‘constricted throat’ but also to the clinical picture of angina (Greek συναγχή, κυναγχή), by which is mostly meant not angina pectoris, but diphtheria (Beekes 2010).

You can deal with fear if you are familiar with it. That is why it is important to talk about it. Fear challenges us to self-development. Seen from this perspective, the encouragement: ‘Courage to fear’ takes on a special meaning (Kast 1996, page 29). If I am flooded with fear and I recognise and accept it, it opens up the possibility for me to withdraw for self-protection. But some people deny fear, so that they do not perceive moderate fear. They deal with fear in a counter-phobic way. (In these cases in which the fear stays unconscious and it is to be distinguished from the strategy where the person feels fear but faces the fearful situation because he is striving for a goal (Fabian 2017)). This may be one reason why Vietnam veterans have significantly higher mortality rates in traffic and poisoning accidents (Bullman et al. 1990).

In Greek philosophy the Stoics, e.g. Epicurus’ ethics teachings, aim at their heart at increasing and consolidating the joy of life by the enjoyment of each day, possibly each moment, in other words ‘seize the day’. For this purpose, it is necessary either to avoid or to overcome all impairments of the peace of mind, which can arise from desires, fear and pain. Constantly savouring the pleasure of life constitutes the art of the Epicurean sage (Konstan 2018).

Many ancient Greek myths are about vanquishing fear. One thinks of Perseus and Medusa. Perseus, a hero of Greek mythology, succeeded with the help of the goddess Athena in slaying Medusa, the ideal embodiment of the image of terror at the sight of which everyone was literally petrified. After completing his deed, he presented the severed head of the Gorgon to Athena, who since then has worn it on her shield as a powerful apotropaic or something used to ward off evil (Gorgoneion). The Perseus myth shows very clearly that the hero of Greek mythology is capable of such extraordinary deeds exclusively in the closest cooperation with his personal guardian deity, i.e. not necessarily by his own power, but on the basis of special qualifications, be it (divine) lineage or special piety, which fit him for divine protection (Cartwright 2012). Throughout the centuries, people have sought to mitigate uncertainty by explaining what frightens them. For by understanding a phenomenon, we take the first step in shedding the feeling of fear or powerlessness, because we come to feel in control of what is happening (Compare Yalom 2010).

In our religion, Christ rises above the level of heroism and promises lasting relief from fear, since he was able to conquer death itself, as the greatest fear factor in human history. In Christianity, however, fear and terror are no longer characterised exclusively as negative powers to which man is helplessly exposed but often even have a catalytic function as a manifestation of wonder (or as we call it in Greek 'thaumazein') at a miracle or heavenly apparition. The decisive factor in overcoming fear and an absolute novelty in Christianity is the principle of hope, which neither mythology nor ancient philosophy implies. And this is consistent with the results of empirical research. Based on the fundamental ideas of Becker (1973), Solomon (2015) and Batthyani (2019) researched how people try to manage their fears when they are aware of their own death. (This research is known as 'Terror Management Theory'.) They concluded that death anxiety is warded off by two mechanisms: firstly, by strengthening one's own self-esteem and, secondly, by increasing one's respective significant social values or worldview (Juckel and Mavrogiorgou 2018).

In philosophy, the existential philosopher Kierkegaard was the first to deal intensively with the subject of fear in his book *The Concept of Anxiety*. He distinguishes between anxiety with an unknown cause and fear based on knowledge of danger. According to Kierkegaard, fear is a basic human feeling. The philosopher draws on the Christian tradition of thought and believes that despite the orthodox view of the redemptive power of the crucifixion and resurrection of Christ, the fear of not being free of original sin remains. He says about fear that this is an adventure that every human being has to go through. They need to have an experience of fear so that subsequently they are not lost when they meet it, either by never having been afraid in the first place or by finding themselves sinking into fear; therefore, whoever has learnt to be afraid in the right way has learnt the highest thing. He compares fear with a feeling of dizziness that arises when one looks into a depth or abyss that threatens to swallow one up. In fear, it is as if one loses one's footing, in which the world one knows loses its familiarity. For Kierkegaard, sin, fear and freedom were linked. In the fear of violating God's commandment, Adam at the same time recognises his freedom of will. Fear brings man in an excellent way before himself and to himself (Kierkegaard 1844; Gron 1996).

Later existential philosophers, such as Heidegger, Jaspers and Sartre, continued this intensive examination of the theme of anxiety. They drew their ideas not only from Kierkegaard's thoughts, but they were also influenced by the two world wars, where the world became extraordinarily threatening. In their teachings, they seek, among other things, an appropriate way of dealing with anxiety and hold the conviction that enduring anxiety, not giving in to it, is the most helpful approach. From this perspective, the person does not sink beneath the weight of anxiety but emerges from it feeling secure. In other words, the philosophers concerned recommend confronting the anxiety, but this is not easy to bring to bear in day-to-day practice with many patients (Kast 2023; Heidegger 1979).

In our modern world, the mechanisms described above (religion and faith, myth, cultural traditions, large communities, etc.) are dwindling more and more, leaving modern people alone without the support and security derived from these structures, confronted with their fears (Fabian 2017).

In the more recent literature, there are many examples where experienced individual fear comes to the fore. Here I would like to mention from the well-known book of Fyodor Dostoevsky *Crime and Punishment* (1866) the dream of Raskolnikov. Raskolnikov, the protagonist of the novel, regresses in a dream and as a small child witnesses the murder of a horse. Afterwards, he wakes up drenched in sweat and wonders if he will really slay an old woman for financial reasons as well, as he planned. Another example is Stefan Zweig's novella *Fear*, where, influenced by Freud's psychoanalysis, he makes fear a direct theme. A psychologically interesting novella illustrates the impact of fear and guilt on a married woman driven by her forbidden desire for adventure in the early twentieth century (Zweig 2021; Ermann 2019). Another instructive example from literature is the book by Tolstoy *Ivan Ilyich*. In this book, a defence form of man's fear of death becomes recognisable, as Yalom says, namely, to believe that one's self is not vulnerable, i.e. is something special. As long as Ivan Ilyich denies his death, he is in severe pain. When he is able to cope with his fear of death with the help of his son and his servant, his pain disappears (Tolstoi 1931, 1960; Yalom 1980). Moreover, in his book *War and Peace*, Tolstoy presents a second mechanism for how people often cope with their fear of death, namely, by believing in a saviour who ensures man's safety and protection. Let us recall Rostov's ecstasy on the battlefield at the thought that the Tsar was near him. Tolstoy writes: '…And Rostov got up, wandered among the bivouac fires and pondered what a happiness it would be to die before the eyes of the Emperor!' (Yalom 1980, page 156).

In the modern visual art, we are often confronted with individual fear in a stark way. For example, the Dutch painter Vincent van Gogh gives us a sense of his existential angst through his painting: *Starry Night*. van Gogh created this painting during an acute schizophrenic episode as Professor Ermann writes (Ermann 2019). Other authors understand his mental symptoms as a consequence of several diagnoses. They postulate a comorbidity of several mental illnesses (Nolen et al. 2020). Edvard Munch, who was confronted with existential and death anxiety due to his life experience, expresses in his painting *The Scream* (1895) how fear can skew a person's sense of them themselves and put them in a state of dramatic shock. Another interesting aspect of the picture is how the two people behind him in the background have turned away from him and do not want to know about his fear, nor by extension probably confront their own.

Climate change is another modern trigger of anxiety. Anxiety in this context arises directly from extreme events, which can lead to PTSD, depression, anxiety disorders or adjustment disorders. However, there are also people who develop anxiety and stress symptoms out of concern about climate change. In spite of this topic being insufficiently researched, the term 'eco anxiety' has become established (Spitzer 2020; Clayton et al. 2021). I suspect that among these people are some who are simply very sensitive and, in my opinion, react quasi-appropriately to the threat of climate change. Is it not understandable, when faced with this danger and what is seen as the world's inadequate response, to develop a fear of the future, especially for young people, because the very existence of our world is threatened? This is particularly the case when they see that modern societies largely deny the consequences of climate change because of barely tolerable feelings such as grief, guilt, envy and powerlessness. We allay and comfort ourselves with feelings of omnipotence that our technological and technical mastery will allow us to deal with the consequences of climate change or in projections such as 'The governments, the oil companies and the industry alone are the bad guys' (Habibi-Kohlen 2020).

Psychoanalysis has also contributed significantly to the understanding of anxiety. In his effort to fathom the deep dimensions of the human soul and its disorders, Freud dealt intensively with the subject of anxiety from the very beginning. He recognised the importance of repressed anxiety as the catalyst in the development of neurosis. Initially, Freud described the anxiety neurosis in 1895, whose origin he saw in the inhibited abreaction of an existing sexual arousal. However, since this biologically based explanation of the anxiety neurosis could not be empirically proven, Freud formulated a concept in his late work (1926), *Inhibitions, Symptoms and Anxiety*, that was based on a mental basis: the ego develops anxiety when it sees itself in a dangerous situation. This fear has the function of a signal to protect the individual from the existing danger by switching on adequate coping mechanisms. If the danger estimated by the individual is assessed as life-threatening, for example, a great deal of strength is mobilised. It is interesting to note, as a study from California showed (Dragos and Tamasescu 2010), that an acute fear reaction increases stress hormones released, whereby the individual is neuroimmunologically better protected against infection and inflammation (as, e.g. T cells are increasingly activated). In neurotic anxiety, however, there is a disproportion between the extent of the objectifiable threat and the fear triggered. These fears are repressed in childhood because they are very conflictual against the background of very ambivalent important relationships. Freud illustrated this form of neurotic anxiety with several analyses of phobias, e.g. 'Analysis of the phobia of a little boy' who developed a phobia of horses. Little Hans shifted his fear of his father, who played 'horses' with him as a child, onto horses and was afraid of being bitten by the animals. The reason for this conflict was his love for his mother and therefore his fear of punishment by his father, whom he otherwise loved. The conflict arises from the very ambivalent feelings towards the father and is resolved by the horse phobia. The neurotic aspect is not his fear itself but the replacement of the father by the horse. Freud's interest was primarily focused on the Oedipus complex and the incest taboo. Panic attacks are interpreted by Freud as well as by later authors (e.g. Fenichel 1946) as the consequence of a defence failure. On the other hand, fear may be overwhelming due to trauma (Freud 1898, 1900, 1905, 1908, 1909, 1912/13, 1916/1917, 1919, 1926).

Later definitions of anxiety distinguish between 'trait' and 'state' anxiety. State anxiety is defined as a temporary reaction to adverse events and trait anxiety as a stable personality feature (Spielberger 1972).

Modern psychoanalytic concepts understand panic attacks not only as the consequence of a defence failure but also as the consequence of a neurobiological vulnerability (De Masi 2004; Rudden et al. 2003). This interplay of innate neurobiological as well as developmental psychological or biographical factors that lead to neurobiological vulnerability has been established by Professor Milrod and her research group as the theoretical basis of panic-focused psychodynamic psychotherapy (PFPP; see Chap. 8. in this book. Milrod and Shear (1991) analysed 35 of over 100 psychodynamic studies and conducted interviews with panic patients on a psychoanalytic basis. Thus they evaluated the following:

1. A prerequisite for panic disorder is neurobiological vulnerability. Neurobiological vulnerability is shown by measuring the activity of the emotion regulation centres in the brain while confronting the person with fear stimuli. Indeed, experimental studies using functional magnetic resonance imaging have shown that the activity of the amygdala nuclei in the brain (which is one of the important centres for emotion regulation) is increased when confronted with stimuli, and the activity of centres in the prefrontal cortex is down-modulated (the prefrontal cortex inhibits affect) (Etkin and Wagner 2007). Moreover, there are studies showing that this neurobiological development occurs in rats when maternal care is deficient. Under these circumstances, altered gene expression occurs (Meany and Szyf 2005).
2. If the child's parents are, for example, unpredictable or prone to outbursts of anger, it leads to an increase in the child's innate anxiety, which makes it more difficult for the child to develop explorative behaviour and autonomy ('trait anxiety').
3. Against this background, they tend to remain dependent on their parents. In this climate of dependency and their parents' tantrums, they often experience being flooded with negative emotions (anger, fear, etc.) themselves. Furthermore, under the influence of their difficult parental relationship, they are unable to form inner supportive ideas of relationships. Instead, they develop images of overpowering, frightening significant others to whom they feel helpless and have a weak self-image. These people protect themselves by avoiding anxiety-provoking situations, thoughts or feelings. This is because they are impaired in coping with negative affects due to their biological and psychological capabilities (in psychodynamic theory we say structural deficits).
4. However, by avoiding such situations and experiencing repeated negative affect, the anxiety of these people is reinforced, i.e. they develop permanent anxiety and are unable to regulate their negative affect well due to their personality structure.
5. If additional stressors occur in the course of their lives, e.g. sexual maturation, illnesses, examinations or separations, the people concerned develop a fear of losing control over themselves and their own lives. If they fail to ward off their fear through avoidance behaviour, they become flooded with it and suffer a first panic attack. The person then starts to catastrophise, which draws their attention to the physical symptoms and avoids the fantasies as well as the feelings that actually scare them (Subric-Wrana et al. 2012).

My personal experience with patients suffering from panic disorder coincides with Ms. Milrod's concept presented here. I have observed that most patients have structural impairments parallel to the neurotic defence against their negative affects.

These are structural impairments in the sense of perceiving affects, differentiating affects, affect intolerance and clear problems regarding self-reflection. In these cases, I prioritise promoting the patient's ability to mentalise right from the beginning of therapy. Namely, I try to make the patient sensitive to mental processes both their own and those of people around them. An important prerequisite is that the patient is able to distance themselves from themselves to a certain extent. The better the mentalisation succeeds, the clearer the existing conflicts become, which tends to give the patient a better chance of developing greater competence to regulate themselves on the basis of improved self-reflection.

References

Askitopoulou, H. (2015). Sleep and Dreams: From Myth to Medicine in Ancient Greece. Journal of Anesthesia History. Volume 1, Issue 3. July 2015, Pages 70–75

Batthyani A (2019). Zur Psychologie einer Grundangst. Karl Alber Verlag. Freiburg, München.

Becker, E. (1973). The Denial of Death. Free Press. London.

Beekes, R. (2010). Etymological Dictionary of Greek (2 Vols). Brill. Leiden-Boston

Bullman, T. A. (Office of Environmental Epidemiology, Dept. of Veterans Affairs, Washington, DC 2006), Kang H. K. & Watanabe K. K. (1990). Proportionate mortality among US Army Vietnam veterans who served in Military Region I. Am J Epidemiology.132:670–4.

Cartwright, M. (2012). Greek Mythology—World History Encyclopedia. https://www.worldhistory.org/Greek_Mythology/

Clayton S, Manning CM, Speiser M. et al (2021): Mental Health and Our Changing Climate: Impacts, Inequities, Responses. American Psychological Association (APA) & ecoAmerica, Washington DC. https://ecoamerica.org/mental-health-and-our-changing-climate-2021-edition/

De Masi F (2004): Psychodynamic of panic attacks. A useful integration of psychoanalysis and neuroscience. International Journal of Psychoanalysis. 85, 311–304.

Dostoevsky, F. (1866). Crime and Punishment. Tranlsated by D. McDuff (1991)

Dragos D & Tamasescu MD. The effect of stress on the defence systems. 2010 Feb 15; 3(1): 10–18. Journal of medicine and life

Ermann, M. (2019). Angst und Angststörungen. Psychoanalytische Konzepte. 2. Auflage. W. Kohlhammer. Stuttgrt.

Etkin A. & Wagner T. D. (2007): Functional neuroimages of anxiety: A metaanalysis of emotional processing in PTSD, social anxiety disordrer, and specific phobia. American journal of psychiatry. 164, 1476–1488.

Fabian E. (2017): Anatomie der Angst. Ängste annehmen und an ihnen wachsen. Stuttgart. Klett-Cotta.

Fenichel O. (1946):The psychoanalytic theory of neurosis. London. Routledge & Kegan Paul.

Freud, S. (1898). Zur Sexualität in der Ätiologie der Neurosen. Wiener klinische Rundschau, 2,4,5 und 7. Alfred Hölder Verlag, Wien.

Freud, S. (1900). Traumdeutung. Gesammelte Werke Band II/III.

Freud, S. (1905). Drei Abhandlungen zur Sexualtheorie. Gesammelte Werke Band V.

Freud, S. (1908). Charakter und Analerotik. Gesammelte Werke Band VII.

Freud, S. (1909). Analyse der Phobie eines 5 jährigen Knabes. Gesammelte Werke Band VII.

Freud, S. (1912/13). Totem und Tabu. Gesammelte Werke Band IX.

Freud, S. (1916/17). Vorlesungen zur Einführung. Gesammelte Werke Band XI.

Freud, S. (1919). Das Unheimliche. Gesammelte Werke Band XII.

Freud, S. (1926). Hemmung, Symptom und Angst. Gesammelte Werke Band XIV.

Gron, A. (1996). Angst bei Soren Kiergegaard. Eine Einführung in sein Denken. Klett-Cotta Verlag. Heidelberg.

Habibi-Kohlen D. (2020): „Klimawandel" und wieso man sich als Psychoanalytiker damit beschäftigen kann Online-Zeitschrift der deutschen Psychoanalytischen Vereinigung DPV.

Heidegger, M. (1979). Sein und Zeit. Max Niemeyer Verlag. Tübingen.

Juckel, G & Mavrogiorgou, P. (2018). Die Angst vor dem Tod und seine Bedeutung für die Psychiatrie.Fortschritte der Neurologie und Psychiatrie; Georg Thieme Verlag KG Stuttgart 86(04): 226–232. https://doi.org/10.1055/s-0043-12391.

Kast V. (1996). Vom Sinn der Angst. Wie Ängste sich festsetzen und wie sie sich verwandeln lassen. Herder. Freiburg.

Kast V. (2023). Vom Sinn der Angst. Wie Ängste sich festsetzen und wie sie sich verwandeln lassen. Herder. Freiburg.

Kierkegaard, S. (1844): Begrebet Angest. Lindhardt og Ringhof.

Konstan, D. (2018). "Epicurus", The Stanford Encyclopedia of Philosophy. Edward N. Zalta. Metaphysics Research Lab, Stanford University

Meany M. J. & Szyf M. (2005): Maternal care as a model for experience-depedent chromatin plasticity? Trends in neuroscience. 28, 456–463.

Milrod, B. & Shear, M.K. (1991): Dynamic treatment of panic disorder. A review. Journal of Nervous and Mental Disease. 179, 741–743.

Nolen WA, van Meekeren E, Voskuil P, van Tilburg W. (2020) New vision on the mental problems of Vincent van Gogh; results from a bottom-up approach using (semi-)structured diagnostic interviews. Int JBipolar Disord 2020 Nov 2:8(1):30. https://doi.org/10.1186/s40345-020-00196-z.

Rudden M., Busch F. N., Milrod B. Singer M., Aronson A., Roiphe J. et al. (2003): Panic disorder and depression. A psychodynamic exploration of comorbidity. International Journal of Psychoanalysis. 84, 997–1015.

Solomon S., Greenberg J., Pyszczynski T. (2015). The worm at the core. Penguin. UK

Spielberger, C. D. (1972): Anxiety: Current Trends in Teory and Research. Academic press. London, New York.

Spitzer M. (2020): Klimawandel: Ursachen, Folgen, Lösungsansätze und Implikationen für das Gesundheitswesen Climate change: Causes, consequences, solutions and public health care implications. Zeitschrift für Evidenz, Fortbildung und Qualität im Gesundheitswesen. Volume 156–157 November 2020

Subric-Wrana, C., Milrod B. & Beutel M. (2012): Panikfokussierte Psychodynamische Psychotherapie. Praxis der psychodynamischen Psychotherapie- analytische und tiefenpsychologisch fundierte Psychotherapie. Hogrefe. Göttingen.

Rudolf, G., Heningsen, P. (2017). Psychotherapeutische Medizin und Psychosomatik. Ein einführendes Lehrbuch auf psychodynamischer Grundlage. Thieme. Stuttgart.

Tolstoy, L. (1931). War and Peace. Modern Library. New York.

Tolstoi, L. (1960). The Death of Ivan Ilych and other Stories. Signet Classics. New York.

Yalom, I. (1980). Existential Psychotherapy. Basis Books, Inc. Publ., New York.

Yalom, I. (2010). Existentielle Psychotherapie. 5 korrigierte Auflage. EHP

Zweig S. (2021). Angst. Novelle. Anaconda Verlag. München.

Neuroendocrine Regulation of Anxiety

Anna Onisiforou, Panos Zanos, and Polymnia Georgiou

Introduction

Anxiety disorders are a debilitating group of mental illnesses with a global prevalence recently estimated at 7% (Baxter et al. 2013). Despite the substantial impairments associated with these disorders, the existing pharmacological treatments are not always effective, indicating the need for continued research into potential alternative effective treatment approaches (Batelaan et al. 2010; Bystritsky 2006; Ginsburg et al. 2011). Neuroendocrine function has long been implicated in anxiety, although the focus on hormonal mediation has traditionally been centered on the activity of the hypothalamic-pituitary-adrenal (HPA) axis (Jacobson 2014; McEwen et al. 2015). In the present chapter, we examine the contributions of the HPA axis and hormones, which have received comparatively less attention in anxiety research. We describe the effects of each of these hormones on the anxious response in both preclinical and clinical research and elaborate on their potential as focal points for the development of novel anxiolytic therapies.

Anxiety disorders are a prevalent mental health issue that can be caused by various factors, including stress and early-life stressors, such as childhood abuse and neglect.

A. Onisiforou · P. Zanos
Department of Psychology, University of Cyprus, Nicosia, Cyprus

P. Georgiou (✉)
Department of Biological Sciences, University of Cyprus, Nicosia, Cyprus

Department of Psychology, University of Wisconsin Milwaukee, Milwaukee, WI, USA
e-mail: georgiop@uwm.edu

C. Charis, G. Panayiotou (eds.), *Anxiety Disorders and Related Conditions*,
https://doi.org/10.1007/978-3-031-56798-8_3

Brain Stress Systems

The HPA Axis in Anxiety

The HPA axis is the main stress response system. It is the neuroendocrine link between perceived stress and physiological reactions to stress (Gerhard 2013). The HPA axis consists of three main components: the hypothalamus, the pituitary gland, and the adrenal glands. When the body is under stress, the paraventricular nucleus (PVN) of the hypothalamus releases corticotropin-releasing factor (CRF), which stimulates the pituitary gland to release adrenocorticotropic hormone (ACTH). ACTH then travels to the adrenal glands, which stimulates the production of cortisol in humans or corticosterone in animals. These hormones are considered stress hormones. Cortisol/corticosterone regulates the body's response to stress by increasing blood sugar levels, suppressing the immune system, and increasing blood pressure.

Abnormal development of the HPA axis can further result in long-term alterations in neuropeptide and neurotransmitter synthesis in the central nervous system, as well as glucocorticoid hormone synthesis in the periphery. Altogether these changes may underlie the development of mood disorders such as anxiety. In fact, heightened activation of the HPA axis results in increased anxiety levels, whereas drugs that inhibit the HPA axis demonstrate anxiolytic effects. Below we discuss in more detail the role of CRF and glucocorticoids in anxiety disorders.

Role of CRF

CRF is a neuropeptide that plays a significant role in the endocrine, autonomic, and behavioral responses to stress (Schulz et al. 1996). It has been widely demonstrated that elevated CRF levels can lead to increased anxiety-like behavior (Bajo et al. 2008; Bruijnzeel et al. 2009; Gafford et al. 2012; Heinrichs et al. 2002; Lukkes et al. 2009; Risbrough et al. 2003; Schulz et al. 1996; Skelton et al. 2000; Vuong et al. 2010). Also, hypersecretion of CRF from hypothalamic as well as from extrahypothalamic neurons was observed in depression and anxiety disorders (Wiersielis et al. 2016). Schulz et al. (1996) found that administration of the anxiolytic chlordiazepoxide blocks the effect of CRF but not the startle-increasing effects of amphetamine or strychnine, suggesting that CRF is involved in anxiety (Schulz et al. 1996). Additionally, elevated levels of CRF are commonly found in the cerebrospinal fluid of patients suffering from depression or anxiety disorders (Bajo et al. 2008). In line with this, central infusions of CRF peptide antagonists, such as a-helical CRF9-41 and D-Phe CRF12-41, induced anxiolytic effects, further supporting the role of CRF in the regulation of anxiety (Dore et al. 2013; Risbrough et al. 2003).

Accumulating evidence supports the hypothesis that the anxiogenic effects of CRF are mediated by type 1 CRF receptors (CRF1Rs), as demonstrated in CRF1R-deficient mice, which show reduced anxiety-like behavior (Bajo et al. 2008). Conversely, CRF2 receptor activation seems to decrease conditioned fear responses while simultaneously increasing unconditioned anxiety-like behavior in the elevated plus maze (Risbrough et al. 2003). Moreover, the CRF1 receptor antagonist R121919 has been shown to attenuate the behavioral and endocrine responses to stress (Gutman et al. 2003), whereas CRF2 receptor antagonism has been shown to reverse increased anxiety-like behavior in rats during amphetamine withdrawal (Vuong et al. 2010).

The amygdala is a key brain region involved in affect-related disorders such as anxiety, and the CRF system plays an important role in the regulation of anxiety in this region (Ji and Neugebauer, 2008). The CRF1 receptor is expressed in the amygdala, particularly in the lateral division of the central nucleus of the amygdala (CeA) (Herman et al. 2016b; Natividad et al. 2017). Studies have shown that CRF1 antagonists have anxiolytic and antidepressant effects (Natividad et al. 2017; Taché 2015). Additionally, CRF1 receptor activation in the amygdala has been shown to be involved in pain-related anxiety-like behavior (Herman et al. 2016b). Furthermore, CRF1 receptors in the amygdala have been implicated in the extrahypothalamic circuits through which CRF contributes to anxiety-like behavior and affective disorders (Natividad et al. 2017).

The CRF1 receptor also plays a significant role in the regulation of anxiety through its expression in the bed nucleus of the stria terminalis (BNST) (Ji et al. 2007; Korosi et al. 2006; Miguel and Nunes-de-Souza 2011; Taché 2015), a region highly involved in the regulation of anxiety. The BNST is a key brain region involved in stress-related anxiety, and CRF1 receptors are expressed in this region (Ji et al. 2007; Korosi et al. 2006). Additionally, downregulation of CRF1 mRNA observed in the substantia nigra might be caused by CRF neurons located in the CeA and the BNST, which also show a clear upregulation of CRF in CRF-overexpressing mice (Korosi et al. 2006). Furthermore, glucocorticoids can potentiate fear via feed-forward regulation of CRF by glucocorticoids in the amygdala and in the BNST (Grillon et al. 2007). Also, CRF-mediated mechanisms in the BNST have been shown to modulate anxiety and nociception (Bajo et al. 2008). Furthermore, the lateral division of the BNST contains a large number of neurons expressing CRF, and chronically enhanced CRF expression within the BNST has been shown to increase anxiety-like behavior in rats (Risbrough et al. 2003).

Evidence supports that CRF2 receptors may also play a role in mediating anxiety-like behavior (D'Anna et al. 2005). Specifically, microinfusion of a CRF1-CRF2 receptor antagonist, but not a specific CRF1 antagonist, into the lateral septum decreased shock-induced freezing, suggesting a role of CRF2 within the lateral septum in mediating anxiety (D'Anna et al. 2005). Additionally, septal administration of antisauvagine-30 reversed CRF-induced anxiogenic behavior (D'Anna et al. 2005). Laudisio et al. (2017) found that CRF and its receptor can be found in the dorsal hippocampus and amygdala, where they induce behavioral alterations found in anxiety and depression (Laudisio et al. 2018). Hence, it can be deduced that CRF2 receptors in the amygdala play a significant role in the regulation of anxiety, potentially serving as effective targets for anxiolytic treatments.

In conclusion, CRF plays a significant role in anxiety disorders, and CRF receptor antagonists have been hypothesized to be useful in treating anxiety disorders.

Further research is needed to fully understand the role of CRF in anxiety and to develop effective treatments for anxiety disorders.

The Role of CRF in the Regulation of Neurotransmitter Systems

There is evidence to suggest that the CRF system may regulate serotonin to mediate anxiety (Magalhaes et al. 2010; Pleil and Skelly 2018; Pomrenze et al. 2019b). The serotonergic system is involved in the regulation of mood and anxiety, and CRF has been shown to modulate serotonin release in the brain (Pomrenze et al. 2019b). Studies have shown that CRF administration increases serotonin release in the amygdala and hippocampus, brain regions involved in anxiety and fear responses (Pleil and Skelly 2018; Pomrenze et al. 2019b). Additionally, CRF1 receptor activation has been shown to increase serotonin release in the dorsal raphe nucleus, a key brain region involved in the regulation of anxiety and mood (Magalhaes et al. 2010). Furthermore, CRF1 receptor antagonists have been shown to decrease serotonin release in the amygdala and hippocampus, suggesting that CRF1 receptors may play a role in the regulation of serotonin release in these regions (Pleil and Skelly 2018; Pomrenze et al. 2019b). Hence, it can be concluded that the CRF system may regulate serotonin to mediate anxiety and that the CRF1 receptor may be a potential therapeutic target for anxiolytic treatments.

Additionally, there is evidence to suggest that the CRF system may regulate GABAergic activity in anxiety disorders (Pomrenze et al. 2019a; Roberto et al. 2010). Studies have shown that CRF administration increases GABA release within the amygdala and induces impairments in GABA(A) receptor-mediated inhibitory transmission, resulting in increased anxiety-like behavior (Gafford et al. 2012; Vuong et al. 2010). The central amygdala (CeA) is a key brain region involved in anxiety and fear responses, and both CRF and GABAergic systems in the CeA have been implicated in anxiety disorders (Roberto et al. 2010). Roberto et al. (2010) found that CRF-induced GABA release in the CeA plays a key role in alcohol dependence, suggesting that CRF may regulate GABAergic activity in this region (Roberto et al. 2010). Additionally, Pomrenze et al. (2019a, b) found that CRF neurons in the CeA project to GABAergic neurons in the BNST, suggesting that CRF may also regulate GABAergic activity in the BNST (Pomrenze et al. 2019a). Thus, it can be concluded that the CRF system may regulate GABAergic activity in anxiety disorders, particularly in the CeA and BNST, and may be a potential target for anxiolytic treatments.

Moreover, there is evidence to suggest that the CRF system may regulate opioidergic activity in anxiety disorders. Bruchas et al. (2009) found that CRF1 receptor activation of the dynorphin/kappa opioid system in the mouse basolateral amygdala mediates anxiety-like behavior (Bruchas et al. 2009). Additionally, Pomrenze et al. (2018) found that CRF neurons in the CeA project to the dlBST, another brain region involved in anxiety, and that the dlBST contains a high density of mu-opioid receptors (Pomrenze et al. 2019b). Additionally, the administration of the CRF1 antagonist antalarmin has been shown to decrease the expression of dynorphin, an endogenous opioid peptide, in the CeA (Hang et al. 2015). This suggests that CRF1 receptor activation of the dynorphin/kappa opioid system in the CeA may mediate anxiety-like behavior and that CRF1 receptor antagonists may have anxiolytic effects by blocking this system (Hang et al. 2015). Hence, it can be concluded that the CRF system may regulate opioidergic activity in anxiety disorders, particularly in the CeA and dlBST, and may be a potential target for anxiolytic treatments.

Role of Glucocorticoids

Exposure to a psychological stressor leads to the activation of the HPA axis which in turn causes the release of glucocorticoids by the adrenal glands (Herman et al. 2016a). Glucocorticoids are a class of steroid hormones that operate as a core component of the HPA axis, and their role on anxiety-like behaviors is multifaceted and profound (Herman et al. 2016a).

Specifically, increased levels of corticosterone have been linked with escalated vigilance, increased arousal, and preparatory responses, closely mirroring the fight-or-flight response (Sapolsky et al. 2000). While this physiological state holds adaptability during acute threats, its persistence can contribute to the development of anxiety-like states when sustained over time (Herman et al. 2016a; Sapolsky et al. 2000).

Interestingly, dysregulation of cortisol levels may also disrupt the equilibrium between the amygdala and prefrontal cortex, amplifying anxiety responses and contributing to impaired emotional regulation (Arnsten 2009; Farooqi et al. 2018; Lupien et al. 2009). Moreover, corticosterone possesses a pivotal control over the hippocampus, a region well known for its involvement in memory processes, learning, and emotional regulation (Harrewijn et al. 2020; Joëls and Baram 2009; Lupien et al. 2009). Chronic stress and elevated corticosterone/cortisol levels have been lint to a reduction in hippocampal neurogenesis (McEwen et al. 2016), a process associated with anxiety modulation, as well as structural alternations. Such impairments in neurogenesis and structural alternations could potentially disrupt critical hippocampal circuits and synaptic plasticity (McEwen et al. 2016), ultimately leading to the amplification of anxiety-like behaviors.

Glucocorticoids exert their effects through binding on the glucocorticoid receptors (J M H M Reul and Kloet 1985). These receptors are expressed in important brain regions that participate in the regulation of anxiety like behaviors, such as the amygdala, hippocampus, and prefrontal cortex (Morimoto et al. 1996). Specifically, peripheral administration or direct administration of glucocorticoid antagonists in the amygdala, hippocampus, and prefrontal cortex induces anxiolytic effects in rodents (Bertholomey et al. 2022; Karst et al. 2005; Reis et al. 2016; Yang et al. 2006). In line with this evidence, genetic and epigenetic factors affect the expression and function of these receptors, resulting in varied responses to stress and anxiety (Mourtzi et al. 2021; Reul et al. 2015). The combinatorial actions between genetic makeup and environmental factors shape an individual's susceptibility to anxiety-related behaviors, providing a glimpse into the complexity of anxiety regulation.

Additionally, glucocorticoids can affect the balance between inhibitory (GABAergic) and excitatory (glutamatergic) neurotransmissions (Cutler et al. 2023; Gulyaeva 2022; Popoli et al. 2011; G.-Y. Wang et al. 2016) which is pivotal in anxiety regulation. Heightened corticosterone levels are implicated in changes to GABA receptor expression and function, which could potentially elevate anxiety-like behaviors (Cutler et al. 2023; Jie et al. 2018; Nuss 2015; G.-Y. Wang et al. 2016). Furthermore, the hormone's influence on glutamate transmission could potentially further exacerbate anxiety responses. Glucocorticoids also interact with serotonin, a neurotransmitter critical for mood regulation (Barr and Forster 2011). Dysregulation of cortisol levels may impact serotonin availability, contributing to mood disturbances and heightened anxiety.

Significantly, the relationship between corticosterone and anxiety-like behaviors is not uniform across sexes. Male and female rodents may display disparate hormonal responses and resultant behavioral outcomes (Baxter et al. 2013; Farhane-Medina et al. 2022; Feng et al. 2011; Frye and Edinger 2004; Kokane and Perrotti 2020; Maeng and Milad 2015). For instance, while manipulation of this system in male rats might lead to increased anxiety-like behaviors, females might not necessarily exhibit the same pattern (Bangasser et al. 2010; Solomon et al. 2012). This recognition of sex-dependent effects underscores the intricate nature of corticosterone's role in anxiety.

Research into glucocorticoid's involvement in anxiety-like behaviors has paved the way for future interventions. Investigations targeting glucocorticoid receptors or pathways involved in its production through pharmacological interventions have been explored to alleviate anxiety-like responses.

The Central Norepinephrine System

Norepinephrine (NE) is a hormone and neurotransmitter that plays a central role in the neuroendocrine regulation of anxiety (Bremner et al. 1996). NE is synthesized by neurons situated in the locus coeruleus of the brainstem, and it is released into the bloodstream in response to stress, initiating the well-known "fight-or-flight" response (Bremner et al. 1996).

NE plays a central role in emotional processing regulation, particularly in fear conditioning. Specifically, within the amygdala, a key player in detecting threats and processing emotions, NE release enhances the encoding of emotional memories linked to fear-inducing stimuli (Bremner et al. 1996). This mechanism can heighten sensitivity to potential dangers and intensify fear responses upon encountering similar situations. NE also affects attention and alertness, contributing to the anxious experience. During stressful events, it enhances vigilance and directs attention toward possible threats (Sciolino and Holmes 2012). This heightened state of alertness often leads to hypervigilance, where individuals become overly focused on potential dangers, driving anxiety levels higher. Importantly, patients with anxiety disorders, such as post-traumatic stress disorder (PTSD), panic disorder, and social anxiety disorder, exhibit abnormalities in NE function (Bremner et al. 2000; Geracioti et al. 2001; Johnson et al. 2015). For instance, individuals with chronic PTSD have been found to have greater central nervous system noradrenergic activity compared to healthy subjects (Geracioti et al. 2001). Similarly, exposure to traumatic memories in patients with PTSD is associated with heightened NE activity, manifesting as intrusive and distressing recollections (Green et al. 2015). In people suffering from panic disorders, abrupt NE surges can trigger severe panic attacks (Bremner et al. 1996). Moreover, alterations in NE receptor binding in specific brain regions, such as the prefrontal cortex, have been associated with PTSD symptoms (Bremner et al. 2000).

Furthermore, NE can also affect the function of the prefrontal cortex which is a region for emotional regulation and higher-order cognitive functions. During stressful and anxiety-filled situations, NE can impede prefrontal cortex activity, resulting in rational decision-making impairments and dysregulation of emotional control (Sciolino and Holmes 2012). This interference can lead to an incapability to effectively manage anxiety-inducing situations. Additionally, the role of NE in memory consolidation contributes to the development and perpetuation of anxiety. For instance, in high anxiety situations, NE facilitates the consolidation of memories tied to anxiety triggers, creating a cycle where specific cues or environments produce anxiety responses, despite the absence of any immediate threats (Bremner et al. 1996).

Importantly, following exposure to stress NE is released by the locus coeruleus, which feeds back to the hypothalamus (McEwen 2007). In response to NE, the hypothalamus releases CRF, initiating the beginning of the stress response (McEwen 2007). A positive feedback loop is created through the interaction between NE and CRF (McEwen 2007), in which NE stimulates the release of CRF, which further activates the locus coeruleus to release more NE (McEwen 2007). This loop amplifies the activation of the HPA axis, leading to the release of ACTH (McEwen 2007), thus prompting the adrenal glands to release cortisol. Once cortisol is released, it signals back to the hypothalamus and anterior pituitary, curtailing further CRF and ACTH secretion (McEwen 2007). Similarly, NE release can be modulated through negative feedback to maintain equilibrium (McEwen 2007). This interaction between the noradrenergic system and the HPA axis extends beyond the physiological responses but also influences behavior and the development of anxiety (McEwen 2007). NE secretion enhances vigilance and concentration, aligning with the body's readiness to respond to potential threats (McEwen 2007). Additionally, cortisol influences energy mobilization and immune function showcasing the adaptive processes operating during stressful situations (McEwen 2007). This interaction between the body's stress systems indicates that both systems might contribute to the development of mood disorders. Indeed, and in line with these findings, excessive or chronic stress can lead to an overactive stress response system, characterized by sustained elevation of NE and cortisol levels (McEwen 2007), resulting in stress-related disorders such as anxiety, depression, and PTSD (McEwen 2007).

Pharmacological interventions targeting the noradrenergic system also support the role of this system in the regulation of anxiety. Specifically, selective serotonin-NE reuptake inhibitors (SNRIs), which inhibit the reuptake of both serotonin and NE, have been used as an alternative to selective serotonin reuptake inhibitors (SSRIs) in patients with anxiety disorders (Dell'Osso et al. 2010). These drugs enhance NE neurotransmission and have been shown to alleviate anxiety symptoms (Dell'Osso et al. 2010). Additionally, other drugs that target the NE system, such as clonidine and prazosin, have shown potential in the treatment of PTSD (Strawn and Geracioti 2008).

In summary, norepinephrine's multifaceted involvement in anxiety encompasses various aspects of the stress response, emotional processing, attention, memory consolidation, and interactions with physiological systems like the HPA axis. Dysregulation of NE pathways contributes to the onset and persistence of anxiety disorders and the effectiveness of SNRIs in their treatment through the modulation of NE neurotransmission, demonstrating the importance of this system and highlighting its importance as a therapeutic target for anxiety disorders.

Role of Neuropeptides

Oxytocin

Oxytocin (OXT) is a nine-amino acid polypeptide hormone, historically recognized as the first sequenced polypeptide hormone. It originated from the supraoptic and paraventricular nuclei of the hypothalamus (Gebert et al. 2018). Initially renowned for its pivotal roles in parturition, lactation, and maternal behavior, OXT has gradually revealed its involvement in an array of functions, encompassing memory modulation, anxiety regulation, mood control, and intricate social behaviors (Myers et al. 2014).

The complex network of OXT pathways modulates an acute stress response, which is initiated by the central nucleus of the amygdala. This initiation triggers localized activation of GABAergic interneurons, further contributing to the regulatory dynamics within this complex neural circuitry. Remarkably, the amygdala governs immediate stress reactions, while the stria terminalis guides the transition to enduring anxiety states, with direct projections from oxytocinergic neurons in the periventricular nucleus into this structure (Love 2018; MacDonald and Feifel 2014). The anterior cingulate cortex emerges as a key facilitator of learning and adaptive social behaviors, thus deepening our comprehension of OXT's intricate regulatory roles (Boccia et al. 2013; Grace et al. 2018).

Widespread oxytocin receptors (OXTR) offer fertile ground for exploration, particularly in unraveling polymorphisms and epigenetic markers linked to OXTR, notably in the context of depression and anxiety. Single nucleotide polymorphisms (SNPs) within the OXTR gene have been intricately linked to depressive patients, while the SNP rs53576 in the third intron of the OXTR gene has shed light on the epigenetic regulation of this gene, extending its implications to adult separation anxiety and even suicide risk (Costa et al. 2017; Myers et al. 2014; Parris et al. 2018).

The intricate interplay between oxytocin and neurotransmitter systems, including serotonin and the HPA axis, results in a dynamic orchestration of neural responses (Acevedo-Rodriguez et al. 2015). Mottolese et al. have elegantly demonstrated the interaction between oxytocin and serotonin, with intranasal oxytocin administration leading to increased serotonin levels across specific brain regions (Mottolese et al. 2014). The convergence of the oxytocinergic and serotoninergic systems is substantiated by the modulation of behavioral responses induced by oxytocin, mediated through serotoninergic receptors, notably the 5HT1A receptor (Broadbear et al. 2014).

Furthermore, the intricate connections between oxytocin and the HPA axis unravel a multifaceted regulatory role. Co-expression of oxytocin and CRF within the PVN underscores the intricate interplay between these systems, leading to central oxytocin administration modulating CRF neuron excitability and neuroendocrine stress response (Love 2018). Beyond these interactions, animal models provide compelling evidence of oxytocin's impact on anxiety-like behaviors and cortisol levels, illuminating its multifaceted regulatory functions (Smith et al. 2016).

The antidepressant-like properties of oxytocin have been unveiled through pioneering studies, as oxytocin administration mirrors the effects of established antidepressants in animal models (Broadbear et al. 2014). Clinical investigations have illuminated the inverse relationship between plasma oxytocin levels and the severity of depression and anxiety symptoms, suggesting its potential therapeutic relevance (Scantamburlo et al. 2007). Oxytocin's influence extends beyond symptoms, as elevated oxytocin levels correlate with reduced central amygdala volume and altered responses to aversive stimuli, providing insight into its complex neurobiological underpinnings (Lancaster et al. 2018).

Yet, amidst the wealth of knowledge, the connection between oxytocin and anxiety symptoms remains enigmatic and context dependent. This phenomenon highlights the intricate "oxytocin paradox" that renders its signaling contextually contingent (Bethlehem et al. 2014). Individual nuances, encompassing factors such as gender, age, and psychosocial functioning, contribute to oxytocin's diverse effects, necessitating comprehensive investigations to unravel the intricate web of its regulation (Gadassi Polack et al. 2021).

While oxytocin's role in anxiety disorders has predominantly been explored within the context of social anxiety disorder, investigations into other subtypes of anxiety disorders offer diverse insights. Specific phobias and panic disorder provide varied outcomes in response to oxytocin administration, highlighting the need for further research in its therapeutic applications (Milrod et al. 2016; Onodera et al. 2015). For instance, in the case of specific phobias, a double-blind, placebo-controlled trial encompassing intranasal oxytocin administration prior to exposure therapy was conducted involving individuals with arachnophobia. Unexpectedly, contrary to initial expectations, the group receiving oxytocin pretreatment exhibited inferior treatment outcomes, along with diminished credibility of the therapeutic intervention and perceptions of the therapeutic alliance, as compared to the placebo-administered group (Milrod et al. 2016). As oxytocin's influence extends to neural activity in areas such as the amygdala, anterior insula, anterior cingulate, and precuneus, regions integral to conscious monitoring of one's surroundings, the significance of contextual framing becomes paramount (Hurlemann 2017). Acknowledging and accounting for this contextual influence is essential to avoid potential unfavorable outcomes in oxytocin-based interventions.

In conclusion, oxytocin's multifaceted roles in anxiety disorders encompass diverse neurobehavioral pathways, genetic influences, and therapeutic interventions. The evolution of our understanding continues to unravel the complexities of oxytocin's impact, promising innovative treatment avenues and offering hope for improved outcomes in individuals grappling with anxiety disorders.

Vasopressin

Vasopressin, also known as the antidiuretic hormone (ADH) or arginine vasopressin (AVP), constitutes a nonapeptide comprising nine amino acids and resides within the class of nonapeptides. Its biosynthesis transpires within the magnocellular cells of the hypothalamic supraoptic nucleus and PVN, followed by the projection of axonal pathways to the posterior pituitary (Caldwell et al. 2008; Young 3rd and Gainer 2003). Upon its subsequent release into the systemic circulation, vasopressin primarily directs its influence toward the renal system and vascular networks. This concerted action orchestrates regulatory dominion over a spectrum of physiological processes, prominently encompassing water reabsorption and vasoconstriction.

Vasopressin manifests amino acid sequences and tertiary structural characteristics that bear a semblance to oxytocin, a phenomenon potentially stemming from the shared genetic provenance of their encoding genes (Zheng et al. 2021). Moreover, it is reasonable to postulate that a complex interplay between oxytocin and vasopressin engenders a contributory role in the modulation of mood and stress responses (Neumann and Landgraf 2012). This neuropeptide engenders interactions with a quartet of distinctive G-protein-coupled receptors: AVPR1A, AVPR1B, and AVPR2 (herein subsequently designated as V1A, V1B, and V2 receptors, respectively), in conjunction with the oxytocin receptor (Hodgson et al. 2014).

The network of AVP receptors, belonging to the seven transmembrane G-protein-coupled receptor (GPCR) superfamilies, orchestrates a multifaceted response within the brain. V1A and V1B receptors are widely distributed in various brain regions, including the olfactory bulb, hippocampus, cerebral cortex, amygdala, caudate putamen, cerebellum, and PVN (Hernando et al. 2001; Koshimizu et al. 2012). Conversely, the V2 receptor predominantly resides within the kidney, modulating regulatory functions such as water reabsorption and vasoconstriction (Bielsky et al. 2004).

The influence of the AVP system on anxiety regulation is manifested through its interaction with receptors localized in the dorsal hippocampus (Joëls and Baram 2009). Notably, the restraint of the AVP system's activity, accomplished via the administration of AVP receptor antagonists or avp gene knockdown, has exhibited the potential to attenuate the release of adrenocorticotropic hormone (ACTH) and corticosterone in response to acute stress paradigms (Koshimizu et al. 2012).

The unique roles of AVP receptors become evident through investigations into specific anxiety-related behaviors. Notably, male mice lacking functional V1A receptors display reduced anxiety-like behavior and impaired social recognition, highlighting the significance of V1A receptors in anxiety modulation (Bielsky et al. 2004; Egashira et al. 2007). Similarly, V1B receptor KO mice exhibit altered aggression levels but maintain normal anxiety levels in certain behavioral tests (Egashira et al. 2005; Wersinger et al. 2002). Interestingly, V1A receptor KO mice display anti-obsessive-compulsive disorder and anti-anxiety effects, as evidenced by their reduced marble-burying behavior (Egashira et al. 2007). In the context of chronic stress, AVP expression patterns differ significantly from those under acute stress, further emphasizing the complex regulatory role of AVP in the hypothalamus (Herman et al. 2008). Chronic exposure to stress leads to a distinct response pattern, with avp mRNA expression increasing above baseline levels, underscoring the involvement of AVP neurons in chronic stress adaptation (Pinnock and Herbert 2001).

The complex interplay between vasopressin and oxytocin has garnered substantial recognition. However, it is noteworthy that vasopressin's scope of interaction extends beyond oxytocin, encompassing engagement with other neuromodulatory systems, including the serotonergic system. Ishizuka et al. undertook a notable inquiry into this interrelationship by employing V1B receptor knockout (KO) mice subjected to treatment with SSRIs and SNRIs, with the objective of elucidating the potential involvement of V1B receptors in the mechanisms of SSRIs (Ishizuka et al. 2010). This investigation encompassed the implementation of the elevated plus-maze and hole-board tests as behavioral assays measuring anxiety-like behaviors in rodents. Notably, the chronic administration of SSRIs to V1B receptor knockout mice did not elicit discernible alterations in behavior, as reflected by measures pertaining to open-arm exploration and head-dipping behavior. In stark contrast, the persistent administration of SNRIs engendered substantial increments in the duration of time spent engaging in open-arm exploration and head-dipping behavior. These compelling findings collectively suggest a plausible mediation role of the V1B receptor in facilitating the anxiolytic effects attributed to 5-HT reuptake inhibitors (Ishizuka et al. 2010).

While the V1B receptor emerges as a factor potentially implicated in depression and anxiety, the V1A receptor subtype appears to be associated with a distinctive manifestation of psychopathology. Notably, Vollebregt et al. reported an observed association between RS3 microsatellite repeats situated within the promoter region of the V1A gene and the presence of extreme childhood aggression (Vollebregt et al. 2021). Expanding beyond receptor-related considerations, it is conceivable that levels of vasopressin play a contributory role in the pathophysiology of anxiety. Pertinently, heightened plasma vasopressin levels have been established in association with symptomatology characteristic of anxiety and depression (Müller et al. 2000). This assertion finds support in human investigations. Noteworthy among them, Goekoop et al. conducted an examination of plasma vasopressin levels within the context of a highly anxious-related subtype of depression, concomitant with a familial history of depression. The outcomes of this study revealed a robust correlation linking anxiety, retardation, and the presence of elevated plasma AVP levels in instances of familial depression with anxiety symptoms (Goekoop et al. 2006).

Despite the availability of various pharmacological agents, the effective treatment of anxiety remains unsatisfactory, and the development of novel antidepressants is a slow process. This impetus underscores the exploration of alternative therapeutic modalities, among which V1B antagonists emerge as a promising avenue (Hodgson et al. 2007; Louis et al. 2006).

This complex interplay between AVP and its receptors underscores their pivotal role in anxiety and mood modulation, offering potential avenues for the development of targeted therapeutic interventions.

Orexins

Orexins (orexin-A and orexin-B), also known as hypocretins, are neuropeptides that are expressed exclusively in the lateral hypothalamic area (LHA) and bind to two G-protein-coupled receptors (GPCRs): orexin-1 receptor (OX1R) and orexin-2 receptor (OX2R) (Wang et al. 2018). Orexin-B has selective affinity for OX2R, while orexin-A binds with high affinity to both OX1R and OX2R (Sakurai et al. 1998). Orexins play a crucial role in the regulation of various physiological functions, including regulating sleep and wakefulness, feeding behavior, arousal and reward, energy homeostasis, and stress (Grafe and Bhatnagar 2018; Inutsuka and Yamanaka 2013; Muschamp et al. 2014; Wang et al. 2018).

Although orexin receptors are expressed exclusively in the LHA, orexin neuron projections reach to diverse brain regions, with the two receptors distributed differentially (Marcus et al. 2001). Interestingly, orexin neuron projections are particularly dense in areas involved in regulation of the stress response system, including the prefrontal cortex and amygdala (Grafe and Bhatnagar 2018). Evidence indicates that dysregulation of orexins is implicated in various stress-related neuropsychiatric disorders, including depression and anxiety disorders (James et al. 2017).

Orexin receptors seem to mediate opposing effects in the modulation of the stress neurocircuitry as activation of OX1R was demonstrated to promote pro-stress responses, while activation of OX2R promotes anti-stress responses (Yaeger et al. 2020). Evidence from animal models indicated that injection with orexin-A in the bed nucleus of the stria terminalis of rats induced anxiety-like behaviors that were dependent on activation of NMDA-type glutamate receptors (Lungwitz et al. 2012). In a rat model of anxiety, stimulation of OX2R promoted resilience to anxiety, by reduced fear conditioning via activation of inhibitory neurons in the amygdala (Staton et al. 2018). Conversely, antagonism of OX2R promoted susceptibility to anxiety (Staton et al. 2018). The role of orexins in anxiety was also demonstrated in humans, as adolescents with anxiety disorder were shown to have higher levels of orexin-A compared to healthy controls (Akça et al. 2020).

Etiological models emphasize the link between apparent fear extinction and anxiety disorders, as the ability to extinct previously fear-inducing stimuli is crucial for the efficacy exposure therapy treatment outcome in anxiety disorders (Mineka and Oehlberg 2008; Raeder et al. 2020). Interestingly, evidence indicates that the orexin system is also involved in the consolidation and extinction of fearful memories (Flores et al. 2014). The exact mechanisms by which orexins modulate fear extinction is ongoing, but recent evidence has shown that orexin-A impairs fear extinction by increasing the expression of the cannabinoid receptor type 2 in the amygdala and 2-arachidonoylglycerol levels (Ten-Blanco et al. 2022).

Anxiety disorder is almost twice more prevalent and more disabling in women than men (McLean et al. 2011). Based on animal studies, female rats exhibit increased expression of orexin mRNA and higher activation of orexin neurons than men, which mediated impaired habituation to repeated stress exposure that was exhibited by female rats (Grafe et al. 2017). Additionally, female rats exhibit higher expression of orexin-A and OX1R in the hypothalamus compared to male rats (Jöhren et al. 2002; Taheri et al. 1999).

In conclusion, orexins, exclusive to the LHA, wield a profound influence on physiological functions, including stress response. Their differential binding to OX1R and OX2R receptors triggers opposing stress-modulating effects. Orexin's complex role in anxiety is evident from animal models to human studies, and its involvement in fear extinction holds a promise for understanding anxiety disorder mechanisms.

Melanocortins

Melanocortins encompass a collection of peptide hormones derived from proopiomelanocortin (POMC), including entities like ACTH; alpha-, beta-, and gamma-melanocyte-stimulating hormones (MSH); beta-endorphin; and corticotropin-like intermediate peptide (CLIP) (Rocha et al. 2019). These hormones have implications across a range of health aspects, including obesity, erectile dysfunction, cachexia, pain, depression, and anxiety (Fosgerau et al. 2014). Their functionality stems from interaction with melanocortin receptors, which comprise five G-protein-coupled receptors (GPCRs) designated as MC1 through MC5 receptors. Among these, MC3R and MC4R, along with their ligand alpha-MSH (and gamma-MSH for MC3R), have been linked to anxiety and depression (Copperi et al. 2022). Melanocortin neurons are mainly situated in the brainstem and the hypothalamus, particularly within the arcuate nucleus (ARC) closely interacting with agouti-related peptide (AgRP) and neuropeptide Y (NPY)-expressing neurons, thus underlining their role in the system (Mountjoy 2010; Nyamugenda et al. 2020). Alpha-MSH has been identified as a suppressor of NPY effects, thereby mitigating its antidepressant impact (Goyal et al. 2006). Administering an alpha-MSH antagonist alongside NPY reveals a synergistic anxiolytic effect (Kokare et al. 2005). Blocking MC4 receptors in the dorsal raphe nucleus (DRN) through alpha-MSH leads to anxiety, depression, and reduced feeding in mice (Bruschetta et al. 2020). The areas most affected by alpha-MSH action include PVN, ARC, and DRN (Kokare et al. 2010). Balancing the melanocortin system, the AgRP functions as a receptor antagonist, inducing an orexigenic effect (Fu and van den Pol 2008). In response to a high-fat diet, chronic administration leads to the attenuation of AgRP's response to anxiety, depression signals, and hunger by curtailing GABAergic outputs from AgRP directed at MC4R. However, GABAergic stimulation combined with 5-HT3R suppression within MC4R neurons in the bed nucleus counteracts the anxiety and depression brought about by high-fat diet (Xia et al. 2021). This combined impact also decreases food intake and subsequently body weight. These findings underscore AgRP's initial role in appetite regulation, followed by the emergence of MC4Rs as a prospective avenue for further exploration in the treatment of anxiety and depression (Chaki and Okubo 2007; Sternson and Atasoy 2014). Specific regulation of proteins impacting the melanocortin system includes the melanocyte-stimulating hormone release-inhibiting factor-1 (MIF-1) and its analog nemifitide. These exhibit limited affinity to μ-opioid receptors, functioning as alpha-MSH release blockers, thus diminishing its inhibitory influence on NPY. While preclinical studies indicate effects in depressive disorders, additional research is imperative to ascertain the efficacy of this particular peptide (Chaki and Okubo 2007; Sternson and Atasoy 2014).

Neuropeptide Y (NPY)

NPY, a neuropeptide hormone consisting of 36 amino acids, exhibits widespread distribution within the central nervous system and maintains connections with the melanocortin system. Notably, NPY is one of the most conserved proteins across evolutionary scales. Historically, NPY levels have shown correlation with affective disorders, with individuals experiencing suicidal depression displaying lowered measured plasma levels (Widerlöv et al. 1988). It is considered an endogenous anxiolytic neuropeptide (Thorsell 2010). It acts on various brain regions important in the regulation of anxiety such as the amygdala, hypothalamus, and locus coeruleus, suggesting its involvement in the integration and transduction of stressful stimuli (Jenck et al. 1997). In agreement with this, it was shown that NPY can attenuate behavioral responses to stress and has anxiolytic effects (Jenck et al. 1997).

Dysregulation of NPY has been observed in stress-related disorders, such as PTSD (Sah et al. 2009). Additionally, in a randomized controlled trial investigating PTSD, it was observed that higher doses of NPY were associated with greater anxiolytic effects (Sayed et al. 2018). Moreover, NPY deficiency enhanced anxiety-like behaviors in zebrafish (Shiozaki et al. 2020). Importantly, accumulating evidence highlights the role of NPY in reducing fear, primarily through actions of exogenous NPY on Y1 receptors (Tasan et al. 2016). In line with this finding, a decrease of fear expression was also observed in Y1 receptor knockout mice (Tasan et al. 2016). Furthermore, other Y receptors may be equally important as Y1. Indeed by acting on Y2 receptors, NPY promotes fear extinction and generates a long-term suppression of fear, two important preconditions that could support cognitive behavioral therapies in human patients (Tasan et al. 2016). The impact of NPY, acting through its receptors, has been extensively reviewed by Morales-Medina et al. culminating in the conclusion that animal models focusing on Y1 and Y2 receptors have provided robust insights into their roles in emotional responses and stress (Morales-Medina et al. 2010). Rats undergoing fear conditioning demonstrated increased NPY immunoreactivity in the nucleus accumbens, amygdala, and hypothalamus suggesting that NPY neurons are responsive to stress (Krysiak et al. 2000). The anti-anxiety drug diazepam reversed fear-induced increases in NPY expression in these regions (Krysiak et al. 2000). These results suggest that endogenous NPY in the NAc, as well as other regions, responds to alleviate fear conditioning.

Additionally, more recently adeno-associated viral vectors (AAV) have been employed to selectively ablate or activate nucleus accumbens NPY neurons to investigate their role in modulating anxiety behavior (Yamada et al. 2020). Employing Cre-dependent diphtheria toxin receptor expression targeted at accumbal NPY neurons, combined with systemic diphtheria toxin administration, yielded manifestations of anxiety behaviors as evidenced by outcomes in open field and elevated plus-maze tests (Yamada et al. 2020). In contrast, the selective activation of accumbal NPY neurons through designer receptors exclusively activated by designer drug (DREADD) technology induced anxiolytic behaviors in mice, consistent with the results from the aforementioned assessments (Yamada et al. 2020). These observations collectively suggest the implication of NPY within the nucleus accumbens in promoting anxiolytic and antidepressant behavioral effects.

In conclusion, NPY is an endogenous anxiolytic neuropeptide that plays a role in the regulation of stress and anxiety-related behaviors. Dysregulation of NPY has been observed in stress-related disorders, and NPY has shown potential as a therapeutic target for anxiety disorders.

Cholecystokinin

Initially identified in the gastrointestinal tract as a digestive peptide hormone, cholecystokinin (CCK) garnered recognition for its involvement in the processing of fats and proteins, by stimulating the pancreas and gallbladder (Grider 1994). Subsequently, CCK emerged as a neurotransmitter dispersed across various regions of the mammalian brain, including the limbic system (Smadja et al. 1997). Its composition varies based on modifications to the 150-amino acid precursor, preprocholecystokinin (Chaudhri et al. 2006). The ubiquity of CCK expression makes it one of the most widely distributed neuropeptides in the brain (Rehfeld 2021). In a seminal clinical trial in 1991, Bradwejn et al. administered CCK tetrapeptide (CCK-4) to individuals with panic disorder, resulting in panic attacks for all participants in the experimental group and surprisingly similar symptoms in a subset of the control group (Bradwejn et al. 1991). Interestingly, it was shown that increased ACTH concentrations were associated with CCK-4-induced panic attacks in panic disorder patients (Ströhle et al. 2000). Another study on human subjects exploring cerebrospinal fluid (CSF) levels of CCK found an inverse relationship between CCK concentrations and susceptibility to anxiety, depression, and suicidal tendencies (Löfberg et al. 1998). Using a knockdown mouse model, Del Boca et al. deduced that diminishing CCK, particularly in the basolateral amygdala, induced anxiolytic and antidepressant-like effects (Del Boca et al. 2012). CCK's involvement in anxiety and depression also extends to social stress-induced instances. Vialou et al. established a mouse model of social defeat stress, revealing that ΔFosB overexpression, a stress susceptibility factor, was mediated through the CCK-B receptor. This connection was reinforced by the effects observed upon infusing CCK-B receptor agonists (Vialou et al. 2014). The correlation between CCK-4 levels and anxiety and depression was repeatedly demonstrated in a mouse model. Furthermore, CCK-4 and NPY counteracted each other's effects on anxiety and depression parameters, indicating their opposing roles (Desai et al. 2014). Despite these findings, as of now, clinical trials have yet to show clinically substantial effects of CCK-B receptor antagonists in humans for mitigating anxiety and depression symptoms (Ballaz et al. 2020). Intriguingly, the intricate nature of CCK's impact on anxiety and depression was revealed by research showing that while acute administration of a CCK-B receptor antagonist produced anxiolytic effects in mice, prolonged use resulted in task reluctance. Remarkably, the restoration of benchmark anxiety levels occurred upon endogenous CCK reactivation of the CCK-B receptor (Ballaz et al. 2020). In conclusion, CCK presents a promising avenue for addressing anxiety and depression, necessitating a more comprehensive collection of clinical trials to facilitate its incorporation into the evidence-based, intricate management of these conditions (Garakani et al. 2020).

Role of Steroid Hormones

Pregnanolones and Pregnenolone

Pregnenolone, pregnenolone sulfate, pregnanolone, and allopregnanolone are neurosteroids synthesized primarily in glial cells, including oligodendrocytes and astrocytes, with possible synthesis occurring in neurons as well (Barbaccia et al. 2001; Baulieu 1981; Paul and Purdy 1992). While pregnenolone and its derivative, pregnenolone sulfate, are synthesized directly from cholesterol via cytochrome P450scc (Hanukoglu and Jefcoate 1980), pregnanolone and allopregnanolone are derived from progesterone, which is a downstream product of pregnenolone (Reddy 2003). These neurosteroids, namely, pregnanolones and pregnenolones, often exert a significant influence on anxiety-related behavior, largely through their interaction with GABAA receptors (Bitran et al. 1991; Engin and Treit 2007; Melchior and Ritzmann 1994; Mòdol et al. 2011; Reddy 2003; Twede et al. 2007). Nevertheless, the effects of these neurosteroids appear to be specific to hormone levels, brain regions, and the behavioral tests conducted.

Pregnenolones have been linked to emotional memory processes, partially through their impact on the lateral septum (LS), a key component of the medial temporal system. This brain region is densely populated with GABAA receptor-containing neurons and is particularly influenced by emotional signals from the amygdala (*No Title* n.d.). Studies involving lesioning or midazolam infusion in the LS have demonstrated a reduction in anxiety-like behavior in rats subjected to a plus-maze test (*No Title* n.d.). Similarly, the injection of pregnanolone into the LS has been reported to decrease anxiety-like behavior (Bitran et al. 1999). Administering pregnenolone intracerebroventricular (i.c.v.) or pregnenolone sulfate i.c.v. into the LS or other limbic structures enhances memory in mice when tested in emotionally charged scenarios, while pregnenolone sulfate proves amnesic in non-emotional paradigms (Flood et al. 1992, 1995). Thus, the differential effects of pregnenolone and pregnenolone sulfate on emotional memory become evident in rodent studies.

Allopregnanolone stands out as a potent positive allosteric modulator of the GABAA receptor, surpassing benzodiazepines in in vitro potency by 20-fold (Majewska et al. 1986). In rats, inhibiting the metabolic conversion of progesterone to allopregnanolone heightens anxiety-related behaviors (Frye and Walf 2002), whereas the introduction of exogenous allopregnanolone generally exhibits anxiolytic effects (Engin and Treit 2007). Human studies echo these findings observed in rodents (Girdler et al. 2001; Sripada et al. 2013). Notably, a functional magnetic resonance imaging study conducted by Sripada et al. (2013) revealed that elevated allopregnanolone levels post-oral pregnenolone administration corresponded to reduced activity in the amygdala and insula. Simultaneously, there was heightened activity in the dorsal medial prefrontal cortex (dmPFC) and enhanced connectivity between the amygdala and dmPFC, aligning with decreased self-reported anxiety. The anxiolytic impact of neurosteroids, while not exclusive to GABAA receptors, is reinforced by evidence demonstrating that blocking these receptors in rats through picrotoxin negates the anxiety-reducing effects of pregnanolone administration (Bitran et al. 1991; Eppolito et al. 2014).

Considering the pronounced involvement of pregnanolones and pregnenolones in anxiety, these neurosteroids hold a promise as potential targets for future pharmacological interventions (Longone et al. 2011). However, the relatively short half-life of allopregnanolone and other inhibitory neurosteroids poses a challenge to their effectiveness in anxiety treatment. Furthermore, exogenous allopregnanolone has been shown to affect ovarian function in rats (Laconi et al. 2012), necessitating alternative strategies for elevating neurosteroid levels. Synthetic analogs like ganaloxone exhibit sedative, anxiolytic, and anticonvulsant effects (Carter et al. 1997). Another approach involves orally administered progesterone, which acts as a prodrug, substantially increasing allopregnanolone and pregnenolone levels in the body (Andréen et al. 2006). This method has demonstrated the ability to enhance nonrapid eye movement (REM) sleep in healthy men (Friess et al. 1997) and REM sleep in postmenopausal women (Schüssler et al. 2008), indicating its potential as a treatment avenue for sleep disturbances frequently accompanying anxiety disorders (Mellman 2006). Additionally, etifoxine, a nonbenzodiazepine anxiolytic drug, has been shown to rapidly stimulate neurosteroid biosynthesis (do Rego et al. 2015), with allopregnanolone possibly contributing to the anxiolytic effects of etifoxine (Ugale et al. 2007). Regardless of the approach chosen, elevating allopregnanolone levels holds a promise as a potential means to alleviate anxiety symptoms.

Progesterone

Progesterone is a hormone that plays a crucial role in the female reproductive system and is involved in various physiological processes. It has been found to impact anxiety-related behaviors through its interaction with the GABAA receptor and modulation of neuronal excitability (Smith et al. 1998).

It was demonstrated that progesterone withdrawal is associated with increased anxiety and seizure susceptibility (Smith et al. 1998). The effects of progesterone on anxiety are mediated by its metabolites as we mentioned before, such as allopregnanolone, which enhances the function of GABA, the brain's major inhibitory neurotransmitter (Smith et al. 1998). The decline in progesterone levels during the menstrual cycle and postpartum period has been also linked to symptoms of anxiety and mood changes (Smith et al. 1998). Progesterone exerts some of its effects through binding on the progesterone receptor, which is a transcription factor. In the brain, the progesterone receptor has been implicated in the regulation of GABAergic tone and anxiety-related behaviors (Tian et al. 2000). Moreover, using a rat model of progesterone withdrawal which mimics the premenstrual and postpartum syndrome, it was demonstrated progesterone withdrawal resulted in increased seizure susceptibility and insensitivity to benzodiazepine sedatives, which are commonly used to treat anxiety (Smith et al. 1998).

However, it is important to note that not all studies have found a direct relationship between progesterone levels and anxiety. Some reports have failed to find a correlation between progesterone levels and state or trait anxiety in women (Hahn et al. 2020). Other factors, such as cortisol levels and interpersonal stress, may also contribute to anxiety symptoms (Hahn et al. 2020).

In conclusion, progesterone and its receptor exhibit a multifaceted role in anxiety. Nevertheless, further research is needed to fully understand the mechanisms underlying the role of progesterone and its receptor in anxiety in order to be explored as a potential therapeutic intervention for its treatment.

Estrogens

While a connection between low endogenous estrogen levels and anxiety symptoms exists (Frye 2009), the impact of estradiol treatment on anxiety relief is not consistently uniform. In rodent models, the outcome of estradiol's influence on anxiety-like behavior seems to hinge on both the dosage administered and the specific behavioral testing paradigm applied (Kastenberger et al. 2012). Diverse studies have yielded disparate results, ranging from reports of estradiol causing heightened anxiety (Mora et al. 1996), diminishing anxiety (Tian et al. 2013), or showing no discernible effect (Walf and Frye 2008). A similar inconsistency is apparent in human studies of estrogen therapy. For instance, estrogen therapy has led to reductions in anxiety symptoms for some postmenopausal women (Gleason et al. 2015), while proving ineffective for others (Demetrio et al. 2011). These conflicting consequences of estradiol on anxiety and related behavior likely stem from the distinct functions of various estrogen receptor (ER) subtypes (Kastenberger et al. 2012).

Research involving the use of an AVV to reduce ERα expression in ovariectomized rats has led to a decrease in anxiety-like behavior (Spiteri et al. 2010). However, treatment with an ERα agonist merely elicits minimal effects on behavior in the open field and elevated plus-maze tests (Lund et al. 2005), and ERα knockout mice did not demonstrate any anxiety-like behaviors in the open field, elevated plus maze, and light-dark box (Georgiou et al. 2019). In contrast, estradiol, via acting at the ERα, normalized postpartum-induced anxiety-like behavior, as tested by the elevated plus maze (Furuta et al. 2013). Moreover, knockdown of the ERα selectively in the posterior-dorsal amygdala of female mice decreased anxiety-like behavior as demonstrated by the increased time spent in the light compartment of the light-dark box (Spiteri et al. 2010), suggesting a possible role of ERα in regulating anxiety behaviors. Thus, further research is required to elucidate the exact role of ERα in anxiety behaviors. Conversely, activating ERβ has demonstrated an ability to alleviate anxiety-like behavior (Lund et al. 2005; Oyola et al. 2012; Walf and Frye 2005). In line with these findings, ERβ knockout mice demonstrated increased anxiety-like behaviors in the open filed and elevated plus-maze tests, a change that was associated with a reduced threshold for the induction of synaptic plasticity in the basolateral amygdala (Krezel et al. 2001). Also, ERβ male but not female knockout mice demonstrated increased susceptibility to develop social interaction deficits, which a core symptom of anxiety following acute, mild stress (Georgiou et al. 2022). Altogether, these findings suggest a clear role of ERβ in the regulation of anxiety. The recently identified G-protein-coupled ER (GPR30), another ER subtype, has also emerged as a factor in anxiety responses, although the precise nature of its impact on anxiety-like behavior remains unclear (Hart et al. 2014; Kastenberger et al. 2012). The varying activation of ERs post-estrogen therapy might account for the conflicting observations concerning estradiol's effects on anxiety-like behavior.

Given the pivotal role of receptor subtypes in the anxiety response, coupled with documented unfavorable effects linked to estrogen therapy (Taylor and Manson 2011), selective ER modulators (SERMs) hold a potential in treating anxiety disorders. SERMs could prove particularly effective in patients with specific ER polymorphisms (Ryan et al. 2011) and those encountering anxiety symptoms closely tied to fluctuating estrogen levels, such as during the premenstrual phase or menopause. Regrettably, as of now, there appears to be a lack of testing SERMs in subjects afflicted with anxiety disorders.

Androgens

Testosterone is a principal androgenic hormone that plays a multifaceted role in the regulation of anxiety. Testosterone's influence on anxiety is marked by complexity, with research revealing connections between testosterone levels and anxiety disorders. It was shown that men with low levels of testosterone experience increased anxiety (Berglund et al. 2011). Similarly, lower salivary testosterone levels were found in women with anxiety disorders, something that was not true in men (Giltay et al. 2012). Another study involving healthy female subjects reported a reduction in unconscious fear, albeit not in conscious anxiety, after sublingual testosterone administration (van Honk et al. 2005). Moreover, Granger et al. (2003) examined the diurnal variation of testosterone in adolescent males and females and found that testosterone levels were associated with individual differences in anxiety symptoms (Granger et al. 2003). The study suggested that testosterone may play a role in the development of anxiety-related behaviors in youth.

Furthermore, the effects of testosterone treatment on mental health in transgender individuals were investigated demonstrating that testosterone treatment in female-to-male transgender people is associated with positive effects on mental health, including reductions in symptoms of anxiety and depression (Davis and St. Amand 2014). These findings suggest that testosterone may have an impact on anxiety symptoms in female-to-male transgender individuals undergoing hormone therapy.

Androgens have a predominant inclination toward eliciting anxiolytic effects in rodent models (Aikey et al. 2002; Carrier et al. 2015; Edinger and Frye 2006), by influencing anxiety-like behavior through a variety of mechanisms. Firstly, the conversion of testosterone to estradiol allows for estradiol to exert the anxiolytic effects discussed earlier. Specifically, inhibition of the conversion of testosterone to estradiol through the use of letrozole, an aromatase inhibitor, induced stress susceptibility via the development of social interaction deficits and anhedonia in male mice (Georgiou et al. 2022). Additionally, Carrier and Kabbaj (2012) conducted experiments on socially isolated male and female rats and found that testosterone had anxiolytic and antidepressant effects in socially isolated male rats but not in females (Carrier and Kabbaj 2012). This suggests that testosterone may have sex-specific effects on anxiety-related behaviors. In agreement, inhibition of hippocampal aromatase with the inhibitor, fadrozole, was shown to abolish the anxiolytic effects of testosterone in male rats that underwent gonadectomy (Carrier et al. 2015). Androgens also contribute to the reduction of anxiety-like behavior by interacting with hippocampal androgen receptors (Edinger and Frye 2006). Furthermore, the conversion to the neuroactive steroid 3a-androstanediol (3a-diol), a positive allosteric modulator of GABAA receptors, permits the mediation of anxiety via the GABAergic system (Aikey et al. 2002). Lastly, 3a-diol has been shown to function through ERβ in male rats, inhibiting HPA axis activity in response to stress (Lund et al. 2006). Despite these robust findings on the anxiolytic impact of androgens in male rodents, sex-related variations might be present in the role of androgens concerning anxiety-like behavior. While there is significantly less literature exploring the effect of androgens on this behavior in female rodents, the treatment with 5a-dihydrotestosterone increases anxiety-like behavior in female rats (Feng et al. 2011). This is in contrast to the anxiolytic outcome of this steroid observed in male rats (Frye and Edinger 2004). Currently, the influence of other androgens, such as 3a-diol, on anxiety-like behavior in females remains unknown.

Importantly, the relationship between androgens and anxiety is multifaceted and can be influenced by various factors, including age, pubertal development, and individual differences. For instance, a study by Boivin et al. (2017) found that pubertal male mice castrated before puberty showed greater anxiety-related behavior during late puberty compared to intact males, while pubertal females were unaffected by hormone injections (Boivin et al. 2017). These findings highlight the complex relationship between hormones, development, age, and anxiety symptoms.

Also, it is important to note that the therapeutic potential of testosterone or other androgens for anxiety disorders is hindered by adverse side effects associated with treatment (Vigen et al. 2013). Subsequent research should aim to establish the safety and effectiveness of alternative androgenic compounds as potential treatment options for anxiety.

Conclusions

The current levels of drug response and remission in patients with anxiety disorders following pharmacological treatment are relatively low (Batelaan et al. 2010; Bystritsky 2006; Ginsburg et al. 2011). Therefore, there is an ongoing need for alternative pharmacotherapies. Within this chapter, substantial evidence has been presented linking various hormones to anxiety, drawn from both clinical and preclinical research. Numerous hormones mentioned earlier exhibit changes in plasma, saliva, or cerebrospinal fluid levels among individuals with anxiety or anxiety disorders (Borrow et al. 2016; Risbrough and Stein 2006; Ströhle et al. 2000). Recent findings concerning neuropeptides OT and AVP also indicate that epigenetic changes in genes related to these hormones might contribute to or result from anxiety and anxiety disorders (Murgatroyd et al. 2009; Ziegler et al. 2015). While the epigenetic regulation of the HPA axis and its involvement in anxiety are well-documented (Lee and Sawa 2014), non-HPA axis hormones have not yet been thoroughly investigated. Additionally, these hormones have not been extensively examined as potential treatments for anxiety disorders in humans. However, from the available limited research, allopregnanolone, SERMs, OT, NPY, and hypocretin hold a promise as targets for pharmacological treatment of anxiety disorders.

It's important to acknowledge that the effectiveness of hormonal therapies for these disorders might vary based on sex. For example, preclinical studies indicate that the androgen 5a-dihydrotestosterone has opposite effects on anxiety-like behavior in male and female rats (Feng et al. 2011; Frye and Edinger 2004), and oxytocin affects female but not male rats after chronic i.c.v. administration (Slattery and Neumann 2010). Despite the significant sex differences in anxiety disorder prevalence and treatment response (Farhane-Medina et al. 2022; Kudwa et al. 2005; Maeng and Milad 2015; McLean et al. 2011), many studies exploring the behavioral effects of the hormones covered in this chapter have not included both sexes, limiting conclusions about their effects in females.

The timing of administering compounds targeting these hormones could also impact their effectiveness, as many of these hormones are influenced by circadian rhythms (Arble et al. 2012; Chaudhri et al. 2006; Hastings 1991; Urbanski 2011).

Interestingly, individuals with anxiety disorders may experience worsened symptoms in the afternoon or evening (Cameron et al. 1986). Female rats tested during the light phase display lower anxiety-like behavior compared to males tested at the same time or females tested during the dark phase (Verma et al. 2010). Few studies have investigated the timing's impact on the administration of specific hormones and anxiety-like behavior. For instance, the anxiolytic effect of testosterone in male mice might be confined to the light phase (Chen et al. 2014). Similarly, mice lacking the NPY receptor Y1 only showed alterations in anxiety-like behavior during the light phase (Karl et al. 2006). It's uncertain if other hormones' anxiolytic effects are similarly confined to the light phase in rodents. Despite the potential challenges of sex and circadian phase, the neuroendocrine system remains an attractive alternative therapeutic avenue for patients with treatment-resistant anxiety disorders. Lastly, although the interplay between the discussed hormones hasn't been fully elucidated, many, if not all, of these hormones interact either directly or indirectly, offering numerous additional mechanisms through which anxiety and anxiety-like behavior could be influenced, warranting further investigation.

References

Acevedo-Rodriguez, A., Mani, S. K., & Handa, R. J. (2015). Oxytocin and Estrogen Receptor β in the Brain: An Overview. *Frontiers in Endocrinology*, *6*, 160. https://doi.org/10.3389/fendo.2015.00160

Aikey, J. L., Nyby, J. G., Anmuth, D. M., & James, P. J. (2002). Testosterone Rapidly Reduces Anxiety in Male House Mice (Mus musculus). *Hormones and Behavior*, *42*(4), 448–460. https://doi.org/10.1006/hbeh.2002.1838

Akça, Ö. F., Uzun, N., & Kılınç, İ. (2020). Orexin A in adolescents with anxiety disorders. *International Journal of Psychiatry in Clinical Practice*. https://doi.org/10.1080/13651501.2019.1711425

Andréen, L., Spigset, O., Andersson, A., Nyberg, S., & Bäckström, T. (2006). Pharmacokinetics of progesterone and its metabolites allopregnanolone and pregnanolone after oral administration of low-dose progesterone. *Maturitas*, *54*(3), 238–244. https://doi.org/10.1016/j.maturitas.2005.11.005

Arble, D. M., Copinschi, G., Vitaterna, M. H., Van Cauter, E., & Turek, F. W. (2012). *Chapter 12 - Circadian Rhythms in Neuroendocrine Systems* (G. Fink, D. W. Pfaff, & J.E.B.T.-H.ofN.Levine(eds.);pp.271–305).AcademicPress.https://doi.org/10.1016/B978-0-12-375097-6.10012-5

Arnsten, A. F. T. (2009). Stress signalling pathways that impair prefrontal cortex structure and function. *Nature Reviews. Neuroscience*, *10*(6), 410–422. https://doi.org/10.1038/nrn2648

Bajo, M., Cruz, M. T., Siggins, G. R., Messing, R., & Roberto, M. (2008). Protein kinase C epsilon mediation of CRF- and ethanol-induced GABA release in central amygdala. *Proceedings of the National Academy of Sciences of the United States of America*, *105*(24), 8410–8415. https://doi.org/10.1073/pnas.0802302105

Ballaz, S. J., Bourin, M., Akil, H., & Watson, S. J. (2020). Blockade of the cholecystokinin CCK-2 receptor prevents the normalization of anxiety levels in the rat. *Progress in Neuro-Psychopharmacology & Biological Psychiatry*, *96*, 109761. https://doi.org/10.1016/j.pnpbp.2019.109761

Bangasser, D. A., Curtis, A., Reyes, B. A. S., Bethea, T. T., Parastatidis, I., Ischiropoulos, H., Van Bockstaele, E. J., & Valentino, R. J. (2010). Sex differences in corticotropin-releasing factor receptor signaling and trafficking: potential role in female vulnerability to stress-related psychopathology. *Molecular Psychiatry*, *15*(9), 877,896-904. https://doi.org/10.1038/mp.2010.66

Barbaccia, M. L., Serra, M., Purdy, R. H., & Biggio, G. (2001). Stress and neuroactive steroids. *International Review of Neurobiology*, *46*, 243–272. https://doi.org/10.1016/s0074-7742(01)46065-x

Barr, J. L., & Forster, G. L. (2011). Serotonergic neurotransmission in the ventral hippocampus is enhanced by corticosterone and altered by chronic amphetamine treatment. *Neuroscience*, *182*, 105–114. https://doi.org/10.1016/j.neuroscience.2011.03.020

Batelaan, N. M., de Graaf, R., Penninx, B. W. J. H., van Balkom, A. J. L. M., Vollebergh, W. A. M., & Beekman, A. T. F. (2010). The 2-year prognosis of panic episodes in the general population. *Psychological Medicine*, *40*(1), 147–157. https://doi.org/10.1017/S0033291709005625

Baulieu, E.-E. (1981). *STEROID HORMONES IN THE BRAIN: SEVERAL MECHANISMS?* (K. Fuxe, J.-Å. Gustafsson, & L. B. T.-S. H. R. of the B. Wetterberg (eds.); pp. 3–14). Pergamon. https://doi.org/10.1016/B978-0-08-026864-4.50007-4

Baxter, A. J., Scott, K. M., Vos, T., & Whiteford, H. A. (2013). Global prevalence of anxiety disorders: a systematic review and meta-regression. *Psychological Medicine*, *43*(5), 897–910. https://doi.org/10.1017/S003329171200147X

Berglund, L. H., Prytz, H. S., Perski, A., & Svartberg, J. (2011). Testosterone levels and psychological health status in men from a general population: the Tromsø study. *The Aging Male: The Official Journal of the International Society for the Study of the Aging Male*, *14*(1), 37–41. https://doi.org/10.3109/13685538.2010.522276

Bertholomey, M. L., Nagarajan, V., Smith, D. M., & Torregrossa, M. M. (2022). Sex- and age-dependent effects of chronic corticosterone exposure on depressive-like, anxiety-like, and fear-related behavior: Role of amygdala glutamate receptors in the rat. *Frontiers in Behavioral Neuroscience*, *16*, 950000. https://doi.org/10.3389/fnbeh.2022.950000

Bethlehem, R. A. I., Baron-Cohen, S., van Honk, J., Auyeung, B., & Bos, P. A. (2014). The oxytocin paradox. *Frontiers in Behavioral Neuroscience*, *8*, 48. https://doi.org/10.3389/fnbeh.2014.00048

Bielsky, I. F., Hu, S.-B., Szegda, K. L., Westphal, H., & Young, L. J. (2004). Profound Impairment in Social Recognition and Reduction in Anxiety-Like Behavior in Vasopressin V1a Receptor Knockout Mice. *Neuropsychopharmacology*, *29*(3), 483–493. https://doi.org/10.1038/sj.npp.1300360

Bitran, D., Dugan, M., Renda, P., Ellis, R., & Foley, M. (1999). Anxiolytic effects of the neuroactive steroid pregnanolone (3 alpha-OH-5 beta-pregnan-20-one) after microinjection in the dorsal hippocampus and lateral septum. *Brain Research*, *850*(1–2), 217–224. https://doi.org/10.1016/s0006-8993(99)02150-2

Bitran, D., Hilvers, R. J., & Kellogg, C. K. (1991). Anxiolytic effects of 3 alpha-hydroxy-5 alpha[beta]-pregnan-20-one: endogenous metabolites of progesterone that are active at the GABAA receptor. *Brain Research*, *561*(1), 157–161. https://doi.org/10.1016/0006-8993(91)90761-j

Boccia, M. L., Petrusz, P., Suzuki, K., Marson, L., & Pedersen, C. A. (2013). Immunohistochemical localization of oxytocin receptors in human brain. *Neuroscience*, *253*, 155–164. https://doi.org/10.1016/j.neuroscience.2013.08.048

Boivin, J. R., Piekarski, D. J., Wahlberg, J. K., & Wilbrecht, L. (2017). Age, sex, and gonadal hormones differently influence anxiety- and depression-related behavior during puberty in mice. *Psychoneuroendocrinology*, *85*, 78–87. https://doi.org/10.1016/j.psyneuen.2017.08.009

Borrow, A. P., Stranahan, A. M., Suchecki, D., & Yunes, R. (2016). Neuroendocrine Regulation of Anxiety: Beyond the Hypothalamic-Pituitary-Adrenal Axis. *Journal of Neuroendocrinology*, *28*(7). https://doi.org/10.1111/jne.12403

Bradwejn, J., Koszycki, D., & Shriqui, C. (1991). Enhanced sensitivity to cholecystokinin tetrapeptide in panic disorder. Clinical and behavioral findings. *Archives of General Psychiatry*, *48*(7), 603–610. https://doi.org/10.1001/archpsyc.1991.01810310021005

Bremner, J. D., Innis, R. B., Southwick, S. M., Staib, L., Zoghbi, S., & Charney, D. S. (2000). Decreased benzodiazepine receptor binding in prefrontal cortex in combat-related posttraumatic stress disorder. *The American Journal of Psychiatry*, *157*(7), 1120–1126. https://doi.org/10.1176/appi.ajp.157.7.1120

Bremner, J. D., Krystal, J. H., Southwick, S. M., & Charney, D. S. (1996). Noradrenergic mechanisms in stress and anxiety: I. Preclinical studies. *Synapse (New York, N.Y.)*, *23*(1), 28–38. https://doi.org/10.1002/(SICI)1098-2396(199605)23:1<28::AID-SYN4>3.0.CO;2-J

Broadbear, J. H., Kabel, D., Tracy, L., & Mak, P. (2014). Oxytocinergic regulation of endogenous as well as drug-induced mood. *Pharmacology, Biochemistry, and Behavior*, *119*, 61–71. https://doi.org/10.1016/j.pbb.2013.07.002

Bruchas, M. R., Land, B. B., Lemos, J. C., & Chavkin, C. (2009). CRF1-R activation of the dynorphin/kappa opioid system in the mouse basolateral amygdala mediates anxiety-like behavior. *PloS One*, *4*(12), e8528. https://doi.org/10.1371/journal.pone.0008528

Bruijnzeel, A. W., Prado, M., & Isaac, S. (2009). Corticotropin-releasing factor-1 receptor activation mediates nicotine withdrawal-induced deficit in brain reward function and stress-induced relapse. *Biological Psychiatry*, *66*(2), 110–117. https://doi.org/10.1016/j.biopsych.2009.01.010

Bruschetta, G., Jin, S., Liu, Z.-W., Kim, J. D., & Diano, S. (2020). MC(4)R Signaling in Dorsal Raphe Nucleus Controls Feeding, Anxiety, and Depression. *Cell Reports*, *33*(2), 108267. https://doi.org/10.1016/j.celrep.2020.108267

Bystritsky, A. (2006). Treatment-resistant anxiety disorders. *Molecular Psychiatry*, *11*(9), 805–814. https://doi.org/10.1038/sj.mp.4001852

Caldwell, H. K., Lee, H.-J., Macbeth, A. H., & Young, W. S. 3rd. (2008). Vasopressin: behavioral roles of an "original" neuropeptide. *Progress in Neurobiology*, *84*(1), 1–24. https://doi.org/10.1016/j.pneurobio.2007.10.007

Cameron, O. G., Lee, M. A., Kotun, J., & McPhee, K. M. (1986). Circadian symptom fluctuations in people with anxiety disorders. *Journal of Affective Disorders*, *11*(3), 213–218. https://doi.org/10.1016/0165-0327(86)90072-8

Carrier, N., & Kabbaj, M. (2012). Testosterone and imipramine have antidepressant effects in socially isolated male but not female rats. *Hormones and Behavior*, *61*(5), 678–685. https://doi.org/10.1016/j.yhbeh.2012.03.001

Carrier, N., Saland, S. K., Duclot, F., He, H., Mercer, R., & Kabbaj, M. (2015). The Anxiolytic and Antidepressant-like Effects of Testosterone and Estrogen in Gonadectomized Male Rats. *Biological Psychiatry*, *78*(4), 259–269. https://doi.org/10.1016/j.biopsych.2014.12.024

Carter, R. B., Wood, P. L., Wieland, S., Hawkinson, J. E., Belelli, D., Lambert, J. J., White, H. S., Wolf, H. H., Mirsadeghi, S., Tahir, S. H., Bolger, M. B., Lan, N. C., & Gee, K. W. (1997). Characterization of the anticonvulsant properties of ganaxolone (CCD 1042; 3alpha-hydroxy-3beta-methyl-5alpha-pregnan-20-one), a selective, high-affinity, steroid modulator of the gamma-aminobutyric acid(A) receptor. *The Journal of Pharmacology and Experimental Therapeutics*, *280*(3), 1284–1295.

Chaki, S., & Okubo, T. (2007). Melanocortin-4 receptor antagonists for the treatment of depression and anxiety disorders. *Current Topics in Medicinal Chemistry*, *7*(11), 1145–1151. https://doi.org/10.2174/156802607780906618

Chaudhri, O., Small, C., & Bloom, S. (2006). Gastrointestinal hormones regulating appetite. *Philosophical Transactions of the Royal Society of London. Series B, Biological Sciences*, *361*(1471), 1187–1209. https://doi.org/10.1098/rstb.2006.1856

Chen, C. V, Brummet, J. L., Lonstein, J. S., Jordan, C. L., & Breedlove, S. M. (2014). New knockout model confirms a role for androgen receptors in regulating anxiety-like behaviors and HPA response in mice. *Hormones and Behavior*, *65*(3), 211–218. https://doi.org/10.1016/j.yhbeh.2014.01.001

Copperi, F., Kim, J. D., & Diano, S. (2022). Melanocortin Signaling Connecting Systemic Metabolism With Mood Disorders. *Biological Psychiatry, 91*(10), 879–887. https://doi.org/10.1016/j.biopsych.2021.05.026

Costa, B., Pini, S., Baldwin, D. S., Silove, D., Manicavasagar, V., Abelli, M., Coppedè, F., & Martini, C. (2017). Oxytocin receptor and G-protein polymorphisms in patients with depression and separation anxiety. *Journal of Affective Disorders, 218*, 365–373. https://doi.org/10.1016/j.jad.2017.03.056

Cutler, A. J., Mattingly, G. W., & Maletic, V. (2023). Understanding the mechanism of action and clinical effects of neuroactive steroids and GABAergic compounds in major depressive disorder. *Translational Psychiatry, 13*(1), 228. https://doi.org/10.1038/s41398-023-02514-2

D'Anna, K. L., Stevenson, S. A., & Gammie, S. C. (2005). Urocortin 1 and 3 impair maternal defense behavior in mice. *Behavioral Neuroscience, 119*(4), 1061–1071. https://doi.org/10.1037/0735-7044.119.4.1061

Davis, S. A., & St. Amand, C. (2014). Effects of Testosterone Treatment and Chest Reconstruction Surgery on Mental Health and Sexuality in Female-To-Male Transgender People. *International Journal of Sexual Health, 26*(2), 113–128. https://doi.org/10.1080/19317611.2013.833152

Del Boca, C., Lutz, P. E., Le Merrer, J., Koebel, P., & Kieffer, B. L. (2012). Cholecystokinin knock-down in the basolateral amygdala has anxiolytic and antidepressant-like effects in mice. *Neuroscience, 218*, 185–195. https://doi.org/10.1016/j.neuroscience.2012.05.022

Dell'Osso, B., Buoli, M., Baldwin, D. S., & Altamura, A. C. (2010). Serotonin norepinephrine reuptake inhibitors (SNRIs) in anxiety disorders: a comprehensive review of their clinical efficacy. *Human Psychopharmacology, 25*(1), 17–29. https://doi.org/10.1002/hup.1074

Demetrio, F. N., Rennó, J. J., Gianfaldoni, A., Gonçalves, M., Halbe, H. W., Filho, A. H. G. V, & Gorenstein, C. (2011). Effect of estrogen replacement therapy on symptoms of depression and anxiety in non-depressive menopausal women: a randomized double-blind, controlled study. *Archives of Women's Mental Health, 14*(6), 479–486. https://doi.org/10.1007/s00737-011-0241-3

Desai, S. J., Borkar, C. D., Nakhate, K. T., Subhedar, N. K., & Kokare, D. M. (2014). Neuropeptide Y attenuates anxiety- and depression-like effects of cholecystokinin-4 in mice. *Neuroscience, 277*, 818–830. https://doi.org/10.1016/j.neuroscience.2014.07.062

do Rego, J. L., Vaudry, D., & Vaudry, H. (2015). The non-benzodiazepine anxiolytic drug etifoxine causes a rapid, receptor-independent stimulation of neurosteroid biosynthesis. *PloS One, 10*(3), e0120473. https://doi.org/10.1371/journal.pone.0120473

Dore, R., Iemolo, A., Smith, K. L., Wang, X., Cottone, P., & Sabino, V. (2013). CRF mediates the anxiogenic and anti-rewarding, but not the anorectic effects of PACAP. *Neuropsychopharmacology: Official Publication of the American College of Neuropsychopharmacology, 38*(11), 2160–2169. https://doi.org/10.1038/npp.2013.113

Edinger, K. L., & Frye, C. A. (2006). Intrahippocampal administration of an androgen receptor antagonist, flutamide, can increase anxiety-like behavior in intact and DHT-replaced male rats. *Hormones and Behavior, 50*(2), 216–222. https://doi.org/10.1016/j.yhbeh.2006.03.003

Egashira, N., Tanoue, A., Higashihara, F., Fuchigami, H., Sano, K., Mishima, K., Fukue, Y., Nagai, H., Takano, Y., Tsujimoto, G., Stemmelin, J., Griebel, G., Iwasaki, K., Ikeda, T., Nishimura, R., & Fujiwara, M. (2005). Disruption of the Prepulse Inhibition of the Startle Reflex in Vasopressin V1b Receptor Knockout Mice: Reversal by Antipsychotic Drugs. *Neuropsychopharmacology, 30*(11), 1996–2005. https://doi.org/10.1038/sj.npp.1300784

Egashira, N., Tanoue, A., Matsuda, T., Koushi, E., Harada, S., Takano, Y., Tsujimoto, G., Mishima, K., Iwasaki, K., & Fujiwara, M. (2007). Impaired social interaction and reduced anxiety-related behavior in vasopressin V1a receptor knockout mice. *Behavioural Brain Research, 178*(1), 123–127. https://doi.org/10.1016/j.bbr.2006.12.009

Engin, E., & Treit, D. (2007). The anxiolytic-like effects of allopregnanolone vary as a function of intracerebral microinfusion site: the amygdala, medial prefrontal cortex, or hippocampus. *Behavioural Pharmacology, 18*(5–6), 461–470. https://doi.org/10.1097/FBP.0b013e3282d28f6f

Eppolito, A. K., Kodeih, H. R., & Gerak, L. R. (2014). Using drug combinations to assess potential contributions of non-GABAA receptors in the discriminative stimulus effects of the neuroactive steroid pregnanolone in rats. *Physiology & Behavior, 137*, 33–41. https://doi.org/10.1016/j.physbeh.2014.07.003

Farhane-Medina, N. Z., Luque, B., Tabernero, C., & Castillo-Mayén, R. (2022). Factors associated with gender and sex differences in anxiety prevalence and comorbidity: A systematic review. *Science Progress, 105*(4), 00368504221135469. https://doi.org/10.1177/00368504221135469

Farooqi, N. A. I., Scotti, M., Lew, J. M., Botteron, K. N., Karama, S., McCracken, J. T., & Nguyen, T.-V. (2018). Role of DHEA and cortisol in prefrontal-amygdalar development and working memory. *Psychoneuroendocrinology, 98*, 86–94. https://doi.org/10.1016/j.psyneuen.2018.08.010

Feng, Y., Shao, R., Weijdegård, B., Wang, T., Johansson, J., Sun, S., Wang, W., Egecioglu, E., Billig, H., & Stener-Victorin, E. (2011). Effects of androgen and leptin on behavioral and cellular responses in female rats. *Hormones and Behavior, 60*(4), 427–438. https://doi.org/10.1016/j.yhbeh.2011.07.012

Flood, J. F., Morley, J. E., & Roberts, E. (1992). Memory-enhancing effects in male mice of pregnenolone and steroids metabolically derived from it. *Proceedings of the National Academy of Sciences of the United States of America, 89*(5), 1567–1571. https://doi.org/10.1073/pnas.89.5.1567

Flood, J. F., Morley, J. E., & Roberts, E. (1995). Pregnenolone sulfate enhances post-training memory processes when injected in very low doses into limbic system structures: the amygdala is by far the most sensitive. *Proceedings of the National Academy of Sciences of the United States of America, 92*(23), 10806–10810. https://doi.org/10.1073/pnas.92.23.10806

Flores, Á., Valls-Comamala, V., Costa, G., Saravia, R., Maldonado, R., & Berrendero, F. (2014). The hypocretin/orexin system mediates the extinction of fear memories. *Neuropsychopharmacology*. https://doi.org/10.1038/npp.2014.146

Fosgerau, K., Raun, K., Nilsson, C., Dahl, K., & Wulff, B. S. (2014). Novel α-MSH analog causes weight loss in obese rats and minipigs and improves insulin sensitivity. *The Journal of Endocrinology, 220*(2), 97–107. https://doi.org/10.1530/JOE-13-0284

Friess, E., Tagaya, H., Trachsel, L., Holsboer, F., & Rupprecht, R. (1997). Progesterone-induced changes in sleep in male subjects. *The American Journal of Physiology, 272*(5 Pt 1), E885-91. https://doi.org/10.1152/ajpendo.1997.272.5.E885

Frye, C A. (2009). Steroids, reproductive endocrine function, and affect. A review. *Minerva Ginecologica, 61*(6), 541–562.

Frye, Cheryl A, & Edinger, K. L. (2004). Testosterone's metabolism in the hippocampus may mediate its anti-anxiety effects in male rats. *Pharmacology, Biochemistry, and Behavior, 78*(3), 473–481. https://doi.org/10.1016/j.pbb.2004.04.019

Frye, Cheryl A, & Walf, A. A. (2002). Changes in progesterone metabolites in the hippocampus can modulate open field and forced swim test behavior of proestrous rats. *Hormones and Behavior, 41*(3), 306–315. https://doi.org/10.1006/hbeh.2002.1763

Fu, L.-Y., & van den Pol, A. N. (2008). Agouti-related peptide and MC3/4 receptor agonists both inhibit excitatory hypothalamic ventromedial nucleus neurons. *The Journal of Neuroscience: The Official Journal of the Society for Neuroscience, 28*(21), 5433–5449. https://doi.org/10.1523/JNEUROSCI.0749-08.2008

Furuta, M., Numakawa, T., Chiba, S., Ninomiya, M., Kajiyama, Y., Adachi, N., Akema, T., & Kunugi, H. (2013). Estrogen, Predominantly via Estrogen Receptor α, Attenuates Postpartum-Induced Anxiety- and Depression-Like Behaviors in Female Rats. *Endocrinology, 154*(10), 3807–3816. https://doi.org/10.1210/en.2012-2136

Gadassi Polack, R., Joormann, J., Orbach, M., Silverman, W. K., & Lebowitz, E. R. (2021). Maternal Depression and Mother-Child Oxytocin Synchrony in Youth with Anxiety Disorders. *Research on Child and Adolescent Psychopathology, 49*(3), 381–392. https://doi.org/10.1007/s10802-020-00744-2

Gafford, G. M., Guo, J.-D., Flandreau, E. I., Hazra, R., Rainnie, D. G., & Ressler, K. J. (2012). Cell-type specific deletion of GABA(A)α1 in corticotropin-releasing factor-containing neurons enhances anxiety and disrupts fear extinction. *Proceedings of the National Academy of Sciences of the United States of America*, *109*(40), 16330–16335. https://doi.org/10.1073/pnas.1119261109

Garakani, A., Murrough, J. W., Freire, R. C., Thom, R. P., Larkin, K., Buono, F. D., & Iosifescu, D. V. (2020). Pharmacotherapy of Anxiety Disorders: Current and Emerging Treatment Options. *Frontiers in Psychiatry*, *11*, 595584. https://doi.org/10.3389/fpsyt.2020.595584

Gebert, D., Auer, M. K., Stieg, M. R., Freitag, M. T., Lahne, M., Fuss, J., Schilbach, K., Schopohl, J., Stalla, G. K., & Kopczak, A. (2018). De-masking oxytocin-deficiency in craniopharyngioma and assessing its link with affective function. *Psychoneuroendocrinology*, *88*, 61–69. https://doi.org/10.1016/j.psyneuen.2017.11.006

Georgiou, P., Mou, T.-C. M., Potter, L. E., An, X., Zanos, P., Patton, M. S., Pultorak, K. J., Clark, S. M., Ngyuyen, V., Powels, C. F., Prokai-Tartai, K., Merchenthaler, I., Prokai, L., McCarthy, M. M., Mathur, B. N., & Gould, T. (2022). Estradiol mediates stress-susceptibility in the male brain. *BioRxiv*, 2022.01.09.475485. https://doi.org/10.1101/2022.01.09.475485

Georgiou, P., Zanos, P., Jenne, C. E., & Gould, T. D. (2019). Sex-specific involvement of estrogen receptors in behavioral responses to stress and psychomotor activation. *Frontiers in Psychiatry*, *10*(FEB), 81. https://doi.org/10.3389/fpsyt.2019.00081

Geracioti, T. D. J., Baker, D. G., Ekhator, N. N., West, S. A., Hill, K. K., Bruce, A. B., Schmidt, D., Rounds-Kugler, B., Yehuda, R., Keck, P. E. J., & Kasckow, J. W. (2001). CSF norepinephrine concentrations in posttraumatic stress disorder. *The American Journal of Psychiatry*, *158*(8), 1227–1230. https://doi.org/10.1176/appi.ajp.158.8.1227

Gerhard, D. (2013). Biological Psychology: An Introduction to Behavioral, Cognitive, and Clinical Neuroscience. In *The Yale Journal of Biology and Medicine* (Vol. 86, Issue 3, pp. 435–436).

Giltay, E. J., Enter, D., Zitman, F. G., Penninx, B. W. J. H., van Pelt, J., Spinhoven, P., & Roelofs, K. (2012). Salivary testosterone: associations with depression, anxiety disorders, and antidepressant use in a large cohort study. *Journal of Psychosomatic Research*, *72*(3), 205–213. https://doi.org/10.1016/j.jpsychores.2011.11.014

Ginsburg, G. S., Kendall, P. C., Sakolsky, D., Compton, S. N., Piacentini, J., Albano, A. M., Walkup, J. T., Sherrill, J., Coffey, K. A., Rynn, M. A., Keeton, C. P., McCracken, J. T., Bergman, L., Iyengar, S., Birmaher, B., & March, J. (2011). Remission after acute treatment in children and adolescents with anxiety disorders: findings from the CAMS. *Journal of Consulting and Clinical Psychology*, *79*(6), 806–813. https://doi.org/10.1037/a0025933

Girdler, S. S., Straneva, P. A., Light, K. C., Pedersen, C. A., & Morrow, A. L. (2001). Allopregnanolone levels and reactivity to mental stress in premenstrual dysphoric disorder. *Biological Psychiatry*, *49*(9), 788–797. https://doi.org/10.1016/s0006-3223(00)01044-1

Gleason, C. E., Dowling, N. M., Wharton, W., Manson, J. E., Miller, V. M., Atwood, C. S., Brinton, E. A., Cedars, M. I., Lobo, R. A., Merriam, G. R., Neal-Perry, G., Santoro, N. F., Taylor, H. S., Black, D. M., Budoff, M. J., Hodis, H. N., Naftolin, F., Harman, S. M., & Asthana, S. (2015). Effects of Hormone Therapy on Cognition and Mood in Recently Postmenopausal Women: Findings from the Randomized, Controlled KEEPS-Cognitive and Affective Study. *PLoS Medicine*, *12*(6), e1001833; discussion e1001833. https://doi.org/10.1371/journal.pmed.1001833

Goekoop, J. G., de Winter, R. P. F., de Rijk, R., Zwinderman, K. H., Frankhuijzen-Sierevogel, A., & Wiegant, V. M. (2006). Depression with above-normal plasma vasopressin: validation by relations with family history of depression and mixed anxiety and retardation. *Psychiatry Research*, *141*(2), 201–211. https://doi.org/10.1016/j.psychres.2005.09.003

Goyal, S. N., Kokare, D. M., Chopde, C. T., & Subhedar, N. K. (2006). Alpha-melanocyte stimulating hormone antagonizes antidepressant-like effect of neuropeptide Y in Porsolt's test in rats. *Pharmacology, Biochemistry, and Behavior*, *85*(2), 369–377. https://doi.org/10.1016/j.pbb.2006.09.004

Grace, S. A., Rossell, S. L., Heinrichs, M., Kordsachia, C., & Labuschagne, I. (2018). Oxytocin and brain activity in humans: A systematic review and coordinate-based meta-analysis of functional MRI studies. *Psychoneuroendocrinology, 96*, 6–24. https://doi.org/10.1016/j.psyneuen.2018.05.031

Grafe, L. A., & Bhatnagar, S. (2018). Orexins and stress. In *Frontiers in Neuroendocrinology*. https://doi.org/10.1016/j.yfrne.2018.06.003

Grafe, L. A., Cornfeld, A., Luz, S., Valentino, R., & Bhatnagar, S. (2017). Orexins Mediate Sex Differences in the Stress Response and in Cognitive Flexibility. *Biological Psychiatry*. https://doi.org/10.1016/j.biopsych.2016.10.013

Granger, D. A., Shirtcliff, E. A., Zahn-Waxler, C., Usher, B., Klimes-Dougan, B., & Hastings, P. (2003). Salivary testosterone diurnal variation and psychopathology in adolescent males and females: individual differences and developmental effects. *Development and Psychopathology, 15*(2), 431–449.

Grider, J. R. (1994). Role of cholecystokinin in the regulation of gastrointestinal motility. *The Journal of Nutrition, 124*(8 Suppl), 1334S-1339S. https://doi.org/10.1093/jn/124.suppl_8.1334S

Grillon, C., Duncko, R., Covington, M. F., Kopperman, L., & Kling, M. A. (2007). Acute stress potentiates anxiety in humans. *Biological Psychiatry, 62*(10), 1183–1186. https://doi.org/10.1016/j.biopsych.2007.06.007

Gulyaeva, N. V. (2022). Neuroendocrine Control of Hyperglutamatergic States in Brain Pathologies: the Effects of Glucocorticoids. *Journal of Evolutionary Biochemistry and Physiology, 58*(5), 1425–1438. https://doi.org/10.1134/S0022093022050131

Gutman, D. A., Owens, M. J., Skelton, K. H., Thrivikraman, K. V, & Nemeroff, C. B. (2003). The corticotropin-releasing factor1 receptor antagonist R121919 attenuates the behavioral and endocrine responses to stress. *The Journal of Pharmacology and Experimental Therapeutics, 304*(2), 874–880. https://doi.org/10.1124/jpet.102.042788

Hahn, A. C., DeBruine, L. M., Pesce, L. A., Diaz, A., Aberson, C. L., & Jones, B. C. (2020). Does women's anxious jealousy track changes in steroid hormone levels? *Psychoneuroendocrinology, 113*, 104553. https://doi.org/10.1016/j.psyneuen.2019.104553

Hang, A., Wang, Y., He, L., & Liu, J. (2015). The role of the dynorphin/κ opioid receptor system in anxiety. *Acta Pharmacologica Sinica, 36*(7), 783–790. https://doi.org/10.1038/aps.2015.32

Hanukoglu, I., & Jefcoate, C. R. (1980). Pregnenolone separation from cholesterol using Sephadex LH-20 mini-columns. *Journal of Chromatography A, 190*(1), 256–262. https://doi.org/10.1016/S0021-9673(00)85545-4

Harrewijn, A., Vidal-Ribas, P., Clore-Gronenborn, K., Jackson, S. M., Pisano, S., Pine, D. S., & Stringaris, A. (2020). Associations between brain activity and endogenous and exogenous cortisol - A systematic review. *Psychoneuroendocrinology, 120*, 104775. https://doi.org/10.1016/j.psyneuen.2020.104775

Hart, D., Nilges, M., Pollard, K., Lynn, T., Patsos, O., Shiel, C., Clark, S. M., & Vasudevan, N. (2014). Activation of the G-protein coupled receptor 30 (GPR30) has different effects on anxiety in male and female mice. *Steroids, 81*, 49–56. https://doi.org/10.1016/j.steroids.2013.11.004

Hastings, M. H. (1991). Neuroendocrine rhythms. *Pharmacology & Therapeutics, 50*(1), 35–71. https://doi.org/10.1016/0163-7258(91)90072-T

Heinrichs, S. C., De Souza, E. B., Schulteis, G., Lapsansky, J. L., & Grigoriadis, D. E. (2002). Brain penetrance, receptor occupancy and antistress in vivo efficacy of a small molecule corticotropin releasing factor type I receptor selective antagonist. *Neuropsychopharmacology: Official Publication of the American College of Neuropsychopharmacology, 27*(2), 194–202. https://doi.org/10.1016/S0893-133X(02)00299-3

Herman, J.P., Flak, J., Jankord, R. (2008). Chronic stress plasticity in the hypothalamic paraventricular nucleus, in: Neumann, I.D., Landgraf, R. (Eds.), *Progress in Brain Research*. Elsevier, pp. 353–364.

Herman, J. P., McKlveen, J. M., Ghosal, S., Kopp, B., Wulsin, A., Makinson, R., Scheimann, J., & Myers, B. (2016a). Regulation of the Hypothalamic-Pituitary-Adrenocortical Stress Response. *Comprehensive Physiology*, *6*(2), 603–621. https://doi.org/10.1002/cphy.c150015

Herman, M. A., Varodayan, F. P., Oleata, C. S., Luu, G., Kirson, D., Heilig, M., Ciccocioppo, R., & Roberto, M. (2016b). Glutamatergic transmission in the central nucleus of the amygdala is selectively altered in Marchigian Sardinian alcohol-preferring rats: Alcohol and CRF effects. *Neuropharmacology*, *102*, 21–31. https://doi.org/10.1016/j.neuropharm.2015.10.027

Hernando, F., Schoots, O., Lolait, S. J., & Burbach, J. P. (2001). Immunohistochemical localization of the vasopressin V1b receptor in the rat brain and pituitary gland: anatomical support for its involvement in the central effects of vasopressin. *Endocrinology*, *142*(4), 1659–1668. https://doi.org/10.1210/endo.142.4.8067

Hodgson, R A, Higgins, G. A., Guthrie, D. H., Lu, S. X., Pond, A. J., Mullins, D. E., Guzzi, M. F., Parker, E. M., & Varty, G. B. (2007). Comparison of the V1b antagonist, SSR149415, and the CRF1 antagonist, CP-154,526, in rodent models of anxiety and depression. *Pharmacology, Biochemistry, and Behavior*, *86*(3), 431–440. https://doi.org/10.1016/j.pbb.2006.12.021

Hodgson, Robert A, Mullins, D., Lu, S. X., Guzzi, M., Zhang, X., Bleickardt, C. J., Scott, J. D., Miller, M. W., Stamford, A. W., Parker, E. M., & Varty, G. B. (2014). Characterization of a novel vasopressin V1b receptor antagonist, V1B-30N, in animal models of anxiety-like and depression-like behavior. *European Journal of Pharmacology*, *730*, 157–163. https://doi.org/10.1016/j.ejphar.2014.02.027

Hurlemann, R. (2017). Oxytocin-Augmented Psychotherapy: Beware of Context. *Neuropsychopharmacology*, *42*(1), 377. https://doi.org/10.1038/npp.2016.188

Inutsuka, A., & Yamanaka, A. (2013). The physiological role of orexin/hypocretin neurons in the regulation of sleep/wakefulness and neuroendocrine functions. In *Frontiers in Endocrinology*. https://doi.org/10.3389/fendo.2013.00018

Ishizuka, Y., Abe, H., Tanoue, A., Kannan, H., & Ishida, Y. (2010). Involvement of vasopressin V1b receptor in anti-anxiety action of SSRI and SNRI in mice. *Neuroscience Research*, *66*(3), 233–237. https://doi.org/10.1016/j.neures.2009.11.004

Jacobson, L. (2014). Hypothalamic-pituitary-adrenocortical axis: neuropsychiatric aspects. *Comprehensive Physiology*, *4*(2), 715–738. https://doi.org/10.1002/cphy.c130036

James, M. H., Campbell, E. J., & Dayas, C. V. (2017). Role of the Orexin/Hypocretin system in stress-related psychiatric disorders. In *Current Topics in Behavioral Neurosciences*. https://doi.org/10.1007/7854_2016_56

Jenck, F., Moreau, J. L., Martin, J. R., Kilpatrick, G. J., Reinscheid, R. K., Monsma, F. J. J., Nothacker, H. P., & Civelli, O. (1997). Orphanin FQ acts as an anxiolytic to attenuate behavioral responses to stress. *Proceedings of the National Academy of Sciences of the United States of America*, *94*(26), 14854–14858. https://doi.org/10.1073/pnas.94.26.14854

Ji, G., Fu, Y., Ruppert, K. A., & Neugebauer, V. (2007). Pain-related anxiety-like behavior requires CRF1 receptors in the amygdala. *Molecular Pain*, *3*, 13. https://doi.org/10.1186/1744-8069-3-13

Ji, G., & Neugebauer, V. (2008). Pro- and anti-nociceptive effects of corticotropin-releasing factor (CRF) in central amygdala neurons are mediated through different receptors. *Journal of Neurophysiology*, *99*(3), 1201–1212. https://doi.org/10.1152/jn.01148.2007

Jie, F., Yin, G., Yang, W., Yang, M., Gao, S., Lv, J., & Li, B. (2018). Stress in Regulation of GABA Amygdala System and Relevance to Neuropsychiatric Diseases. *Frontiers in Neuroscience*, *12*, 562. https://doi.org/10.3389/fnins.2018.00562

Joëls, M., & Baram, T. Z. (2009). The neuro-symphony of stress. In *Nature reviews. Neuroscience* (Vol. 10, Issue 6, pp. 459–466). https://doi.org/10.1038/nrn2632

Johnson, P. L., Molosh, A., Fitz, S. D., Arendt, D., Deehan, G. A., Federici, L. M., Bernabe, C., Engleman, E. A., Rodd, Z. A., Lowry, C. A., & Shekhar, A. (2015). Pharmacological depletion of serotonin in the basolateral amygdala complex reduces anxiety and disrupts fear conditioning. *Pharmacology, Biochemistry, and Behavior*, *138*, 174–179. https://doi.org/10.1016/j.pbb.2015.09.021

Jöhren, O., Neidert, S. J., Kummer, M., & Dominiak, P. (2002). Sexually dimorphic expression of prepro-orexin mRNA in the rat hypothalamus. *Peptides*. https://doi.org/10.1016/S0196-9781(02)00052-9

Karl, T., Burne, T. H. J., & Herzog, H. (2006). Effect of Y1 receptor deficiency on motor activity, exploration, and anxiety. *Behavioural Brain Research, 167*(1), 87–93. https://doi.org/10.1016/j.bbr.2005.08.019

Karst, H., Berger, S., Turiault, M., Tronche, F., Schütz, G., & Joëls, M. (2005). Mineralocorticoid receptors are indispensable for nongenomic modulation of hippocampal glutamate transmission by corticosterone. *Proceedings of the National Academy of Sciences of the United States of America, 102*(52), 19204–19207. https://doi.org/10.1073/pnas.0507572102

Kastenberger, I., Lutsch, C., & Schwarzer, C. (2012). Activation of the G-protein-coupled receptor GPR30 induces anxiogenic effects in mice, similar to oestradiol. *Psychopharmacology, 221*(3), 527–535. https://doi.org/10.1007/s00213-011-2599-3

Kokane, S. S., & Perrotti, L. I. (2020). Sex Differences and the Role of Estradiol in Mesolimbic Reward Circuits and Vulnerability to Cocaine and Opiate Addiction. *Frontiers in Behavioral Neuroscience, 14*, 74. https://doi.org/10.3389/fnbeh.2020.00074

Kokare, Dadasaheb M, Dandekar, M. P., Singru, P. S., Gupta, G. L., & Subhedar, N. K. (2010). Involvement of alpha-MSH in the social isolation induced anxiety- and depression-like behaviors in rat. *Neuropharmacology, 58*(7), 1009–1018. https://doi.org/10.1016/j.neuropharm.2010.01.006

Kokare, Dadasaheb Mahadeo, Dandekar, M. P., Chopde, C. T., & Subhedar, N. (2005). Interaction between neuropeptide Y and alpha-melanocyte stimulating hormone in amygdala regulates anxiety in rats. *Brain Research, 1043*(1–2), 107–114. https://doi.org/10.1016/j.brainres.2005.02.038

Korosi, A., Veening, J. G., Kozicz, T., Henckens, M., Dederen, J., Groenink, L., van der Gugten, J., Olivier, B., & Roubos, E. W. (2006). Distribution and expression of CRF receptor 1 and 2 mRNAs in the CRF over-expressing mouse brain. *Brain Research, 1072*(1), 46–54. https://doi.org/10.1016/j.brainres.2005.12.034

Koshimizu, T., Nakamura, K., Egashira, N., Hiroyama, M., Nonoguchi, H., & Tanoue, A. (2012). Vasopressin V1a and V1b receptors: from molecules to physiological systems. *Physiological Reviews, 92*(4), 1813–1864. https://doi.org/10.1152/physrev.00035.2011

Krezel, W., Dupont, S., Krust, A., Chambon, P., & Chapman, P. F. (2001). Increased anxiety and synaptic plasticity in estrogen receptor beta -deficient mice. *Proceedings of the National Academy of Sciences of the United States of America, 98*(21), 12278–12282. https://doi.org/10.1073/pnas.221451898

Krysiak, R., Obuchowicz, E., & Herman, Z. S. (2000). Conditioned fear-induced changes in neuropeptide Y-like immunoreactivity in rats: the effect of diazepam and buspirone. *Neuropeptides, 34*(3), 148–157. https://doi.org/10.1054/npep.2000.0804

Kudwa, A. E., Bodo, C., Gustafsson, J.-A., & Rissman, E. F. (2005). A previously uncharacterized role for estrogen receptor beta: defeminization of male brain and behavior. *Proceedings of the National Academy of Sciences of the United States of America, 102*(12), 4608–4612. https://doi.org/10.1073/pnas.0500752102

Laconi, M. R., Chavez, C., Cavicchia, J. C., Fóscolo, M., Sosa, Z., Yunes, R. F., & Cabrera, R. J. (2012). Allopregnanolone alters the luteinizing hormone, prolactin, and progesterone serum levels interfering with the regression and apoptosis in rat corpus luteum. *Hormone and Metabolic Research = Hormon- Und Stoffwechselforschung = Hormones et Metabolisme, 44*(8), 632–638. https://doi.org/10.1055/s-0032-1314834

Lancaster, K., Goldbeck, L., Pournajafi-Nazarloo, H., Connelly, J. J., Carter, C. S., & Morris, J. P. (2018). The Role of Endogenous Oxytocin in Anxiolysis: Structural and Functional Correlates. *Biological Psychiatry. Cognitive Neuroscience and Neuroimaging, 3*(7), 618–625. https://doi.org/10.1016/j.bpsc.2017.10.003

Laudisio, A., Antonelli Incalzi, R., Gemma, A., Giovannini, S., Lo Monaco, M. R., Vetrano, D. L., Padua, L., Bernabei, R., & Zuccalà, G. (2018). Use of proton-pump inhibitors is associated with depression: a population-based study. *International Psychogeriatrics*, *30*(1), 153–159. https://doi.org/10.1017/S1041610217001715

Lee, R. S., & Sawa, A. (2014). Environmental stressors and epigenetic control of the hypothalamic-pituitary-adrenal axis. *Neuroendocrinology*, *100*(4), 278–287. https://doi.org/10.1159/000369585

Löfberg, C., Ågren, H., Harro, J., & Oreland, L. (1998). Cholecystokinin in CSF from depressed patients: possible relations to severity of depression and suicidal behaviour. *European Neuropsychopharmacology*, *8*(2), 153–157. https://doi.org/10.1016/S0924-977X(97)00046-1

Longone, P., di Michele, F., D'Agati, E., Romeo, E., Pasini, A., & Rupprecht, R. (2011). Neurosteroids as neuromodulators in the treatment of anxiety disorders. *Frontiers in Endocrinology*, *2*, 55. https://doi.org/10.3389/fendo.2011.00055

Louis, C., Cohen, C., Depoortère, R., & Griebel, G. (2006). Antidepressant-like effects of the corticotropin-releasing factor 1 receptor antagonist, SSR125543, and the vasopressin 1b receptor antagonist, SSR149415, in a DRL-72 s schedule in the rat. *Neuropsychopharmacology: Official Publication of the American College of Neuropsychopharmacology*, *31*(10), 2180–2187. https://doi.org/10.1038/sj.npp.1301036

Love, T. M. (2018). The impact of oxytocin on stress: the role of sex. *Current Opinion in Behavioral Sciences*, *23*, 136–142. https://doi.org/10.1016/j.cobeha.2018.06.018

Lukkes, J., Vuong, S., Scholl, J., Oliver, H., & Forster, G. (2009). Corticotropin-releasing factor receptor antagonism within the dorsal raphe nucleus reduces social anxiety-like behavior after early-life social isolation. *The Journal of Neuroscience: The Official Journal of the Society for Neuroscience*, *29*(32), 9955–9960. https://doi.org/10.1523/JNEUROSCI.0854-09.2009

Lund, T. D., Hinds, L. R., & Handa, R. J. (2006). The androgen 5alpha-dihydrotestosterone and its metabolite 5alpha-androstan-3beta, 17beta-diol inhibit the hypothalamo-pituitary-adrenal response to stress by acting through estrogen receptor beta-expressing neurons in the hypothalamus. *The Journal of Neuroscience: The Official Journal of the Society for Neuroscience*, *26*(5), 1448–1456. https://doi.org/10.1523/JNEUROSCI.3777-05.2006

Lund, T. D., Rovis, T., Chung, W. C. J., & Handa, R. J. (2005). Novel Actions of Estrogen Receptor-β on Anxiety-Related Behaviors. *Endocrinology*, *146*(2), 797–807. https://doi.org/10.1210/en.2004-1158

Lungwitz, E. A., Molosh, A., Johnson, P. L., Harvey, B. P., Dirks, R. C., Dietrich, A., Minick, P., Shekhar, A., & Truitt, W. A. (2012). Orexin-A induces anxiety-like behavior through interactions with glutamatergic receptors in the bed nucleus of the stria terminalis of rats. *Physiology and Behavior*. https://doi.org/10.1016/j.physbeh.2012.05.019

Lupien, S. J., McEwen, B. S., Gunnar, M. R., & Heim, C. (2009). Effects of stress throughout the lifespan on the brain, behaviour and cognition. *Nature Reviews Neuroscience*, *10*(6), 434–445. https://doi.org/10.1038/nrn2639

MacDonald, K., & Feifel, D. (2014). Oxytocin's role in anxiety: a critical appraisal. *Brain Research*, *1580*, 22–56. https://doi.org/10.1016/j.brainres.2014.01.025

Maeng, L. Y., & Milad, M. R. (2015). Sex differences in anxiety disorders: Interactions between fear, stress, and gonadal hormones. *Hormones and Behavior*, *76*, 106–117. https://doi.org/10.1016/j.yhbeh.2015.04.002

Magalhaes, A. C., Holmes, K. D., Dale, L. B., Comps-Agrar, L., Lee, D., Yadav, P. N., Drysdale, L., Poulter, M. O., Roth, B. L., Pin, J.-P., Anisman, H., & Ferguson, S. S. G. (2010). CRF receptor 1 regulates anxiety behavior via sensitization of 5-HT2 receptor signaling. *Nature Neuroscience*, *13*(5), 622–629. https://doi.org/10.1038/nn.2529

Majewska, M. D., Harrison, N. L., Schwartz, R. D., Barker, J. L., & Paul, S. M. (1986). Steroid hormone metabolites are barbiturate-like modulators of the GABA receptor. *Science (New York, N.Y.)*, *232*(4753), 1004–1007. https://doi.org/10.1126/science.2422758

Marcus, J. N., Aschkenasi, C. J., Lee, C. E., Chemelli, R. M., Saper, C. B., Yanagisawa, M., & Elmquist, J. K. (2001). Differential expression of Orexin receptors 1 and 2 in the rat brain. *Journal of Comparative Neurology*. https://doi.org/10.1002/cne.1190

McEwen, B. S. (2007). Physiology and neurobiology of stress and adaptation: central role of the brain. *Physiological Reviews*, *87*(3), 873–904. https://doi.org/10.1152/physrev.00041.2006

McEwen, B. S., Gray, J. D., & Nasca, C. (2015). 60 YEARS OF NEUROENDOCRINOLOGY: Redefining neuroendocrinology: stress, sex and cognitive and emotional regulation. *The Journal of Endocrinology*, *226*(2), T67-83. https://doi.org/10.1530/JOE-15-0121

McEwen, B. S., Nasca, C., & Gray, J. D. (2016). Stress Effects on Neuronal Structure: Hippocampus, Amygdala, and Prefrontal Cortex. *Neuropsychopharmacology: Official Publication of the American College of Neuropsychopharmacology*, *41*(1), 3–23. https://doi.org/10.1038/npp.2015.171

McLean, C. P., Asnaani, A., Litz, B. T., & Hofmann, S. G. (2011). Gender differences in anxiety disorders: Prevalence, course of illness, comorbidity and burden of illness. *Journal of Psychiatric Research*. https://doi.org/10.1016/j.jpsychires.2011.03.006

Melchior, C. L., & Ritzmann, R. F. (1994). Pregnenolone and pregnenolone sulfate, alone and with ethanol, in mice on the plus-maze. *Pharmacology Biochemistry and Behavior*, *48*(4), 893–897. https://doi.org/10.1016/0091-3057(94)90197-X

Mellman, T. A. (2006). Sleep and anxiety disorders. *The Psychiatric Clinics of North America*, *29*(4), 1047–1058; abstract x. https://doi.org/10.1016/j.psc.2006.08.005

Miguel, T. T., & Nunes-de-Souza, R. L. (2011). Anxiogenic and antinociceptive effects induced by corticotropin-releasing factor (CRF) injections into the periaqueductal gray are modulated by CRF1 receptor in mice. *Hormones and Behavior*, *60*(3), 292–300. https://doi.org/10.1016/j.yhbeh.2011.06.004

Milrod, B., Altemus, M., Gross, C., Busch, F., Silver, G., Christos, P., Stieber, J., & Schneier, F. (2016). Adult separation anxiety in treatment nonresponders with anxiety disorders: delineation of the syndrome and exploration of attachment-based psychotherapy and biomarkers. *Comprehensive Psychiatry*, *66*, 139–145. https://doi.org/10.1016/j.comppsych.2016.01.004

Mineka, S., & Oehlberg, K. (2008). The relevance of recent developments in classical conditioning to understanding the etiology and maintenance of anxiety disorders. *Acta Psychologica*. https://doi.org/10.1016/j.actpsy.2007.11.007

Mòdol, L., Darbra, S., & Pallarès, M. (2011). Neurosteroids infusion into the CA1 hippocampal region on exploration, anxiety-like behaviour and aversive learning. *Behavioural Brain Research*, *222*(1), 223–229. https://doi.org/10.1016/j.bbr.2011.03.058

Mora, S., Dussaubat, N., & Díaz-Véliz, G. (1996). Effects of the estrous cycle and ovarian hormones on behavioral indices of anxiety in female rats. *Psychoneuroendocrinology*, *21*(7), 609–620. https://doi.org/10.1016/s0306-4530(96)00015-7

Morales-Medina, J. C., Dumont, Y., & Quirion, R. (2010). A possible role of neuropeptide Y in depression and stress. *Brain Research*, *1314*, 194–205. https://doi.org/10.1016/j.brainres.2009.09.077

Morimoto, M., Morita, N., Ozawa, H., Yokoyama, K., & Kawata, M. (1996). Distribution of glucocorticoid receptor immunoreactivity and mRNA in the rat brain: an immunohistochemical and in situ hybridization study. *Neuroscience Research*, *26*(3), 235–269. https://doi.org/10.1016/s0168-0102(96)01105-4

Mottolese, R., Redouté, J., Costes, N., Le Bars, D., & Sirigu, A. (2014). Switching brain serotonin with oxytocin. *Proceedings of the National Academy of Sciences of the United States of America*, *111*(23), 8637–8642. https://doi.org/10.1073/pnas.1319810111

Mountjoy, K. G. (2010). Distribution and function of melanocortin receptors within the brain. *Advances in Experimental Medicine and Biology*, *681*, 29–48. https://doi.org/10.1007/978-1-4419-6354-3_3

Mourtzi, N., Sertedaki, A., & Charmandari, E. (2021). Glucocorticoid Signaling and Epigenetic Alterations in Stress-Related Disorders. *International Journal of Molecular Sciences*, *22*(11). https://doi.org/10.3390/ijms22115964

Müller, M. B., Landgraf, R., & Keck, M. E. (2000). Vasopressin, major depression, and hypothalamic-pituitary-adrenocortical desensitization. *Biological Psychiatry*, *48*(4), 330–333. https://doi.org/10.1016/s0006-3223(00)00886-6

Murgatroyd, C., Patchev, A. V, Wu, Y., Micale, V., Bockmühl, Y., Fischer, D., Holsboer, F., Wotjak, C. T., Almeida, O. F. X., & Spengler, D. (2009). Dynamic DNA methylation programs persistent adverse effects of early-life stress. *Nature Neuroscience*, *12*(12), 1559–1566. https://doi.org/10.1038/nn.2436

Muschamp, J. W., Hollander, J. A., Thompson, J. L., Voren, G., Hassinger, L. C., Onvani, S., Kamenecka, T. M., Borgland, S. L., Kenny, P. J., & Carlezon, W. A. (2014). Hypocretin (orexin) facilitates reward by attenuating the antireward effects of its cotransmitter dynorphin in ventral tegmental area. *Proceedings of the National Academy of Sciences of the United States of America*. https://doi.org/10.1073/pnas.1315542111

Myers, A. J., Williams, L., Gatt, J. M., McAuley-Clark, E. Z., Dobson-Stone, C., Schofield, P. R., & Nemeroff, C. B. (2014). Variation in the oxytocin receptor gene is associated with increased risk for anxiety, stress and depression in individuals with a history of exposure to early life stress. *Journal of Psychiatric Research*, *59*, 93–100. https://doi.org/10.1016/j.jpsychires.2014.08.021

Natividad, L. A., Buczynski, M. W., Herman, M. A., Kirson, D., Oleata, C. S., Irimia, C., Polis, I., Ciccocioppo, R., Roberto, M., & Parsons, L. H. (2017). Constitutive Increases in Amygdalar Corticotropin-Releasing Factor and Fatty Acid Amide Hydrolase Drive an Anxious Phenotype. *Biological Psychiatry*, *82*(7), 500–510. https://doi.org/10.1016/j.biopsych.2017.01.005

Neumann, I. D., & Landgraf, R. (2012). Balance of brain oxytocin and vasopressin: implications for anxiety, depression, and social behaviors. *Trends in Neurosciences*, *35*(11), 649–659. https://doi.org/10.1016/j.tins.2012.08.004

No Title. (n.d.). https://link.springer.com/chapter/10.1007/978-1-4612-1302-4_9

Nuss, P. (2015). Anxiety disorders and GABA neurotransmission: a disturbance of modulation. *Neuropsychiatric Disease and Treatment*, *11*, 165–175. https://doi.org/10.2147/NDT.S58841

Nyamugenda, E., Griffin, H., Russell, S., Cooney, K. A., Kowalczyk, N. S., Islam, I., Phelan, K. D., & Baldini, G. (2020). Selective Survival of Sim1/MC4R Neurons in Diet-Induced Obesity. *IScience*, *23*(5), 101114. https://doi.org/10.1016/j.isci.2020.101114

Onodera, M., Ishitobi, Y., Tanaka, Y., Aizawa, S., Masuda, K., Inoue, A., Oshita, H., Okamoto, K., Kawashima, C., Nakanishi, M., Hirakawa, H., Ninomiya, T., Maruyama, Y., Kanehisa, M., Higuma, H., & Akiyoshi, J. (2015). Genetic association of the oxytocin receptor genes with panic, major depressive disorder, and social anxiety disorder. In *Psychiatric genetics* (Vol. 25, Issue 5, p. 212). https://doi.org/10.1097/YPG.0000000000000096

Oyola, M. G., Portillo, W., Reyna, A., Foradori, C. D., Kudwa, A., Hinds, L., Handa, R. J., & Mani, S. K. (2012). Anxiolytic effects and neuroanatomical targets of estrogen receptor-β (ERβ) activation by a selective ERβ agonist in female mice. *Endocrinology*, *153*(2), 837–846. https://doi.org/10.1210/en.2011-1674

Parris, M. S., Grunebaum, M. F., Galfalvy, H. C., Andronikashvili, A., Burke, A. K., Yin, H., Min, E., Huang, Y.-Y., & Mann, J. J. (2018). Attempted suicide and oxytocin-related gene polymorphisms. *Journal of Affective Disorders*, *238*, 62–68. https://doi.org/10.1016/j.jad.2018.05.022

Paul, S. M., & Purdy, R. H. (1992). Neuroactive steroids. *FASEB Journal: Official Publication of the Federation of American Societies for Experimental Biology*, *6*(6), 2311–2322.

Pinnock, S. B., & Herbert, J. (2001). Corticosterone differentially modulates expression of corticotropin releasing factor and arginine vasopressin mRNA in the hypothalamic paraventricular nucleus following either acute or repeated restraint stress. *The European Journal of Neuroscience*, *13*(3), 576–584. https://doi.org/10.1046/j.0953-816x.2000.01406.x

Pleil, K. E., & Skelly, M. J. (2018). CRF modulation of central monoaminergic function: Implications for sex differences in alcohol drinking and anxiety. *Alcohol (Fayetteville, N.Y.)*, *72*, 33–47. https://doi.org/10.1016/j.alcohol.2018.01.007

Pomrenze, M. B., Giovanetti, S. M., Maiya, R., Gordon, A. G., Kreeger, L. J., & Messing, R. O. (2019a). Dissecting the Roles of GABA and Neuropeptides from Rat Central Amygdala CRF Neurons in Anxiety and Fear Learning. *Cell Reports*, *29*(1), 13-21.e4. https://doi.org/10.1016/j.celrep.2019.08.083

Pomrenze, M. B., Tovar-Diaz, J., Blasio, A., Maiya, R., Giovanetti, S. M., Lei, K., Morikawa, H., Hopf, F. W., & Messing, R. O. (2019b). A Corticotropin Releasing Factor Network in the Extended Amygdala for Anxiety. *The Journal of Neuroscience: The Official Journal of the Society for Neuroscience*, *39*(6), 1030–1043. https://doi.org/10.1523/JNEUROSCI.2143-18.2018

Popoli, M., Yan, Z., McEwen, B. S., & Sanacora, G. (2011). The stressed synapse: the impact of stress and glucocorticoids on glutamate transmission. *Nature Reviews. Neuroscience*, *13*(1), 22–37. https://doi.org/10.1038/nrn3138

Raeder, F., Merz, C. J., Margraf, J., & Zlomuzica, A. (2020). The association between fear extinction, the ability to accomplish exposure and exposure therapy outcome in specific phobia. *Scientific Reports*. https://doi.org/10.1038/s41598-020-61004-3

Reddy, D. S. (2003). Pharmacology of endogenous neuroactive steroids. *Critical Reviews in Neurobiology*, *15*(3–4), 197–234. https://doi.org/10.1615/critrevneurobiol.v15.i34.20

Rehfeld, J. F. (2021). Cholecystokinin and Panic Disorder: Reflections on the History and Some Unsolved Questions. *Molecules (Basel, Switzerland)*, *26*(18). https://doi.org/10.3390/molecules26185657

Reis, F. M. C. V, Almada, R. C., Fogaça, M. V, & Brandão, M. L. (2016). Rapid Activation of Glucocorticoid Receptors in the Prefrontal Cortex Mediates the Expression of Contextual Conditioned Fear in Rats. *Cerebral Cortex*, *26*(6), 2639–2649. https://doi.org/10.1093/cercor/bhv103

Reul, J M H M, & Kloet, E. R. D. E. (1985). Two Receptor Systems for Corticosterone in Rat Brain: Microdistribution and Differential Occupation. *Endocrinology*, *117*(6), 2505–2511. https://doi.org/10.1210/endo-117-6-2505

Reul, Johannes M H M, Collins, A., Saliba, R. S., Mifsud, K. R., Carter, S. D., Gutierrez-Mecinas, M., Qian, X., & Linthorst, A. C. E. (2015). Glucocorticoids, epigenetic control and stress resilience. *Neurobiology of Stress*, *1*, 44–59. https://doi.org/10.1016/j.ynstr.2014.10.001

Risbrough, V. B., Hauger, R. L., Pelleymounter, M. A., & Geyer, M. A. (2003). Role of corticotropin releasing factor (CRF) receptors 1 and 2 in CRF-potentiated acoustic startle in mice. *Psychopharmacology*, *170*(2), 178–187. https://doi.org/10.1007/s00213-003-1535-6

Risbrough, V. B., & Stein, M. B. (2006). Role of corticotropin releasing factor in anxiety disorders: a translational research perspective. *Hormones and Behavior*, *50*(4), 550–561. https://doi.org/10.1016/j.yhbeh.2006.06.019

Roberto, M., Cruz, M. T., Gilpin, N. W., Sabino, V., Schweitzer, P., Bajo, M., Cottone, P., Madamba, S. G., Stouffer, D. G., Zorrilla, E. P., Koob, G. F., Siggins, G. R., & Parsons, L. H. (2010). Corticotropin releasing factor-induced amygdala gamma-aminobutyric Acid release plays a key role in alcohol dependence. *Biological Psychiatry*, *67*(9), 831–839. https://doi.org/10.1016/j.biopsych.2009.11.007

Rocha, A., Godino-Gimeno, A., & Cerdá-Reverter, J. M. (2019). Evolution of proopiomelanocortin. *Vitamins and Hormones*, *111*, 1–16. https://doi.org/10.1016/bs.vh.2019.05.008

Ryan, J., Scali, J., Carrière, I., Scarabin, P.-Y., Ritchie, K., & Ancelin, M.-L. (2011). Estrogen receptor gene variants are associated with anxiety disorders in older women. *Psychoneuroendocrinology*, *36*(10), 1582–1586. https://doi.org/10.1016/j.psyneuen.2011.04.011

Sah, R., Ekhator, N. N., Strawn, J. R., Sallee, F. R., Baker, D. G., Horn, P. S., & Geracioti, T. D. J. (2009). Low cerebrospinal fluid neuropeptide Y concentrations in posttraumatic stress disorder. *Biological Psychiatry*, *66*(7), 705–707. https://doi.org/10.1016/j.biopsych.2009.04.037

Sakurai, T., Amemiya, A., Ishii, M., Matsuzaki, I., Chemelli, R. M., Tanaka, H., Williams, S. C., Richardson, J. A., Kozlowski, G. P., Wilson, S., Arch, J. R. S., Buckingham, R. E., Haynes, A. C., Carr, S. A., Annan, R. S., McNulty, D. E., Liu, W. S., Terrett, J. A., Elshourbagy, N. A., … Yanagisawa, M. (1998). Orexins and orexin receptors: A family of hypothalamic neuropeptides and G protein-coupled receptors that regulate feeding behavior. *Cell*. https://doi.org/10.1016/S0092-8674(00)80949-6

Sapolsky, R. M., Romero, L. M., & Munck, A. U. (2000). How Do Glucocorticoids Influence Stress Responses? Integrating Permissive, Suppressive, Stimulatory, and Preparative Actions*. *Endocrine Reviews*, *21*(1), 55–89. https://doi.org/10.1210/edrv.21.1.0389

Sayed, S., Van Dam, N. T., Horn, S. R., Kautz, M. M., Parides, M., Costi, S., Collins, K. A., Iacoviello, B., Iosifescu, D. V, Mathé, A. A., Southwick, S. M., Feder, A., Charney, D. S., & Murrough, J. W. (2018). A Randomized Dose-Ranging Study of Neuropeptide Y in Patients with Posttraumatic Stress Disorder. *International Journal of Neuropsychopharmacology, 21*(1), 3–11. https://doi.org/10.1093/ijnp/pyx109

Scantamburlo, G., Hansenne, M., Fuchs, S., Pitchot, W., Maréchal, P., Pequeux, C., Ansseau, M., & Legros, J. J. (2007). Plasma oxytocin levels and anxiety in patients with major depression. *Psychoneuroendocrinology, 32*(4), 407–410. https://doi.org/10.1016/j.psyneuen.2007.01.009

Schulz, D. W., Mansbach, R. S., Sprouse, J., Braselton, J. P., Collins, J., Corman, M., Dunaiskis, A., Faraci, S., Schmidt, A. W., Seeger, T., Seymour, P., Tingley, F. D. 3rd, Winston, E. N., Chen, Y. L., & Heym, J. (1996). CP-154,526: a potent and selective nonpeptide antagonist of corticotropin releasing factor receptors. *Proceedings of the National Academy of Sciences of the United States of America, 93*(19), 10477–10482. https://doi.org/10.1073/pnas.93.19.10477

Schüssler, P., Kluge, M., Yassouridis, A., Dresler, M., Held, K., Zihl, J., & Steiger, A. (2008). Progesterone reduces wakefulness in sleep EEG and has no effect on cognition in healthy postmenopausal women. *Psychoneuroendocrinology, 33*(8), 1124–1131. https://doi.org/10.1016/j.psyneuen.2008.05.013

Sciolino, N. R., & Holmes, P. V. (2012). Exercise offers anxiolytic potential: a role for stress and brain noradrenergic-galaninergic mechanisms. *Neuroscience and Biobehavioral Reviews, 36*(9), 1965–1984. https://doi.org/10.1016/j.neubiorev.2012.06.005

Shiozaki, K., Kawabe, M., Karasuyama, K., Kurachi, T., Hayashi, A., Ataka, K., Iwai, H., Takeno, H., Hayasaka, O., Kotani, T., Komatsu, M., & Inui, A. (2020). Neuropeptide Y deficiency induces anxiety-like behaviours in zebrafish (Danio rerio). *Scientific Reports, 10*(1), 5913. https://doi.org/10.1038/s41598-020-62699-0

Skelton, K. H., Nemeroff, C. B., Knight, D. L., & Owens, M. J. (2000). Chronic administration of the triazolobenzodiazepine alprazolam produces opposite effects on corticotropin-releasing factor and urocortin neuronal systems. *The Journal of Neuroscience: The Official Journal of the Society for Neuroscience, 20*(3), 1240–1248. https://doi.org/10.1523/JNEUROSCI.20-03-01240.2000

Slattery, D. A., & Neumann, I. D. (2010). Chronic icv oxytocin attenuates the pathological high anxiety state of selectively bred Wistar rats. *Neuropharmacology, 58*(1), 56–61. https://doi.org/10.1016/j.neuropharm.2009.06.038

Smadja, C., Ruiz, F., Coric, P., Fournié-Zaluski, M. C., Roques, B. P., & Maldonado, R. (1997). CCK-B receptors in the limbic system modulate the antidepressant-like effects induced by endogenous enkephalins. *Psychopharmacology, 132*(3), 227–236. https://doi.org/10.1007/s002130050340

Smith, A. S., Tabbaa, M., Lei, K., Eastham, P., Butler, M. J., Linton, L., Altshuler, R., Liu, Y., & Wang, Z. (2016). Local oxytocin tempers anxiety by activating GABAA receptors in the hypothalamic paraventricular nucleus. *Psychoneuroendocrinology, 63*, 50–58. https://doi.org/10.1016/j.psyneuen.2015.09.017

Smith, S. S., Gong, Q. H., Hsu, F. C., Markowitz, R. S., ffrench-Mullen, J. M., & Li, X. (1998). GABA(A) receptor alpha4 subunit suppression prevents withdrawal properties of an endogenous steroid. *Nature, 392*(6679), 926–930. https://doi.org/10.1038/31948

Solomon, M. B., Furay, A. R., Jones, K., Packard, A. E. B., Packard, B. A., Wulsin, A. C., & Herman, J. P. (2012). Deletion of forebrain glucocorticoid receptors impairs neuroendocrine stress responses and induces depression-like behavior in males but not females. *Neuroscience, 203*, 135–143. https://doi.org/10.1016/j.neuroscience.2011.12.014

Spiteri, T., Musatov, S., Ogawa, S., Ribeiro, A., Pfaff, D. W., & Ågmo, A. (2010). The role of the estrogen receptor α in the medial amygdala and ventromedial nucleus of the hypothalamus in social recognition, anxiety and aggression. *Behavioural Brain Research, 210*(2), 211–220. https://doi.org/10.1016/j.bbr.2010.02.033

Sripada, R. K., Marx, C. E., King, A. P., Rampton, J. C., Ho, S. S., & Liberzon, I. (2013). Allopregnanolone elevations following pregnenolone administration are associated with enhanced activation of emotion regulation neurocircuits. *Biological Psychiatry*, *73*(11), 1045–1053. https://doi.org/10.1016/j.biopsych.2012.12.008

Staton, C. D., Yaeger, J. D. W., Khalid, D., Haroun, F., Fernandez, B. S., Fernandez, J. S., Summers, B. K., Summers, T. R., Sathyanesan, M., Newton, S. S., & Summers, C. H. (2018). Orexin 2 receptor stimulation enhances resilience, while orexin 2 inhibition promotes susceptibility, to social stress, anxiety and depression. *Neuropharmacology*. https://doi.org/10.1016/j.neuropharm.2018.09.016

Sternson, S. M., & Atasoy, D. (2014). Agouti-related protein neuron circuits that regulate appetite. *Neuroendocrinology*, *100*(2–3), 95–102. https://doi.org/10.1159/000369072

Strawn, J. R., & Geracioti, T. D. J. (2008). Noradrenergic dysfunction and the psychopharmacology of posttraumatic stress disorder. *Depression and Anxiety*, *25*(3), 260–271. https://doi.org/10.1002/da.20292

Ströhle, A., Holsboer, F., & Rupprecht, R. (2000). Increased ACTH Concentrations Associated with Cholecystokinin Tetrapeptide-Induced Panic Attacks in Patients with Panic Disorder. *Neuropsychopharmacology*, *22*(3), 251–256. https://doi.org/10.1016/S0893-133X(99)00115-3

Taché, Y. (2015). Corticotrophin-releasing factor 1 activation in the central amygdale and visceral hyperalgesia. *Neurogastroenterology and Motility: The Official Journal of the European Gastrointestinal Motility Society*, *27*(1), 1–6. https://doi.org/10.1111/nmo.12495

Taheri, S., Mahmoodi, M., Opacka-Juffry, J., Ghatei, M. A., & Bloom, S. R. (1999). Distribution and quantification of immunoreactive orexin A in rat tissues. *FEBS Letters*. https://doi.org/10.1016/S0014-5793(99)01030-3

Tasan, R. O., Verma, D., Wood, J., Lach, G., Hörmer, B., de Lima, T. C. M., Herzog, H., & Sperk, G. (2016). The role of Neuropeptide Y in fear conditioning and extinction. *Neuropeptides*, *55*, 111–126. https://doi.org/10.1016/j.npep.2015.09.007

Taylor, H. S., & Manson, J. E. (2011). Update in hormone therapy use in menopause. *The Journal of Clinical Endocrinology and Metabolism*, *96*(2), 255–264. https://doi.org/10.1210/jc.2010-0536

Ten-Blanco, M., Flores, Á., Pereda-Pérez, I., Piscitelli, F., Izquierdo-Luengo, C., Cristino, L., Romero, J., Hillard, C. J., Maldonado, R., Di Marzo, V., & Berrendero, F. (2022). Amygdalar CB2 cannabinoid receptor mediates fear extinction deficits promoted by orexin-A/hypocretin-1. *Biomedicine and Pharmacotherapy*. https://doi.org/10.1016/j.biopha.2022.112925

Thorsell, A. (2010). Brain neuropeptide Y and corticotropin-releasing hormone in mediating stress and anxiety. *Experimental Biology and Medicine (Maywood, N.J.)*, *235*(10), 1163–1167. https://doi.org/10.1258/ebm.2010.009331

Tian, J., Kim, S., Heilig, E., & Ruderman, J. V. (2000). Identification of XPR-1, a progesterone receptor required for Xenopus oocyte activation. *Proceedings of the National Academy of Sciences of the United States of America*, *97*(26), 14358–14363. https://doi.org/10.1073/pnas.250492197

Tian, Z., Wang, Y., Zhang, N., Guo, Y.-Y., Feng, B., Liu, S.-B., & Zhao, M.-G. (2013). Estrogen receptor GPR30 exerts anxiolytic effects by maintaining the balance between GABAergic and glutamatergic transmission in the basolateral amygdala of ovariectomized mice after stress. *Psychoneuroendocrinology*, *38*(10), 2218–2233. https://doi.org/10.1016/j.psyneuen.2013.04.011

Twede, V., Tartaglia, A. L., Covey, D. F., & Bamber, B. A. (2007). The neurosteroids dehydroepiandrosterone sulfate and pregnenolone sulfate inhibit the UNC-49 GABA receptor through a common set of residues. *Molecular Pharmacology*, *72*(5), 1322–1329. https://doi.org/10.1124/mol.107.034058

Ugale, R. R., Sharma, A. N., Kokare, D. M., Hirani, K., Subhedar, N. K., & Chopde, C. T. (2007). Neurosteroid allopregnanolone mediates anxiolytic effect of etifoxine in rats. *Brain Research*, *1184*, 193–201. https://doi.org/10.1016/j.brainres.2007.09.041

Urbanski, H. F. (2011). Role of Circadian Neuroendocrine Rhythms in the Control of Behavior and Physiology. *Neuroendocrinology*, *93*(4), 211–222. https://doi.org/10.1159/000327399

van Honk, J., Peper, J. S., & Schutter, D. J. L. G. (2005). Testosterone reduces unconscious fear but not consciously experienced anxiety: implications for the disorders of fear and anxiety. *Biological Psychiatry*, *58*(3), 218–225. https://doi.org/10.1016/j.biopsych.2005.04.003

Verma, P., Hellemans, K. G. C., Choi, F. Y., Yu, W., & Weinberg, J. (2010). Circadian phase and sex effects on depressive/anxiety-like behaviors and HPA axis responses to acute stress. *Physiology & Behavior*, *99*(3), 276–285. https://doi.org/10.1016/j.physbeh.2009.11.002

Vialou, V., Bagot, R. C., Cahill, M. E., Ferguson, D., Robison, A. J., Dietz, D. M., Fallon, B., Mazei-Robison, M., Ku, S. M., Harrigan, E., Winstanley, C. A., Joshi, T., Feng, J., Berton, O., & Nestler, E. J. (2014). Prefrontal cortical circuit for depression- and anxiety-related behaviors mediated by cholecystokinin: role of ΔFosB. *The Journal of Neuroscience: The Official Journal of the Society for Neuroscience*, *34*(11), 3878–3887. https://doi.org/10.1523/JNEUROSCI.1787-13.2014

Vigen, R., O'Donnell, C. I., Barón, A. E., Grunwald, G. K., Maddox, T. M., Bradley, S. M., Barqawi, A., Woning, G., Wierman, M. E., Plomondon, M. E., Rumsfeld, J. S., & Ho, P. M. (2013). Association of Testosterone Therapy With Mortality, Myocardial Infarction, and Stroke in Men With Low Testosterone Levels. *JAMA*, *310*(17), 1829–1836. https://doi.org/10.1001/jama.2013.280386

Vollebregt, O., Koyama, E., Zai, C. C., Shaikh, S. A., Lisoway, A. J., Kennedy, J. L., & Beitchman, J. H. (2021). Evidence for association of vasopressin receptor 1A promoter region repeat with childhood onset aggression. *Journal of Psychiatric Research*, *140*, 522–528. https://doi.org/10.1016/j.jpsychires.2021.05.062

Vuong, S. M., Oliver, H. A., Scholl, J. L., Oliver, K. M., & Forster, G. L. (2010). Increased anxiety-like behavior of rats during amphetamine withdrawal is reversed by CRF2 receptor antagonism. *Behavioural Brain Research*, *208*(1), 278–281. https://doi.org/10.1016/j.bbr.2009.11.036

Walf, A. A., & Frye, C. A. (2005). ERβ-Selective Estrogen Receptor Modulators Produce Antianxiety Behavior when Administered Systemically to Ovariectomized Rats. *Neuropsychopharmacology*, *30*(9), 1598–1609. https://doi.org/10.1038/sj.npp.1300713

Walf, A. A., & Frye, C. A. (2008). Parity and estrogen-administration alter affective behavior of ovariectomized rats. *Physiology & Behavior*, *93*(1–2), 351–356. https://doi.org/10.1016/j.physbeh.2007.09.002

Wang, C., Wang, Q., Ji, B., Pan, Y., Xu, C., Cheng, B., Bai, B., & Chen, J. (2018). The Orexin/Receptor System: Molecular Mechanism and Therapeutic Potential for Neurological Diseases. In *Frontiers in Molecular Neuroscience*. https://doi.org/10.3389/fnmol.2018.00220

Wang, G.-Y., Zhu, Z.-M., Cui, S., & Wang, J.-H. (2016). Glucocorticoid Induces Incoordination between Glutamatergic and GABAergic Neurons in the Amygdala. *PloS One*, *11*(11), e0166535. https://doi.org/10.1371/journal.pone.0166535

Wersinger, S. R., Ginns, E. I., O'Carroll, A.-M., Lolait, S. J., & Young, W. S. 3rd. (2002). Vasopressin V1b receptor knockout reduces aggressive behavior in male mice. *Molecular Psychiatry*, *7*(9), 975–984. https://doi.org/10.1038/sj.mp.4001195

Widerlöv, E., Lindström, L. H., Wahlestedt, C., & Ekman, R. (1988). Neuropeptide Y and peptide YY as possible cerebrospinal fluid markers for major depression and schizophrenia, respectively. *Journal of Psychiatric Research*, *22*(1), 69–79. https://doi.org/10.1016/0022-3956(88)90030-1

Wiersielis, K. R., Wicks, B., Simko, H., Cohen, S. R., Khantsis, S., Baksh, N., Waxler, D. E., & Bangasser, D. A. (2016). Sex differences in corticotropin releasing factor-evoked behavior and activated networks. *Psychoneuroendocrinology*, *73*, 204–216. https://doi.org/10.1016/j.psyneuen.2016.07.007

Xia, G., Han, Y., Meng, F., He, Y., Srisai, D., Farias, M., Dang, M., Palmiter, R. D., Xu, Y., & Wu, Q. (2021). Reciprocal control of obesity and anxiety-depressive disorder via a GABA and serotonin neural circuit. *Molecular Psychiatry*, *26*(7), 2837–2853. https://doi.org/10.1038/s41380-021-01053-w

Yaeger, J. D. W., Krupp, K. T., Gale, J. J., & Summers, C. H. (2020). Counterbalanced microcircuits for Orx1 and Orx2 regulation of stress reactivity. *Medicine in Drug Discovery*. https://doi.org/10.1016/j.medidd.2020.100059

Yamada, S., Islam, M. S., van Kooten, N., Bovee, S., Oh, Y.-M., Tsujimura, A., Watanabe, Y., & Tanaka, M. (2020). Neuropeptide Y neurons in the nucleus accumbens modulate anxiety-like behavior. *Experimental Neurology, 327*, 113216. https://doi.org/10.1016/j.expneurol.2020.113216

Yang, Y.-L., Chao, P.-K., & Lu, K.-T. (2006). Systemic and Intra-Amygdala Administration of Glucocorticoid Agonist and Antagonist Modulate Extinction of Conditioned Fear. *Neuropsychopharmacology, 31*(5), 912–924. https://doi.org/10.1038/sj.npp.1300899

Young, W. S. 3rd, & Gainer, H. (2003). Transgenesis and the study of expression, cellular targeting and function of oxytocin, vasopressin and their receptors. *Neuroendocrinology, 78*(4), 185–203. https://doi.org/10.1159/000073702

Zheng, H., Lim, J. Y., Kim, Y., Jung, S. T., & Hwang, S. W. (2021). The role of oxytocin, vasopressin, and their receptors at nociceptors in peripheral pain modulation. *Frontiers in Neuroendocrinology, 63*, 100942. https://doi.org/10.1016/j.yfrne.2021.100942

Ziegler, C., Dannlowski, U., Bräuer, D., Stevens, S., Laeger, I., Wittmann, H., Kugel, H., Dobel, C., Hurlemann, R., Reif, A., Lesch, K.-P., Heindel, W., Kirschbaum, C., Arolt, V., Gerlach, A. L., Hoyer, J., Deckert, J., Zwanzger, P., & Domschke, K. (2015). Oxytocin receptor gene methylation: converging multilevel evidence for a role in social anxiety. *Neuropsychopharmacology: Official Publication of the American College of Neuropsychopharmacology, 40*(6), 1528–1538. https://doi.org/10.1038/npp.2015.2

Slow Breathing for Anxiety: A Critical Perspective Towards Personalization

Elke Vlemincx and Gabriela Cortez-Vázquez

Breathing practices are increasingly popular to improve physical and mental health, and wellbeing (Clarke et al. 2018). A huge number of stand-alone breathing apps exist, and breathing is a fundamental element of popular mind-body practices, such as yoga, qigong, meditation and mindfulness. In stark contrast to the appeal and widespread use of breathing practices, scientific research documenting the effectivity of breathing interventions shows inconsistency and inconclusiveness of findings (Courtois et al. 2020; Gholamrezaei et al. 2021; Jafari et al. 2017, 2020; Meuret et al. 2003). Furthermore, a solid understanding of the causal mechanisms underlying the effects of breathing on health and wellbeing is lacking (Jafari et al. 2017).

Since recent systematic reviews and meta-analyses have summarized the effects of breathing practices to reduce anxiety, stress and depression, and improve mood and wellbeing (Banushi et al. 2023; Fincham et al. 2023; Hamasaki 2020; Zaccaro et al. 2018), the aim of this chapter is not to give an exhaustive overview of the evidence on breathing interventions for anxiety. Rather, we aim to provide a critical perspective on the role of breathing practices for anxiety, drawing from findings on a broad range of physiological and self-report outcomes. First, we will briefly summarize different types of breathing practices that are popular to manage anxiety. Second, since slow breathing is by far the most studied breathing practice for

E. Vlemincx (✉)
Department of Health Sciences, Vrije Universiteit Amsterdam, Amsterdam, The Netherlands

Health Psychology, KU Leuven, Leuven, Belgium

Amsterdam Public Health Research Institute, Amsterdam, The Netherlands

Amsterdam Movement Sciences Research Institute, Amsterdam, The Netherlands
e-mail: e.vlemincx@vu.nl

G. Cortez-Vázquez
Department of Health Sciences, Vrije Universiteit Amsterdam, Amsterdam, The Netherlands

Amsterdam Public Health Research Institute, Amsterdam, The Netherlands

C. Charis, G. Panayiotou (eds.), *Anxiety Disorders and Related Conditions*,
https://doi.org/10.1007/978-3-031-56798-8_4

anxiety, we will elaborate on one key assumed mechanism underlying the anxiety-reducing effects of slow breathing. Third, we will give a concise synopsis of the effects of slow breathing to reduce self-reported anxiety. Fourth, the crux of this chapter will highlight the research gaps and challenges in understanding the working mechanisms of slow breathing for anxiety and, more broadly, health and wellbeing. Finally, we will propose opportunities for the personalization and individual tailoring of breathing practices. We emphasize that the cited literature is not exhaustive, but merely exemplary to support the discussions in this chapter.

Common Breathing Practices

Overall, breathing practices can be classified into two broad categories. Breath awareness aims to increase attention to and awareness of the sensation and act of breathing. Examples include mindful breathing and breath meditation. Breath control or breath work focuses on the voluntarily manipulation of specific breathing parameters, such as breathing frequency (e.g. slow breathing (Evaristo et al. 2020; Huang et al. 2019; Laudenslager et al. 2015; Newman Van Denburg 2020; Rosenberg and Hamiel 2021; Teng et al. 2018)); breathing volume (e.g. taking a few deep breaths (Alberts et al. 2020)); chest vs. abdominal breathing (e.g. diaphragmatic breathing (Atilgan and Tuncer 2021; Evaristo et al. 2020; Fiskin and Sahin 2018; Teng et al. 2018; Thomas et al. 2003)); mouth vs. nasal breathing (e.g. pursed lip breathing (Atilgan and Tuncer 2021; Valenza et al. 2014), left, right or alternate nostril breathing (Kamath et al. 2017; Mahendru et al. 2021; Sureka et al. 2014)); inhalation-exhalation ratio (Van Diest et al. 2014), with or without breath holds or pauses (e.g. extended exhalation (Dhruva et al. 2012; Rosenberg and Hamiel 2021; Sureka et al. 2014), box breathing (Balban et al. 2023)); and levels of exhaled carbon dioxide (e.g. exhaled carbon dioxide biofeedback (Kim et al. 2012; Meuret et al. 2008, 2010; Wollburg et al. 2011)).

Undoubtedly, the most researched breathing practice is slow breathing, which is defined as breathing slower than 10 breaths per minute (Zaccaro et al. 2018), as compared to a normal breathing frequency ranging from 12 to 20 breaths per minute with an overall average of 14–15 breaths per minute. In the literature, slow breathing is also referred to as slow deep breathing, slow diaphragmatic breathing, resonant frequency breathing or heart coherence breathing, for example. Several techniques can be applied to achieve slow breathing, such as breath counting, paced breathing (a person voluntarily matches their breathing to a pacer indicating an imposed breathing rhythm) or biofeedback (a person learns to change their breathing rhythm using feedback indicating whether their objectively measured breathing matches the instructed breathing rhythm).

Conveniently, slow breathing is proposed as a one-size-fits-all intervention for physical and mental health and wellbeing, including hypertension (Cernes and Zimlichman 2015; Mahtani et al. 2016); respiratory disorders (Bruton et al. 2018; Meuret and Ritz 2010; Ritz et al. 2014); panic disorder (Meuret and Ritz 2010);

anxiety, stress and depression (Fincham et al. 2023; Zaccaro et al. 2018); pain (Jafari et al. 2017); and relaxation (Van Diest et al. 2014; Zaccaro et al. 2018). While slow breathing is often defined as breathing less than ten breaths per minute, the most common targeted breathing frequency is six breaths per minute. Below, we discuss the core psychophysiological mechanism by which slow breathing and especially slow breathing at six breaths per minute may elicit these beneficial effects, for example, reducing anxiety.

A Key Psychophysiological Mechanism of Slow Breathing: Vagally Mediated Heart Rate Variability

Slow breathing has been shown to improve autonomic regulation by increasing heart rate variability. Heart rate variability refers to the fluctuations in time between successive heart beats and has been proposed as a transdiagnostic biobehavioural marker (Beauchaine and Thayer 2015; Heiss et al. 2021). While low heart rate variability has been associated with physical and mental illness and ill-being, including anxiety and anxiety disorders (Beauchaine and Thayer 2015; Chalmers et al. 2014; Cheng et al. 2022; Friedman 2007; Heiss et al. 2021), higher heart rate variability has been associated with improved autonomic regulation, prefrontal control, flexibility and self-regulation (Appelhans and Luecken 2006; Holzman and Bridgett 2017; Thayer et al. 2009). Increasing heart rate variability (e.g. by heart rate variability biofeedback and slow breathing) has been shown to reduce anxiety symptoms (Lehrer et al. 2020).

One mechanism[1] by which slow breathing increases heart rate variability is resonance. When breathing at a slow, individual resonant breathing frequency (approximately between 4.5 and 6.5 breaths per minute), breathing and heart rate fluctuations synchronize, and respiratory sinus arrhythmia maximizes (Russo et al. 2017; Vaschillo et al. 2004, 2006). Respiratory sinus arrhythmia is the phenomenon of cardiorespiratory coupling by which heart rate increases during inhalation and decreases during exhalation (Berntson et al. 1993; Hirsch and Bishop 1981). The increase in respiratory sinus arrhythmia during slow breathing is mediated by the vagus nerve, part of the parasympathetic nervous system (Lehrer et al. 2020), and thus slow breathing close to the individual resonant frequency increases vagally mediated heart rate variability specifically (Laborde et al. 2022a). Given that vagally mediated heart rate variability is widely implicated in autonomic regulation, executive functions and affective regulation (Thayer et al. 2009), breathing practices enhancing vagally mediated heart rate variability, such as slow breathing, have been proposed as alternatives and supplements to traditional anxiety treatments (Jerath et al. 2015).

[1] For a full review of the physiological effects of slow breathing, see (Russo et al. 2017).

While extended evidence exists on the effects of slow breathing on vagally mediated heart rate variability, it has been hypothesized that breath awareness (Gerritsen and Band 2018) and other forms of breath control, including diaphragmatic breathing (Hamasaki 2020) and alternate nostril breathing (Subramanian 2016; Telles et al. 2014), may also increase vagally mediated heart rate variability, through different mechanisms. However, so far, empirical evidence for these effects is scarce. Furthermore, despite the well-established effects of slow breathing on physiological mechanisms, the effects on self-reported outcomes of health are conflicting (Courtois et al. 2020; Gholamrezaei et al. 2021; Jafari et al. 2017, 2020; Meuret et al. 2003).

Effects of Slow Breathing on Self-Reported Anxiety

Recent systematic reviews and meta-analyses have summarized the causal effects of breath control on self-reported stress, anxiety and depression (Fincham et al. 2023); associations between slow breathing and psycho(physio)logical outcomes, including anxiety (Zaccaro et al. 2018); and effects of breathing interventions for anxiety disorders (Banushi et al. 2023). Here we will briefly discuss the studied effects of slow breathing on self-reported anxiety derived from randomized controlled evidence specifically.

Studies investigating the anxiety effects of slow breathing as the main intervention component have examined various populations, including healthy participants (with elevated stress) (Laudenslager et al. 2015; Newman Van Denburg 2020; Novaes et al. 2020; Rosenberg and Hamiel 2021; Shehab 2021) and a wide variety of patients (including patients with psychiatric disorders (Sureka et al. 2014), panic disorder specifically (de Ruiter et al. 1989; Hibbert and Chan 1989; Ito et al. 1996; Kim et al. 2012; Meuret et al. 2008, 2010; Wollburg et al. 2011), asthma (Evaristo et al. 2020), cardiovascular disease (Teng et al. 2018), cancer (Dhruva et al. 2012), gestational diabetes (Fiskin and Sahin 2018), overactive bladder syndrome (Huang et al. 2019) and inflammatory bowel disease (Gerbarg et al. 2015)) and caregivers of patients (James et al. 2021; Laudenslager et al. 2015). In these studies, slow breathing is often embedded in comprehensive interventions focusing on Eastern-oriented mind-body practices (e.g. Pranayama, Ujjayi, Bhastrika, Sudarshan Kriya, Qigong) (Dhruva et al. 2012; Gerbarg et al. 2015; Novaes et al. 2020; Sureka et al. 2014), heart rate variability biofeedback (Herhaus et al. 2022; James et al. 2021; Shehab 2021), psychosocial stress interventions (Laudenslager et al. 2015) including cognitive restructuring (de Ruiter et al. 1989; Hibbert and Chan 1989) or usual care (Teng et al. 2018). Also, control groups are very diverse, ranging from wait-list controls (Dhruva et al. 2012; Shehab 2021; Sureka et al. 2014) to care-as-usual (Laudenslager et al. 2015; Newman Van Denburg 2020; Teng et al. 2018), alternative treatment (e.g. graded exposure in panic disorder (de Ruiter et al. 1989), cognitive training (Meuret et al. 2010), psychoeducation (Gerbarg et al. 2015; Hibbert and Chan 1989; Rosenberg and Hamiel 2021)), music (Huang et al. 2019; Newman Van Denburg

2020), other cognitive activities (Novaes et al. 2020) or sham biofeedback (Herhaus et al. 2022). In light of the diversity in study methodologies, the reported results on the effectivity of slow breathing on anxiety are mixed, ranging from larger decreases after slow breathing than control (Dhruva et al. 2012; Fiskin and Sahin 2018; Gerbarg et al. 2015; Laudenslager et al. 2015; Novaes et al. 2020; Sureka et al. 2014; Teng et al. 2018) to no significant differences (de Ruiter et al. 1989; Evaristo et al. 2020; Herhaus et al. 2022; Hibbert and Chan 1989; Huang et al. 2019; Newman Van Denburg 2020; Rosenberg and Hamiel 2021; Shehab 2021) or even (non-significant) increases (James et al. 2021) in anxiety.

Interestingly, slow breathing in anxiety disorders has been mainly studied in panic disorder (Banushi et al. 2023; Meuret et al. 2003), and slow breathing interventions in panic disorder patients have used more patient-specific techniques. For example, slow breathing has been integrated in more comprehensive breathing training, in which slow breathing practice is preceded by voluntary hyperventilation with or without cognitive restructuring of the sensations of hyperventilation (de Ruiter et al. 1989; Hibbert and Chan 1989; Ito et al. 1996). Other slow breathing interventions have used capnometry-assisted respiratory training (i.e. respiratory training by means of biofeedback of exhaled carbon dioxide levels and respiration rate). As panic disorder patients often show fast chest breathing, frequent deep breaths and even hyperventilation, capnometry-assisted respiratory training includes gradual decreases of breathing rate with a focus on abdominal breathing, instructions to avoid deep breaths and biofeedback of exhaled carbon dioxide levels (Meuret et al. 2001, 2008, 2010; Meuret and Ritz 2010). Randomized controlled evidence has shown moderate to large reductions in hyperventilation, panic disorder severity and anxiety sensitivity in panic disorder patients receiving capnometry-assisted respiratory training, compared to a wait-list control (Meuret et al. 2008) but not compared to cognitive training (Meuret et al. 2010). Yet, findings suggest that changes in breathing unidirectionally predicted panic disorder severity and preceded cognitive improvements including symptom appraisal and perceived control (Meuret et al. 2010). However, other studies investigating the effects of capnometry-assisted respiratory training have shown no differences in anxiety when lowering exhaled carbon dioxide levels by slow deep paced breathing compared to raising exhaled carbon dioxide levels by slow shallow paced breathing (at the same breathing frequency of nine breaths per minute) (Kim et al. 2012; Wollburg et al. 2011).

In sum, the effects of slow breathing on anxiety in a broad range of populations are mostly small and conflicting (Fincham et al. 2023; Meuret et al. 2003; Zaccaro et al. 2018). Below, we discuss an overview of factors that may contribute to the inconclusiveness of findings.

Research Gaps and Challenges in Investigating Anxiety Effects of Slow Breathing Interventions

While the physiological and psychological effects of slow breathing have been studied extensively in a wide variety of populations, important research gaps remain and our understanding of the effects of breathing interventions remains limited. These research gaps are associated with specific challenges in studying the effects of breathing that complicate teasing out the isolated effects of specific breath control instructions and clarifying which mechanisms underlie the effects. Below, we address some important research gaps and associated challenges.

Causal Effects Not Explained by Other Mechanisms Than Slow Breathing

The majority of studies investigating breathing interventions involve observational research comparing physiological and self-report indices before breathing exercises with those during or after (Zaccaro et al. 2018). While some studies have investigated the effects of breathing interventions using randomized cross-over designs (Busch et al. 2012), the impact of these studies relies on the assumption that the effects of slow breathing can be 'washed out', or slow breathing can be 'unlearned', which may not be feasible. More randomized controlled trials are essential to conclude on causal effects of breathing interventions (Fincham et al. 2023; Zaccaro et al. 2018). However, even experimental research struggles with major challenges.

Experimental studies have compared breathing interventions to a variety of control groups. Most studies compare the effects of breathing interventions to inactive control conditions, including quiet sitting while breathing spontaneously, wait-list controls, standard care or care-as-usual. Since studies comparing breathing interventions to inactive control conditions cannot be easily blinded to participants or experimenters, self-reported effects of breathing exercises could possibly be explained by *expectation or demand effects*. This is particularly problematic given potentially strong lay assumptions that exist about the associations between affect and relaxation, on the one hand, and slow breathing or deep breaths, on the other hand (Danvers et al. 2021; Teigen 2008). Indeed, researchers have questioned whether breathing exercises add more than a placebo effect (Garssen et al. 1992). If blinding is not feasible, efforts may be made to standardize expectations of breathing instructions, e.g. by a cover story (Szulczewski and Rynkiewicz 2018) or providing a more detailed context of potential positive and negative effects of various breathing instructions (Vlemincx et al. 2016).

Also, active control conditions are diverse, including paced breathing at the individual's intrinsic respiration rate, paced breathing at a fixed rate within normal ranges (e.g. 12–15 breaths per min), paced fast breathing, music listening, attention or cognitive tasks (e.g. breath counting, crosswords), psychoeducation or sham biofeedback. These different comparison conditions attempt to control for various potentially confounding factors that are inherently associated with slow breathing practices. Examples of these confounding factors include breathing patterns other than frequency, increased breath awareness and cognitive, task-related aspects of slow breathing, as discussed below.

First, studies investigating slow breathing exercises often lack detailed information on the *specific breathing instructions* given. Instructions on respiratory volume, diaphragmatic breathing, nasal inhalation, pursed lip exhalation and inhalation-exhalation ratio with or without breath holds or pauses may importantly influence physiological and subjective effects. While it may not be possible to methodologically control for these different breathing influences, transparency on the given breathing instructions and (at least intermittently) monitoring of breathing patterns are essential, and even statistically controlling for the recorded breathing patterns may be feasible and informative. While evidence on the effects of breath control of other breathing parameters than frequency is rather limited and conflicting, researchers have hypothesized on the roles of occasional deep breaths (Vlemincx et al. 2013, 2022), diaphragmatic breathing (Atilgan and Tuncer 2021; Evaristo et al. 2020; Fiskin and Sahin 2018; Hamasaki 2020; Teng et al. 2018; Thomas et al. 2003), nostril breathing (Kamath et al. 2017; Subramanian et al. 2016; Telles et al. 2014), pursed lip breathing (Atilgan and Tuncer 2021; Srimookda et al. 2021; Valenza et al. 2014) and changes in inhalation-exhalation ratio (Bae et al. 2021; Dhruva et al. 2012; Lin et al. 2014; Rosenberg and Hamiel 2021; Sureka et al. 2014; Van Diest et al. 2014) for affect, emotion and mood regulation. For example, some studies suggest that extended exhalation or low inhalation-exhalation ratio increases vagally mediated heart rate variability and self-reported relaxation (Bae et al. 2021; Van Diest et al. 2014), while other studies suggest that equal inhalation-exhalation time increases heart rate variability more than low inhalation-exhalation ratio, and changes in inhalation-exhalation ratio are unrelated to self-reported relaxation (Lin et al. 2014). Similarly, some studies indicate that deep breaths may reduce stress (Vlemincx et al. 2012a, 2016, 2017) or increase positive affect (Balban et al. 2023), while others indicate that deep breaths may inhibit stress and anxiety reduction (Meuret et al. 2001; Vlemincx et al. 2010). These findings illustrate that more research is needed on the isolated effects of slow breathing and the contribution of breathing parameters other than breathing frequency.

Second, breathing exercises inherently increase *attention to and awareness of breathing* and *distraction* from other potentially ongoing stressors, threats or other aversive states. Therefore, disentangling the effects of slow breathing independent of increased attention, awareness and distraction may be important, yet challenging. Recent studies have attempted to directly compare breath work to increased breath awareness conditions, such as mindfulness meditation (Balban et al. 2023) and mindful breathing (Vlemincx 2023; Vlemincx et al. 2019). These comparisons show that the superiority effects of breath work over mindful breathing may be limited for subjective outcomes (Balban et al. 2023; Vlemincx 2023; Vlemincx et al. 2019) (with the exception of cyclic sighing (Balban et al. 2023)). For physiological effects, however, slow breathing may be superior to mindful breathing, as slow breathing increases heart rate variability more than mindful breathing (Vlemincx 2023; Vlemincx et al. 2019). Interestingly, these findings illustrate the lack of correspondence between physiological and self-reported effects of breath work when confounding factors of attention, awareness and distraction are controlled for.

Third, breath control techniques are often *demanding* and involve tasks in which practitioners are able to actively take *control* of their breathing (such as biofeedback) or, conversely, hand over control to an imposed breathing rhythm (such as paced breathing). Slow breathing techniques such as paced breathing and respiratory biofeedback require extended cognitive resources as they are (difficult) tasks which may distract from ongoing aversive states and affect feelings of control. So these task-related cognitions and associated effects of distraction and feelings of control may potentially explain the effects of slow breathing interventions. Researchers have attempted to control for these effects with control groups that involve cognitive engagement or distraction, such as crosswords or puzzles (Novaes et al. 2020), music (Huang et al. 2019; Newman Van Denburg 2020), paced breathing at other frequencies than slow breathing (Courtois et al. 2020; Jafari et al. 2020) or sham biofeedback (Herhaus et al. 2022).

In sum, we discussed some potentially essential confounding factors in experimental research investigating slow breathing interventions. Importantly, however, whether to control for these factors depends on the research question of interest. So careful consideration of the effects of interest is required to set up a research protocol that matches the research question. The list above merely serves as food for thought when designing slow breathing intervention studies. Below we address more research gaps in the literature on anxiety effects of slow breathing.

Training Effects, Long-Lasting Effects and Transferability

Little is known about the training effects of slow breathing. It is generally assumed that executing slow breathing exercises requires practice. However, it is not clear how much training is required to execute breath control correctly and how to measure that. Moreover, while the acute physiological effects of slow breathing are instantaneous, it remains unknown how much training is required to gain changes in subjective feelings of stress or anxiety. Recent data show that breath work (i.e. cyclic sighing) compared to breath meditation results in higher positive affect after a period of approximately 15 days of 5 minutes of daily practice (Balban et al. 2023). Also in a sample of women with gestational diabetes, who practised diaphragmatic breathing daily for 5 minutes over 30 days, significant reductions in depression, anxiety and stress were found after 15 days (Fiskin and Sahin 2018).

The duration of studied breathing interventions differs largely, from single 10-minute sessions of breath work (e.g. Kamath et al. 2017) to daily practice over the period of 1 month (e.g. Alberts et al. 2020; Balban et al. 2023; Fiskin and Sahin 2018; Shehab 2021), 6–8 weeks (e.g. Atilgan and Tuncer 2021; Sureka et al. 2014) or 12 weeks (e.g. Huang et al. 2019). In addition, long-term follow-up measurements post-intervention are limited. Few studies have reported long-term (3-, 6- and 12-month follow-up) effects of slow breathing on anxiety in asthma and panic disorder (Evaristo et al. 2020; Meuret et al. 2008; Thomas et al. 2003). Moreover, the physiological effects of breathing exercises exhibit mostly during the practice of the breathing exercises, but evidence for the transferability of physiological effects to baselines, reactivity to stress or threat, and/or recovery from stress or threat, while not performing the breathing exercise, is low. Increases in baroreflex gain across sessions have been reported in healthy persons (Lehrer et al. 2003), but these findings have not been replicated. In persons with hypertension, some studies have shown slow breathing to reduce blood pressure, probably due to increases in baroreflex sensitivity (Cernes and Zimlichman 2015), while other studies show mixed results (Mahtani et al. 2016). More research investigating the integration of slow breathing exercises in daily life in heterogeneous populations, with exposure to real-life perceived stress and threat, is needed to increase the transferability of slow breathing effects.

Altogether, this raises the question of which conditions of breath work may lead to more long-lasting and transferable effects. In the next paragraph, we will elaborate further on this discussion.

Comparison of Different Breathing Techniques

To impose slow breathing, a variety of breathing techniques have been used, including paced breathing (with or without heart rate variability biofeedback), respiratory biofeedback and breath counting. The comparative effects of these different breathing techniques have not been systematically examined, while the underlying mechanisms and resulting breathing patterns may differ largely between them. During paced breathing, participants are asked to match their inhalation and exhalation time with a visual, auditory, and/or tactile pacer to a specific slow inhalation-exhalation rhythm. This way, attention is oriented both externally (to the pacer) and internally (to breathing). Successful paced breathing results in fixed (i.e. very regular) breathing patterns with little latitude for variations in breathing. During respiratory biofeedback, participants are given visual, auditory, and/or tactile animated feedback of their breathing rhythm, which they learn to adjust to an instructed breathing rhythm. Respiratory biofeedback allows participants to breathe spontaneously, and adjustment of breathing is established via a learning process. Attention is oriented both externally (to the animated feedback) and internally (to breathing). Relatedly, research found no evidence for differences between slow paced breathing with and without heart rate variability biofeedback, with the exception that slow paced breathing with heart rate variability biofeedback was experienced as more pleasant (Laborde et al. 2022b).

More recently, the use of virtual reality (VR) has been investigated as a method to induce slow breathing. VR may potentially have important advantages over

2D-paced breathing or biofeedback. VR involves an immersive experience, often with reinforcing stimuli and gamification elements, which enhance an embodied experience. This may increase motivation to perform breathing exercises, decrease the perceived difficulty to adjust breathing and increase internal bodily focus, attention and awareness. However, a systematic review and meta-analysis have shown that VR breathing interventions are not superior to non-VR alternatives in reducing anxiety, stress, depression or improving mood, nor are they liked or evaluated better by participants (Cortez-Vázquez et al., 2024).

Overall, future research on the comparison between different breathing techniques could increase our understanding of the mechanisms and breathing patterns underlying the effects of slow breathing.

Adherence and Compliance

Many slow breathing interventions rely on independent home practice of the participants. However, mostly, no systematic data are available on adherence to the instructed breathing practice. Most researchers report that they 'encouraged' participants to practise daily, twice daily or a fixed number of times per week, but have no real insight into whether participants adhered to these instructions. Some device-guided slow breathing tools allow to record usage of the device and may provide adherence data. In a study investigating the effects of slow breathing through biofeedback (as part of a psychosocial stress intervention) in caregivers of stem cell transplant patients, adherence was low (Laudenslager et al. 2015). Participants were asked to practise slow breathing four to five times per week for 15 minutes. Only 16% of participants used the device consistently (Laudenslager et al. 2015).

In addition, it is unclear to what extent participants comply with slow breathing practices and perform them correctly. While some lab studies monitored and analysed breathing during the breathing practice (for example, Meuret et al. 2008; Van Diest et al. 2014; Vlemincx 2023; Vlemincx et al. 2019), most studies do not report on recording of breathing. Without at least monitoring breathing, it is unknown whether participants complied with the breathing instructions, whether the breathing instructions were performed correctly and how deviations from the intended intervention affect results. Furthermore, it is unclear which factors influence adherence to and compliance with breathing instructions, such as motivation, enjoyment, interest, experience, competence, self-efficacy, effort, benefits and fit into daily life.

Adverse Events and Side Effects

Slow breathing interventions are commonly suggested as a safer alternative to medication (e.g. anxiolytic medication, hypertension medication) (Jerath et al. 2015; Mahtani et al. 2016). However, while mostly unreported, it seems very plausible that adverse side effects may occur during slow breathing (Landman et al. 2013, 2014; Mahtani et al. 2016; Meuret et al. 2003). Next, we will discuss different reasons why slow breathing interventions may have adverse physiological and psychological effects.

First, it has been shown that imposing breathing patterns, in the laboratory, outside the context of relaxation, stress or anxiety reduction, an intervention or treatment, is experienced as difficult and effortful (Vlemincx et al. 2012b). Moreover, in the same study, participants report feeling more tense and less relaxed during imposed breathing compared to spontaneous breathing. This could imply that the context of the research, the instructions and the expectation and demand effects may be critical in the resulting effects.

Second, slow breathing most often results in compensatory techniques, of which deep breathing is very common. When first practising slow breathing, it is rather difficult to adopt an adaptive breathing pattern, balancing respiratory frequency and volume, chest vs. abdominal breathing and mouth vs. nasal breathing. Participants may overcompensate a slow breathing frequency, by breathing too deeply, potentially causing hyperventilation (Meuret et al. 2003; Szulczewski 2019). Hyperventilation often co-occurs with feelings of dyspnoea or shortness of breath. In a study in patients with type 2 diabetes mellitus and hypertension, 2 of 21 patients in a device-guided slow breathing intervention withdrew from the intervention due to shortness of breath (Landman et al. 2013, 2014; Mahtani et al. 2016). In the latter study, slow breathing instructions consisted of reducing breathing rate below ten breaths per minute by respiratory music biofeedback. Hyperventilation effects may even be more common and severe when reducing breathing frequency to the resonant frequency range of 4.5–6.5 breaths per minute. Taking into account the risk of hyperventilation, it may be important to take measures to avoid hyperventilation (Fiskin and Sahin 2018), for example, by monitoring exhaled carbon dioxide (Meuret et al. 2008; Meuret and Ritz 2010; Ritz et al. 2014) or symptoms of hyperventilation or by specific anti-hyperventilation instructions (Szulczewski 2019).

Third, slow breathing may induce relaxation-induced anxiety (Heide and Borkovec 1984), especially in persons with high trait anxiety sensitivity or worry. Slow breathing involves deviations in respiration and respiratory sensations from normal. These differences in somatic sensations may induce worry and anxiety (de Ruiter et al. 1989; Hibbert and Chan 1989). Furthermore, adhering to an imposed breathing rhythm involves a loss of control, which may be anxiety-inducing.

Finally, slow breathing is often imposed by means of paced breathing, which is fixed-rate, regular breathing. The set timing of each inhalation and exhalation is identical to the next. This is in stark contrast with spontaneous breathing, which is biologically variable. Studies have shown that a lack of biological variation in the breathing pattern is associated with reduced lung compliance and gas exchange efficiency (Mutch et al. 2000, 2007; Wysocki et al. 2006), which may elicit breathing symptoms, such as chest tightness and breathlessness.

Overall, it seems that adverse side effects of slow breathing practices are plausible. Reporting of adverse events, quantitatively or qualitatively, is essential to increase our understanding of side effects of slow breathing and the consequences for the implementation of slow breathing in research and practice.

Towards Personalized Breathing Interventions for Anxiety

So far, slow breathing is presented as a one-size-fits-all intervention for physical health (e.g. hypertension (Cernes and Zimlichman 2015; Mahtani et al. 2016), respiratory disorders (Bruton et al. 2018; Meuret and Ritz 2010; Ritz et al. 2014)) and mental health and wellbeing (e.g. panic disorder (Meuret and Ritz 2010); anxiety, stress and depression (Fincham et al. 2023; Zaccaro et al. 2018); pain (Jafari et al. 2017); relaxation (Van Diest et al. 2014; Zaccaro et al. 2018)). Yet, evidence on the effectivity of slow breathing is mixed. One explanation is that we don't understand sufficiently how, why and under which conditions slow breathing may be effective. While there is extensive support for the acute mechanism of vagally mediated heart rate variability, the long-term physiological effects and the subjective effects of slow breathing appear to be more complex.

The inconsistency of findings, the limited evidence for the transferability of physiological benefits to everyday life, the dissociation between physiological and self-reported effects and the possibility of adverse side effects suggest that slow breathing may benefit from a more personalized, tailored approach. Such personalization or tailoring could be based on (1) individual traits, (2) individual breathing patterns, and (3) individual preferences in the execution and implementation of breathing exercises in daily life (Fig. 1).

First, *individual traits* may provide indications to tailor breathing practices. For example, for individuals who show high anxiety sensitivity and thus easily feel anxious in response to (changes in) bodily sensations associated with fear or anxiety, attention to breathing and changes in breathing patterns may require more caution. For example, (more gradual) interoceptive exposure to changes in breathing

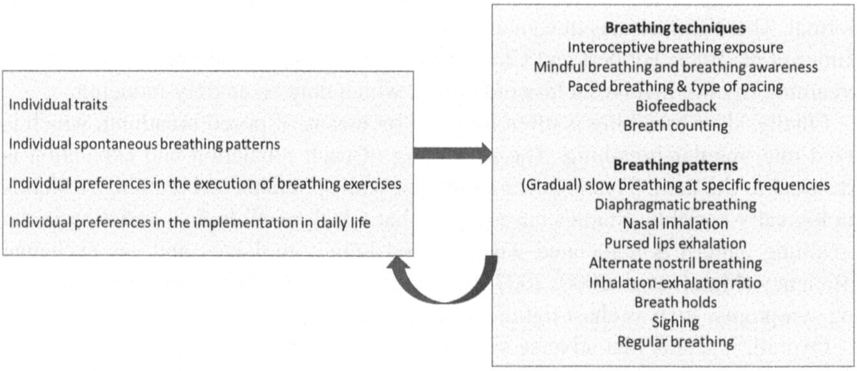

Fig. 1 Personal tailoring of breathing interventions

sensations may be advised to learn that these changes are not harmful. In persons with high interoceptive attention or awareness, it may be important to check the persons' appraisals of changes in interoceptive sensations in response to slow breathing. In persons with a high need for control, it may be beneficial to choose biofeedback techniques over paced breathing, such that persons can remain in control of the breathing patterns they adopt to slow breathing. All this may reduce or prevent relaxation-induced anxiety and associated physiological adverse side effects (e.g. feelings of shortness of breath, heart palpitations).

Second, breathing practices could benefit from tailoring based on *individual spontaneous breathing patterns*. For example, individuals who show fast, highly irregular, and/or predominantly chest breathing may benefit more from slow, regular, and/or diaphragmatic breathing, respectively. Persons with very high respiration rates and tendencies to hyperventilate may do better with more gradual decreases in respiration rate, supported by capnometry biofeedback or anti-hyperventilation instructions. For persons who tend to hyperventilate due to excessive sighing, instructions to avoid deep breaths may be more effective. This way, specific dysfunctional breathing patterns can be counteracted by specific breathing instructions that avoid hyperventilation and associated symptoms and thus adverse side effects. To avoid adverse compensatory breathing patterns, it would be recommended to monitor breathing patterns on a continuous basis and to adjust where necessary.

Finally, qualitative research has shown that the search for *individual preferences in the execution and implementation of breathing exercises in everyday life* requires reflection and flexibility (Donker et al. n.d.). To make slow breathing work in their lives, persons consider individual preferences for specific breathing patterns, reflecting on breathing frequency, inhalation-exhalation ratio with or without breath holds, diaphragmatic breathing, nasal inhalation, pursed lip exhalation, breathing regularity and the type of pacing (Donker et al. n.d.). In addition, individual preferences in the implementation of breathing practice in daily life play a major role in the maintenance of the breathing practice. Persons consider the duration and moment of practice, as well as the environment when practising (Donker et al. n.d.). Furthermore, breathing practices seem easier to implement in less stressful periods in life, while they may be needed more when life is stressful. Therefore, it is key to integrate breathing exercises during anticipation of and recovery from stressful events or challenges. While it may not be feasible or adaptive to practise slow breathing during acute stressful events, it may help integrate breathing exercises during periods of chronic stress.

The search for individually preferred breathing patterns and their tailored implementation in daily life may enhance the transferability and feasibility of breathing practices in everyday life. Key is to learn what works for an individual in any specific situation. This requires a continuous reflection and evaluation of what works and doesn't work for an individual person, and flexible adjusting. Importantly, this implies the consideration that breathing exercises may not work well at all for some persons or for some situations. Additionally, this requires letting go of the perception that breathing exercises should work universally and especially the assumption that breathing exercises should work because they work for others. Altogether, the personal tailoring of slow breathing practices based on personal traits, spontaneous breathing patterns and preferences may increase their effectiveness, transferability and safety, as well as the feasibility of their implementation in daily life.

Conclusion

Despite the popularity of slow breathing for anxiety, its effectivity remains unclear. We have argued that the inconclusiveness of findings may be associated with methodological challenges in slow breathing research. We have discussed that changes in self-reported anxiety may be due to demand and expectation effects, changes in respiratory parameters other than breathing frequency, increased attention to and awareness of breathing, distraction and cognitive engagement. Moreover, the potential roles of training, transferability, different breathing techniques, adherence, compliance and adverse side effects of slow breathing are understudied. Rather than considering slow breathing as a one-size-fits-all intervention for anxiety, we suggest that individual tailoring of breathing practices and personalization may importantly contribute to the effectivity of slow breathing.

References

Alberts, N. M., Leisenring, W. M., Flynn, J. S., Whitton, J., Gibson, T. M., Jibb, L., McDonald, A., Ford, J., Moraveji, N., Dear, B. F., Krull, K. R., Robison, L. L., Stinson, J. N., & Armstrong, G. T. (2020). Wearable Respiratory Monitoring and Feedback for Chronic Pain in Adult Survivors of Childhood Cancer: A Feasibility Randomized Controlled Trial From the Childhood Cancer Survivor Study. *JCO Clinical Cancer Informatics*, *4*, 1014–1026. https://doi.org/10.1200/CCI.20.00070

Appelhans, B. M., & Luecken, L. J. (2006). Heart Rate Variability as an Index of Regulated Emotional Responding. *Review of General Psychology*, *10*(3), 229–240. https://doi.org/10.1037/1089-2680.10.3.229

Atilgan, E. D., & Tuncer, A. (2021). The effects of breathing exercises in mothers of children with special health care needs:A randomized controlled trial. *Journal of Back and Musculoskeletal Rehabilitation*, *34*(5), 795–804. https://doi.org/10.3233/BMR-200327

Bae, D., Matthews, J. J. L., Chen, J. J., & Mah, L. (2021). Increased exhalation to inhalation ratio during breathing enhances high-frequency heart rate variability in healthy adults. *Psychophysiology*, *58*(11), e13905. https://doi.org/10.1111/psyp.13905

Balban, M. Y., Neri, E., Kogon, M. M., Weed, L., Nouriani, B., Jo, B., Holl, G., Zeitzer, J. M., Spiegel, D., & Huberman, A. D. (2023). Brief structured respiration practices enhance mood and reduce physiological arousal. *Cell Reports Medicine*, *4*(1). https://doi.org/10.1016/j.xcrm.2022.100895

Banushi, B., Brendle, M., Ragnhildstveit, A., Murphy, T., Moore, C., Egberts, J., & Robison, R. (2023). Breathwork Interventions for Adults with Clinically Diagnosed Anxiety Disorders: A Scoping Review. *Brain Sciences*, *13*(2), Article 2. https://doi.org/10.3390/brainsci13020256

Beauchaine, T. P., & Thayer, J. F. (2015). Heart rate variability as a transdiagnostic biomarker of psychopathology. *International Journal of Psychophysiology*, *98*(2, Part 2), 338–350. https://doi.org/10.1016/j.ijpsycho.2015.08.004

Berntson, G. G., Cacioppo, J. T., & Quigley, K. S. (1993). Respiratory sinus arrhythmia: Autonomic origins, physiological mechanisms, and psychophysiological implications. *Psychophysiology, 30*(2), 183–196. https://doi.org/10.1111/j.1469-8986.1993.tb01731.x

Bruton, A., Lee, A., Yardley, L., Raftery, J., Arden-Close, E., Kirby, S., Zhu, S., Thiruvothiyur, M., Webley, F., Taylor, L., Gibson, D., Yao, G., Stafford-Watson, M., Versnel, J., Moore, M., George, S., Little, P., Djukanovic, R., Price, D., … Thomas, M. (2018). Physiotherapy breathing retraining for asthma: A randomised controlled trial. *The Lancet Respiratory Medicine, 6*(1), 19–28. https://doi.org/10.1016/S2213-2600(17)30474-5

Busch, V., Magerl, W., Kern, U., Haas, J., Hajak, G., & Eichhammer, P. (2012). The Effect of Deep and Slow Breathing on Pain Perception, Autonomic Activity, and Mood Processing—An Experimental Study. *Pain Medicine, 13*(2), 215–228. https://doi.org/10.1111/j.1526-4637.2011.01243.x

Cernes, R., & Zimlichman, R. (2015). RESPeRATE: The role of paced breathing in hypertension treatment. *Journal of the American Society of Hypertension, 9*(1), 38–47. https://doi.org/10.1016/j.jash.2014.10.002

Chalmers, J. A., Quintana, D. S., Abbott, M. J.-A., & Kemp, A. H. (2014). Anxiety Disorders are Associated with Reduced Heart Rate Variability: A Meta-Analysis. *Frontiers in Psychiatry, 5*, 80. https://doi.org/10.3389/fpsyt.2014.00080

Cheng, Y.-C., Su, M.-I., Liu, C.-W., Huang, Y.-C., & Huang, W.-L. (2022). Heart rate variability in patients with anxiety disorders: A systematic review and meta-analysis. *Psychiatry and Clinical Neurosciences, 76*(7), 292–302. https://doi.org/10.1111/pcn.13356

Clarke, T. C., Barnes, P. M., Black, L. I., Stussman, B. J., & Nahin, R. L. (2018). Use of Yoga, Meditation, and Chiropractors Among U.S. Adults Aged 18 and Over. *NCHS Data Brief, 325*, 1–8.

Cortez-Vázquez, G., Adriaanse, M., Burchell, G. L., Ostelo, R., Panayiotou, G., & Vlemincx, E. (2024). Virtual Reality Breathing Interventions for Mental Health: A Systematic Review and Meta-Analysis of Randomized Controlled Trials. Applied Psychophysiology and Biofeedback. https://doi.org/10.1007/s10484-023-09611-4

Courtois, I., Gholamrezaei, A., Jafari, H., Lautenbacher, S., Diest, I. V., Oudenhove, L. V., & Vlaeyen, J. W. S. (2020). Respiratory Hypoalgesia? The Effect of Slow Deep Breathing on Electrocutaneous, Thermal, and Mechanical Pain. *The Journal of Pain, 21*(5), 616–632. https://doi.org/10.1016/j.jpain.2019.10.002

Danvers, A. F., Milek, A., Tackman, A. M., Kaplan, D. M., Robbins, M. L., Poslinelli, A., Moseley, S., Raison, C. L., Sbarra, D., & Mehl, M. R. (2021). Is frequent sighing an indicator of dispositional negative emotionality? A multi-sample, multi-measure naturalistic-observation study. *Journal of Research in Personality, 90*, 104046. https://doi.org/10.1016/j.jrp.2020.104046

de Ruiter, C., Rijken, H., Kraaimaat, F., & Garssen, B. (1989). Breathing retraining, exposure and a combination of both, in the treatment of panic disorder with agoraphobia. *Behaviour Research and Therapy, 27*(6), 647–655. https://doi.org/10.1016/0005-7967(89)90148-4

Dhruva, A., Miaskowski, C., Abrams, D., Acree, M., Cooper, B., Goodman, S., & Hecht, F. M. (2012). Yoga Breathing for Cancer Chemotherapy–Associated Symptoms and Quality of Life: Results of a Pilot Randomized Controlled Trial. *The Journal of Alternative and Complementary Medicine, 18*(5), 473–479. https://doi.org/10.1089/acm.2011.0555

Donker, M. H., Berger, S., Flederus, A., & Vlemincx, E. (n.d.). Exploring the implementation of slow breathing exercises in daily life: A qualitative study. *In Preparation.*

Evaristo, K. B., Mendes, F. A. R., Saccomani, M. G., Cukier, A., Carvalho-Pinto, R. M., Rodrigues, M. R., Santaella, D. F., Saraiva-Romanholo, B. M., Martins, M. A., & Carvalho, C. R. F. (2020). Effects of Aerobic Training Versus Breathing Exercises on Asthma Control: A Randomized Trial. *The Journal of Allergy and Clinical Immunology: In Practice, 8*(9), 2989-2996.e4. https://doi.org/10.1016/j.jaip.2020.06.042

Fincham, G. W., Strauss, C., Montero-Marin, J., & Cavanagh, K. (2023). Effect of breathwork on stress and mental health: A meta-analysis of randomised-controlled trials. *Scientific Reports, 13*(1), Article 1. https://doi.org/10.1038/s41598-022-27247-y

Fiskin, G., & Sahin, N. H. (2018). Effect of diaphragmatic breathing exercise on psychological parameters in gestational diabetes: A randomised controlled trial. *European Journal of Integrative Medicine*, *23*, 50–56. https://doi.org/10.1016/j.eujim.2018.09.006

Friedman, B. H. (2007). An autonomic flexibility–neurovisceral integration model of anxiety and cardiac vagal tone. *Biological Psychology*, *74*(2), 185–199. https://doi.org/10.1016/j.biopsycho.2005.08.009

Garssen, B., de Ruiter, C., & van Dyck, R. (1992). Breathing retraining: A rational placebo? *Clinical Psychology Review*, *12*(2), 141–153. https://doi.org/10.1016/0272-7358(92)90111-K

Gerbarg, P. L., Jacob, V. E., Stevens, L., Bosworth, B. P., Chabouni, F., DeFilippis, E. M., Warren, R., Trivellas, M., Patel, P. V., Webb, C. D., Harbus, M. D., Christos, P. J., Brown, R. P., & Scherl, E. J. (2015). The Effect of Breathing, Movement, and Meditation on Psychological and Physical Symptoms and Inflammatory Biomarkers in Inflammatory Bowel Disease: A Randomized Controlled Trial. *Inflammatory Bowel Diseases*, *21*(12), 2886–2896. https://doi.org/10.1097/MIB.0000000000000568

Gerritsen, R. J. S., & Band, G. P. H. (2018). Breath of Life: The Respiratory Vagal Stimulation Model of Contemplative Activity. *Frontiers in Human Neuroscience*, *12*. https://doi.org/10.3389/fnhum.2018.00397

Gholamrezaei, A., Diest, I. V., Aziz, Q., Vlaeyen, J. W. S., & Oudenhove, L. V. (2021). Psychophysiological responses to various slow, deep breathing techniques. *Psychophysiology*, *58*(2), e13712. https://doi.org/10.1111/psyp.13712

Hamasaki, H. (2020). Effects of Diaphragmatic Breathing on Health: A Narrative Review. *Medicines*, *7*(10), 65. https://doi.org/10.3390/medicines7100065

Heide, F. J., & Borkovec, T. D. (1984). Relaxation-induced anxiety: Mechanisms and theoretical implications. *Behaviour Research and Therapy*, *22*(1), 1–12. https://doi.org/10.1016/0005-7967(84)90027-5

Heiss, S., Vaschillo, B., Vaschillo, E. G., Timko, C. A., & Hormes, J. M. (2021). Heart rate variability as a biobehavioral marker of diverse psychopathologies: A review and argument for an "ideal range." *Neuroscience and Biobehavioral Reviews*, *121*, 144–155. https://doi.org/10.1016/j.neubiorev.2020.12.004

Herhaus, B., Siepmann, M., Kahaly, G. J., Conrad, R., & Petrowski, K. (2022). Effect of a Biofeedback Intervention on Heart Rate Variability in Individuals With Panic Disorder: A Randomized Controlled Trial. *Psychosomatic Medicine*, *84*(2), 199. https://doi.org/10.1097/PSY.0000000000001031

Hibbert, G. A., & Chan, M. (1989). Respiratory Control: Its Contribution to the Treatment of Panic Attacks: A Controlled Study. *The British Journal of Psychiatry*, *154*(2), 232–236. https://doi.org/10.1192/bjp.154.2.232

Hirsch, J. A., & Bishop, B. (1981). Respiratory sinus arrhythmia in humans: How breathing pattern modulates heart rate. *American Journal of Physiology-Heart and Circulatory Physiology*, *241*(4), H620–H629. https://doi.org/10.1152/ajpheart.1981.241.4.H620

Holzman, J. B., & Bridgett, D. J. (2017). Heart rate variability indices as bio-markers of top-down self-regulatory mechanisms: A meta-analytic review. *Neuroscience & Biobehavioral Reviews*, *74*, 233–255. https://doi.org/10.1016/j.neubiorev.2016.12.032

Huang, A. J., Grady, D., Mendes, W. B., Hernandez, C., Schembri, M., & Subak, L. L. (2019). A Randomized Controlled Trial of Device Guided, Slow-Paced Respiration in Women with Overactive Bladder Syndrome. *Journal of Urology*, *202*(4), 787–794. https://doi.org/10.1097/JU.0000000000000328

Ito, L. M., Noshirvani, H., Başoğlu, M., & Marks, I. M. (1996). Does Exposure to Internal Cues Enhance Exposure to External Cues in Agoraphobia with Panic? A Pilot Controlled Study of Self-Exposure. *Psychotherapy and Psychosomatics*, *65*(1), 24–28.

Jafari, H., Courtois, I., Van den Bergh, O., Vlaeyen, J. W. S., & Van Diest, I. (2017). Pain and respiration: A systematic review. *Pain*, *158*(6), 995–1006. https://doi.org/10.1097/j.pain.0000000000000865

Jafari, H., Gholamrezaei, A., Franssen, M., Oudenhove, L. V., Aziz, Q., Bergh, O. V. den, Vlaeyen, J. W. S., & Diest, I. V. (2020). Can Slow Deep Breathing Reduce Pain? An Experimental Study Exploring Mechanisms. *The Journal of Pain*, *21*(9), 1018–1030. https://doi.org/10.1016/j.jpain.2019.12.010

James, T. A., James, D., & Larkey, L. K. (2021). Heart-focused breathing and perceptions of burden in Alzheimer's caregivers: An online randomized controlled pilot study. *Geriatric Nursing*, *42*(2), 397–404. https://doi.org/10.1016/j.gerinurse.2021.02.006

Jerath, R., Crawford, M. W., Barnes, V. A., & Harden, K. (2015). Self-regulation of breathing as a primary treatment for anxiety. *Applied Psychophysiology and Biofeedback*, *40*(2), 107–115. https://doi.org/10.1007/s10484-015-9279-8

Kamath, A., Urval, R. P., & Shenoy, A. K. (2017). Effect of Alternate Nostril Breathing Exercise on Experimentally Induced Anxiety in Healthy Volunteers Using the Simulated Public Speaking Model: A Randomized Controlled Pilot Study. *BioMed Research International*, *2017*. https://doi.org/10.1155/2017/2450670

Kim, S., Wollburg, E., & Roth, W. T. (2012). Opposing Breathing Therapies for Panic Disorder: A Randomized Controlled Trial of Lowering vs Raising End-Tidal Pco_2. *The Journal of Clinical Psychiatry*, *73*(07), 931–939. https://doi.org/10.4088/JCP.11m07068

Laborde, S., Allen, M. S., Borges, U., Dosseville, F., Hosang, T. J., Iskra, M., Mosley, E., Salvotti, C., Spolverato, L., Zammit, N., & Javelle, F. (2022a). Effects of voluntary slow breathing on heart rate and heart rate variability: A systematic review and a meta-analysis. *Neuroscience & Biobehavioral Reviews*, *138*, 104711. https://doi.org/10.1016/j.neubiorev.2022.104711

Laborde, S., Allen, M. S., Borges, U., Iskra, M., Zammit, N., You, M., Hosang, T., Mosley, E., & Dosseville, F. (2022b). Psychophysiological effects of slow-paced breathing at six cycles per minute with or without heart rate variability biofeedback. *Psychophysiology*, *59*(1), e13952. https://doi.org/10.1111/psyp.13952

Landman, G. W. D., Drion, I., van Hateren, K. J. J., van Dijk, P. R., Logtenberg, S. J. J., Lambert, J., Groenier, K. H., Bilo, H. J. G., & Kleefstra, N. (2013). Device-Guided Breathing as Treatment for Hypertension in Type 2 Diabetes Mellitus: A Randomized, Double-blind, Sham-Controlled Trial. *JAMA Internal Medicine*, *173*(14), 1346–1350. https://doi.org/10.1001/jamainternmed.2013.6883

Landman, G. W. D., van Hateren, K. J. J., van Dijk, P. R., Logtenberg, S. J. J., Houweling, S. T., Groenier, K. H., Bilo, H. J. G., & Kleefstra, N. (2014). Efficacy of Device-Guided Breathing for Hypertension in Blinded, Randomized, Active-Controlled Trials: A Meta-analysis of Individual Patient Data. *JAMA Internal Medicine*, *174*(11), 1815–1821. https://doi.org/10.1001/jamainternmed.2014.4336

Laudenslager, M. L., Simoneau, T. L., Kilbourn, K., Natvig, C., Philips, S., Spradley, J., Benitez, P., McSweeney, P., & Mikulich-Gilbertson, S. K. (2015). A randomized control trial of a psychosocial intervention for caregivers of allogeneic hematopoietic stem cell transplant patients: Effects on distress. *Bone Marrow Transplantation*, *50*(8), Article 8. https://doi.org/10.1038/bmt.2015.104

Lehrer, P., Kaur, K., Sharma, A., Shah, K., Huseby, R., Bhavsar, J., & Zhang, Y. (2020). Heart Rate Variability Biofeedback Improves Emotional and Physical Health and Performance: A Systematic Review and Meta Analysis. *Applied Psychophysiology and Biofeedback*. https://doi.org/10.1007/s10484-020-09466-z

Lehrer, P. M., Vaschillo, E., Vaschillo, B., Lu, S.-E., Eckberg, D. L., Edelberg, R., Shih, W. J., Lin, Y., Kuusela, T. A., Tahvanainen, K. U. O., & Hamer, R. M. (2003). Heart Rate Variability Biofeedback Increases Baroreflex Gain and Peak Expiratory Flow: *Psychosomatic Medicine*, *65*(5), 796–805. https://doi.org/10.1097/01.PSY.0000089200.81962.19

Lin, I. M., Tai, L. Y., & Fan, S. Y. (2014). Breathing at a rate of 5.5breaths per minute with equal inhalation-to-exhalation ratio increases heart rate variability. *International Journal of Psychophysiology*, *91*(3), 206–211. https://doi.org/10.1016/j.ijpsycho.2013.12.006

Mahendru, K., Pandit, A., Singh, V., Choudhary, N., Mohan, A., & Bhatnagar, S. (2021). Effect of Meditation and Breathing Exercises on the Well-being of Patients with SARS-CoV-2 Infection under Institutional Isolation: A Randomized Control Trial. *Indian Journal of Palliative Care*, *27*(4), 490–494. https://doi.org/10.25259/IJPC_40_21

Mahtani, K. R., Beinortas, T., Bauza, K., & Nunan, D. (2016). Device-Guided Breathing for Hypertension: A Summary Evidence Review. *Current Hypertension Reports*, *18*(4), 33. https://doi.org/10.1007/s11906-016-0631-z

Meuret, A. E., & Ritz, T. (2010). Hyperventilation in panic disorder and asthma: Empirical evidence and clinical strategies. *International Journal of Psychophysiology*, *78*(1), 68–79. https://doi.org/10.1016/j.ijpsycho.2010.05.006

Meuret, A. E., Rosenfield, D., Seidel, A., Bhaskara, L., & Hofmann, S. G. (2010). Respiratory and Cognitive Mediators of Treatment Change in Panic Disorder: Evidence for Intervention Specificity. *Journal of Consulting and Clinical Psychology*, *78*(5), 691–704. https://doi.org/10.1037/a0019552

Meuret, A. E., Wilhelm, F. H., Ritz, T., & Roth, W. T. (2003). Breathing Training for Treating Panic Disorder: Useful Intervention or Impediment? *Behavior Modification*, *27*(5), 731–754. https://doi.org/10.1177/0145445503256324

Meuret, A. E., Wilhelm, F. H., Ritz, T., & Roth, W. T. (2008). Feedback of end-tidal pCO2 as a therapeutic approach for panic disorder. *Journal of Psychiatric Research*, *42*(7), 560–568. https://doi.org/10.1016/j.jpsychires.2007.06.005

Meuret, A. E., Wilhelm, F. H., & Roth, W. T. (2001). Respiratory Biofeedback-Assisted Therapy in Panic Disorder. *Behavior Modification*, *25*(4), 584–605. https://doi.org/10.1177/0145445501254006

Mutch, W. A. C., Buchman, T. G., Girling, L. G. Bs. (Hons), Walker, E. K.-Y., McManus, B. M., & Graham, M. R. M. (2007). Biologically variable ventilation improves gas exchange and respiratory mechanics in a model of severe bronchospasm. *Critical Care Medicine*, *35*(7), 1749–1755. https://doi.org/10.1097/01.CCM.0000269039.61615.A1

Mutch, W. A. C., Harms, S., Ruth Graham, M., Kowalski, S. E., Girling, L. G., & Lefevre, G. R. (2000). Biologically Variable or Naturally Noisy Mechanical Ventilation Recruits Atelectatic Lung. *American Journal of Respiratory and Critical Care Medicine*, *162*(1), 319–323. https://doi.org/10.1164/ajrccm.162.1.9903120

Newman Van Denburg, A. (2020). *A Controlled Breathing Intervention for Women Undergoing MRI-Guided Breast Biopsy: A Randomized Controlled Trial.* https://dukespace.lib.duke.edu/dspace/handle/10161/21478

Novaes, M. M., Palhano-Fontes, F., Onias, H., Andrade, K. C., Lobão-Soares, B., Arruda-Sanchez, T., Kozasa, E. H., Santaella, D. F., & de Araujo, D. B. (2020). Effects of Yoga Respiratory Practice (Bhastrika pranayama) on Anxiety, Affect, and Brain Functional Connectivity and Activity: A Randomized Controlled Trial. *Frontiers in Psychiatry*, *11*. https://www.frontiersin.org/articles/10.3389/fpsyt.2020.00467

Ritz, T., Rosenfield, D., Steele, A. M., Millard, M. W., & Meuret, A. E. (2014). Controlling Asthma by Training of Capnometry-Assisted Hypoventilation (CATCH) vs Slow Breathing: A Randomized Controlled Trial. *Chest*, *146*(5), 1237–1247. https://doi.org/10.1378/chest.14-0665

Rosenberg, A., & Hamiel, D. (2021). Reducing Test Anxiety and Related Symptoms Using a Biofeedback Respiratory Practice Device: A Randomized Control Trial. *Applied Psychophysiology and Biofeedback*, *46*(1), 69–82. https://doi.org/10.1007/s10484-020-09494-9

Russo, M. A., Santarelli, D. M., & O'Rourke, D. (2017). The physiological effects of slow breathing in the healthy human. *Breathe*, *13*(4), 298–309. https://doi.org/10.1183/20734735.009817

Shehab, A. A. S. (2021). *A Randomized Controlled Trial of Psychological Outcomes of Mobile Guided Resonant Frequency Breathing in Young Adults with Elevated Stress During the COVID-19 Pandemic.*

Srimookda, N., Saensom, D., Mitsungnern, T., Kotruchin, P., & Ruaisungnoen, W. (2021). The effects of breathing training on dyspnea and anxiety among patients with acute heart failure at emergency department. *International Emergency Nursing*, *56*, 101008. https://doi.org/10.1016/j.ienj.2021.101008

Subramanian, R. K., P.R, D., & P., S. (2016). Alternate Nostril Breathing at Different Rates and its Influence on Heart Rate Variability in Non Practitioners of Yoga. *Journal of Clinical and Diagnostic Research : JCDR, 10*(1), CM01–CM02. https://doi.org/10.7860/JCDR/2016/15287.7094

Sureka, P., Govil, S., Dash, D., Dash, C., Kumar, M., & Singhal, V. (2014). Effect of Sudarshan Kriya on male prisoners with non psychotic psychiatric disorders: A randomized control trial. *Asian Journal of Psychiatry, 12*, 43–49. https://doi.org/10.1016/j.ajp.2014.06.010

Szulczewski, M. T. (2019). An Anti-hyperventilation Instruction Decreases the Drop in End-tidal CO2 and Symptoms of Hyperventilation During Breathing at 0.1 Hz. *Applied Psychophysiology and Biofeedback, 44*(3), 247–256. https://doi.org/10.1007/s10484-019-09438-y

Szulczewski, M. T., & Rynkiewicz, A. (2018). The effects of breathing at a frequency of 0.1 Hz on affective state, the cardiovascular system, and adequacy of ventilation. *Psychophysiology, 55*(12), e13221. https://doi.org/10.1111/psyp.13221

Teigen, K. H. (2008). Is a sigh "just a sigh"? Sighs as emotional signals and responses to a difficult task. *Scandinavian Journal of Psychology, 49*(1), 49–57. https://doi.org/10.1111/j.1467-9450.2007.00599.x

Telles, S., Sharma, S. K., & Balkrishna, A. (2014). Blood Pressure and Heart Rate Variability during Yoga-Based Alternate Nostril Breathing Practice and Breath Awareness. *Medical Science Monitor Basic Research, 20*, 184–193. https://doi.org/10.12659/MSMBR.892063

Teng, H.-C., Yeh, M.-L., & Wang, M.-H. (2018). Walking with controlled breathing improves exercise tolerance, anxiety, and quality of life in heart failure patients: A randomized controlled trial. *European Journal of Cardiovascular Nursing, 17*(8), 717–727. https://doi.org/10.1177/1474515118778453

Thayer, J. F., Hansen, A. L., Saus-Rose, E., & Johnsen, B. H. (2009). Heart Rate Variability, Prefrontal Neural Function, and Cognitive Performance: The Neurovisceral Integration Perspective on Self-regulation, Adaptation, and Health. *Annals of Behavioral Medicine, 37*(2), 141–153. https://doi.org/10.1007/s12160-009-9101-z

Thomas, M., McKinley, R. K., Freeman, E., Foy, C., Prodger, P., & Price, D. (2003). Breathing retraining for dysfunctional breathing in asthma: A randomised controlled trial. *Thorax, 58*(2), 110–115. https://doi.org/10.1136/thorax.58.2.110

Valenza, M. C., Valenza-Peña, G., Torres-Sánchez, I., González-Jiménez, E., Conde-Valero, A., & Valenza-Demet, G. (2014). Effectiveness of controlled breathing techniques on anxiety and depression in hospitalized patients with COPD: A randomized clinical Trial. *Respiratory Care, 59*(2), 209–215. https://doi.org/10.4187/respcare.02565

Van Diest, I., Verstappen, K., Aubert, A. E., Widjaja, D., Vansteenwegen, D., & Vlemincx, E. (2014). Inhalation/Exhalation Ratio Modulates the Effect of Slow Breathing on Heart Rate Variability and Relaxation. *Applied Psychophysiology and Biofeedback, 39*(3–4), 171–180. https://doi.org/10.1007/s10484-014-9253-x

Vaschillo, E. G., Vaschillo, B., & Lehrer, P. M. (2006). Characteristics of resonance in heart rate variability stimulated by biofeedback. *Applied Psychophysiology and Biofeedback, 31*(2), 129–142. https://doi.org/10.1007/s10484-006-9009-3

Vaschillo, E., Vaschillo, B., & Lehrer, P. (2004). Heartbeat synchronizes with respiratory rhythm only under specific circumstances. *Chest, 126*(4), 1385–1386; author reply 1386-1387. https://doi.org/10.1378/chest.126.4.1385-a

Vlemincx, E. (2023). *Breathing-induced relaxation: A direct comparison between slow breathing and mindful breathing*. Emotions 2023.

Vlemincx, E., Abelson, J. L., Lehrer, P. M., Davenport, P. W., Van Diest, I., & Van den Bergh, O. (2013). Respiratory variability and sighing: A psychophysiological reset model. *Biological Psychology, 93*(1), 24–32. https://doi.org/10.1016/j.biopsycho.2012.12.001

Vlemincx, E., Meulders, M., & Abelson, J. L. (2017). Sigh rate during emotional transitions: More evidence for a sigh of relief. *Biological Psychology, 125*, 163–172. https://doi.org/10.1016/j.biopsycho.2017.03.005

Vlemincx, E., Nasir, S. M., & Du Rietz Burke, E. (2019). *The relaxation effects of slow breathing beyond breathing awareness*. 26th Annual Meeting of the International Society for the Advancement of Respiratory Psychophysiology (ISARP).

Vlemincx, E., Severs, L., & Ramirez, J.-M. (2022). The psychophysiology of the sigh: II: The sigh from the psychological perspective. *Biological Psychology*, *173*, 108386. https://doi.org/10.1016/j.biopsycho.2022.108386

Vlemincx, E., Taelman, J., Van Diest, I., & Van den Bergh, O. (2010). Take a deep breath: The relief effect of spontaneous and instructed sighs. *Physiology & Behavior*, *101*(1), 67–73. https://doi.org/10.1016/j.physbeh.2010.04.015

Vlemincx, E., Van Diest, I., & Van den Bergh, O. (2012a). A sigh following sustained attention and mental stress: Effects on respiratory variability. *Physiology & Behavior*, *107*(1), 1–6. https://doi.org/10.1016/j.physbeh.2012.05.013

Vlemincx, E., Van Diest, I., & Van Den Bergh, O. (2012b). Imposing Respiratory Variability Patterns. *Applied Psychophysiology and Biofeedback*, *37*(3), 153–160. https://doi.org/10.1007/s10484-012-9187-0

Vlemincx, E., Van Diest, I., & Van den Bergh, O. (2016). A sigh of relief or a sigh to relieve: The psychological and physiological relief effect of deep breaths. *Physiology & Behavior*, *165*, 127–135. https://doi.org/10.1016/j.physbeh.2016.07.004

Wollburg, E., Roth, W. T., & Kim, S. (2011). Effects of Breathing Training on Voluntary Hypo- and Hyperventilation in Patients with Panic Disorder and Episodic Anxiety. *Applied Psychophysiology and Biofeedback*, *36*(2), 81–91. https://doi.org/10.1007/s10484-011-9150-5

Wysocki, M., Cracco, C., Teixeira, A. M., Mercat, A., Diehl, J.-L., Lefort, Y., Derenne, J.-P., & Similowski, T. (2006). Reduced breathing variability as a predictor of unsuccessful patient separation from mechanical ventilation. *Critical Care Medicine*, *34*(8), 2076–2083. https://doi.org/10.1097/01.CCM.0000227175.83575.E9

Zaccaro, A., Piarulli, A., Laurino, M., Garbella, E., Menicucci, D., Neri, B., & Gemignani, A. (2018). How Breath-Control Can Change Your Life: A Systematic Review on Psycho-Physiological Correlates of Slow Breathing. *Frontiers in Human Neuroscience*, *12*. https://doi.org/10.3389/fnhum.2018.00353

Pharmacological Treatment of Anxiety Disorders: Current and Novel Targets

Andreas Chatzittofis

Introduction

Normal-adaptive anxiety has the purpose to alert and prepare the individual as a response to a potential threat. However, anxiety becomes pathological and maladaptive if it is permanent with limited control of the individual resulting in negative consequences in the function during daily activities. Anxiety responses include emotional, physical cognitive, and behavioral symptoms to the potential danger/threat.

On the other hand, fear is the instinctual emotional response to an imminent threat with high evolutionary value but also related to anxiety disorders especially when chronic, disproportional, and affecting normal functioning (Penninx et al. 2021).

The current classification of anxiety disorders, according to the *Diagnostic and Statistical Manual of Mental Disorders Fifth Edition (DSM-5)* and the latest edition of the International Statistical Classification of Diseases and Related Health Problems (ICD-11), includes panic disorder with or without agoraphobia (PD), phobias, social anxiety disorder (SAD), and generalized anxiety disorder (GAD) (*Diagnostic and Statistical Manual of Mental Disorders: DSM-5* 2013; WHO 2019). However, post-traumatic stress disorder (PTSD) and obsessive-compulsive disorder (OCD) are now listed in a different category after the revision of the two classification systems. Considering that the treatment of these disorders has long followed the treatment of anxiety disorders and anxiety symptoms are also core symptoms of OCD and PTSD with some overlapping neurobiology, we include in this chapter the pharmacological treatment of OCD and PTSD as well.

A. Chatzittofis (✉)
Medical School, University of Cyprus, Nicosia, Cyprus
e-mail: chatzittofis.andreas@ucy.ac.cy

C. Charis, G. Panayiotou (eds.), *Anxiety Disorders and Related Conditions*,
https://doi.org/10.1007/978-3-031-56798-8_5

Anxiety disorders are the most prevalent psychiatric disorders, with estimated life prevalence up to 30% and women being more frequently affected compared to men (Penninx et al. 2021). Specific phobias are the most prevalent among anxiety disorders, followed by panic disorder, social phobia, and generalized anxiety disorder. Anxiety disorders are highly comorbid with other psychiatric disorders, mainly depression but also substance use disorders. The high comorbidity increases the burden of disease and treatment resistance requiring increasing resources.

In addition, anxiety disorders are undertreated with estimates that around 20% of individuals with anxiety disorders seeking professional help and of those about 50% received medication (Alonso and Lépine 2007). The underrecognition and undertreatment of anxiety disorders are higher in low-income countries with less healthcare resources (Alonso et al. 2018).

Clinical Significance and Anxiety Symptoms

As a full description of the phenomenology of anxiety disorders and differential diagnosis is beyond the scope of this chapter, we will only mention some important elements of the clinical representation of anxiety disorders.

Although categorical diagnostic criteria in the form of symptoms are clinically relevant and required to set a diagnosis of anxiety disorder, the boundaries between normal reactions and pathological can sometimes be indistinct. Characteristics of the disorder are duration, persistence, and importantly degree of functional impairment and crucial element of the clinical judgment. For example, a specific phobia for snakes might cause minimal to none impairment in a rural environment, whereas claustrophobia (i.e., elevators) might have an important impact on daily life.

Symptoms, especially physical presentations, are also not pathognomonic for certain anxiety disorders nor other somatic diseases; thus shortness of breath, sweating, palpitations, fatigue, and nausea can indicate not only panic attack but also problems of the heart, lungs, or other organs (Penninx et al. 2021). It is very important to identify cognitive anxiety symptoms as well as behavioral changes such as avoidance of social interaction that together might indicate different anxiety disorders, i.e., panic disorder (if, e.g., the cognitive explanation is the fear for panic attacks) or social anxiety disorder (if the cognitive explanation is the fear to be judged by others). In difficult diagnostic cases, the clinician should use validated structured or semi-structured clinical interviews and validated scales to measure the severity of symptoms and monitor treatment. Finally, as more than 50% of individuals with anxiety disorders have depressive symptoms or other comorbidities including somatic illness, a thorough examination is required to both identify and treat complicated cases (Lamers et al. 2011).

Pathophysiology

The current model of the pathophysiology and the etiology of anxiety disorders includes a genetic predisposition in the form of vulnerability for anxiety disorders evident through brain dysfunction and the influence of environmental/psychosocial factors, including exposure to childhood adversity and traumatic and stressful events through lifetime (Penninx et al. 2021).

Although no individual biomarker has been found for anxiety disorders, there is a large amount of genetical, neuroimage, neurochemical, and neurophysiological data regarding anxiety disorders (Bandelow et al. 2016, 2017). Heritability of anxiety disorders ranges from 30 to 50% making family history very important. Although specific genes have been suggested to be implicated such as TMEM132D, HTR2A, NPSR1, and MAOA, genome-wide association studies are still inconclusive and show a genetic overlap between most mental disorders (Bandelow et al. 2016). Likewise, epigenetic studies are at its infancy in anxiety disorders, and at the moment no genetic nor epigenetic application can be used in clinical praxis. In contrast, there is a lot of research in basic neuroscience showing that attention, memory, learning, and emotion are involved in the development of anxiety disorders. Especially processes of learning include conditioning, extinction, and memory reconsolidation (Duits et al. 2015; Monfils and Holmes 2018).

Additionally, regarding neuroimaging, there has been both structural and functional studies on decision-making, threat responding, attention bias, and acute and prolonged stress responses (Bandelow et al. 2016). The implication of the peripheral, neurophysiologic, hormonal, and autonomic system response has been evaluated. Although some biomarkers such as error-related negativity seem promising, there is still lack of validated useful biomarkers (Bandelow et al. 2017).

Anxiety disorders are proposed to have developmental origins, starting with vulnerability in childhood and adolescence (Kalin 2017; Pine and Fox 2015). Temperament traits such as heightened emotional sensitivity, defensive responding to threat exposure, and behavioral inhibition, (i.e., reduced movement and vocalization in the presence of novelty) are considered anxiety risk markers. These, in combination with environmental factors such as stressful life events, childhood adversity, and overprotective parenting minimizing children's opportunities to adapt to environmental stressors contribute to the development of anxiety disorders.

Prevention and Treatment of Anxiety Disorders

Regarding prevention, most studies conducted included psychoeducation or a combination of cognitive behavioral therapy (CBT) with minimal results (Moreno-Peral et al. 2017). The question of the efficacy of specific intervention, population targets, cost-effectiveness, and potential long-lasting effects remains to be answered.

Aside from pharmacotherapy, different types of psychotherapy, mainly cognitive behavioral therapy (CBT), have been shown to be effective for the treatment of anxiety disorders and are considered first-line treatment (Bandelow et al. 2015). These short-term psychotherapies usually involve exposure to the feared stimuli, stopping of avoidance behavior, and cognitive restructuring. Newer delivery forms of psychotherapy include telephone, Internet, and use of virtual reality.

In addition, in a recent meta-analysis of randomized controlled trials, pharmacotherapy was shown to have higher effect size than psychotherapies with patients receiving psychotherapy reporting less severe anxiety symptoms compared to those receiving pharmacotherapy (Bandelow et al. 2015). In this chapter we will focus on established pharmacotherapy as well as novel approaches and promising compounds for further evaluation of their effectiveness.

Pharmacotherapy

General Treatment Principles and Recommendations

The treatment approach should include psychotherapy, pharmacotherapy, and other interventions which should be selected after consideration of individual characteristics such as psychiatric history, previous applied treatments, symptom severity, comorbidities, availability and cost of treatment methods, and the patient's preference. For some disorders such as specific phobia, separation anxiety disorder, and selective mutism, there is scarce evidence for pharmacological treatments. For specific phobias exposure therapy can be applied. In general, pharmacotherapy is considered a first-line treatment for anxiety disorders, and the recommendations in this chapter are based on treatment guidelines for anxiety disorders (Baldwin et al. 2014; Bandelow et al. 2012). A full review on novel pharmacological targets is already published (Sartori and Singewald 2019).

There are several factors, such as non-response to psychotherapy, chronic courses or complex conditions, and depression comorbidity, which might prioritize treatment with medication. *Initial disease severity* moderates the effect of the drug with a better effect in more severe disorders. These have been shown for both size panic disorder and generalized anxiety disorder (de Vries et al. 2018).

Patient education about their symptoms, treatment alternatives, and expected treatment outcome is required by the treating physician. Especially, information regarding contraindications, possible adverse effects, interactions, and safety warnings has to be given in a patient-friendly way to ensure understanding and informed consent. In addition, patient preparation for early and, most importantly, transitional side effects (such as the most common for selective serotonin reuptake inhibitors (SSRIs) and selective serotonin-norepinephrine reuptake inhibitors (SNRIs)) gives the opportunity to increase adherence to the treatment plan resulting in favorable treatment response. Regarding patients with anxiety disorders, initial feelings of nervousness and anxiety symptoms with exacerbation of in panic attacks in the first weeks after starting treatment have the risk to lead to discontinuation of the medication. Medication has also an important *placebo effect* that can be manipulated in favor of the patient with simple techniques such as presenting the medication in a positive way and *managing patients' expectations* (Enck et al. 2013). Other more complex techniques such as "conditioning" can also be applied to benefit the patient (Enck et al. 2013). Although doses in the lower part of the therapeutic range of anxiety medication lead to treatment response, higher doses to the upper limit of the standard dose range are necessary for some patients.

Other considerations include the consideration of the *gender* and the *weight of the patient* as most dosing recommendations, retrieved from studies, are based on males and persons with an average weight. Pharmacokinetics should also be considered, especially when there is comorbidity with other illnesses such as severe renal or hepatic impairment requiring dosage adjustment. For example, in severe hepatic impairment, pregabalin, with renal clearance, is considered a good alternative.

Anxiety disorders are usually treated in the community except for cases with increased suicide risk and severe comorbidity, (e.g., with major depression, personality disorders, substance use disorder) where inpatient treatment is advised.

Selective Serotonin Reuptake Inhibitors (SSRIs) and Selective Serotonin-Norepinephrine Reuptake Inhibitors (SNRIs)

Selective serotonin reuptake inhibitors (SSRIs) and serotonin-noradrenaline reuptake inhibitors (SNRIs) are effective for anxiety disorders including social anxiety disorder, panic disorder, and generalized anxiety disorder (Bighelli et al. 2018; Curtiss et al. 2017; Gomez et al. 2018; Melaragno 2021). Although there are individual differences between medications, the effects seem to be class related; thus all SSRIs and SNRIs are considered effective. These medications have a positive benefit/risk ratio with the onset of their effect having a latency of 2–4 weeks, during which adverse effects may be more pronounced. Starting with a lower dose of the drug is proposed to minimize the initial side effects during the first weeks of treatment. SSRIs are considered to be more tolerable than SNRIs, but there is a large individual variability on the tolerability of these drugs (Cipriani et al. 2009). After discontinuation of the treatment with an SSRI or SNRI, discontinuation symptoms may occur, most commonly with paroxetine and venlafaxine compared to other SSRIs.

Pregabalin

Pregabalin is effective for generalized anxiety disorder, through acting at the alpha-2-delta subunit and thus blocking of voltage-gated calcium channels in GABA receptors (Baldwin et al. 2013). Onset of the effects can be earlier compared to that of SSRIs/SNRIs. Pregabalin has also shown a favorable safety profile, primarily cleared through the kidneys and not subjected to hepatic metabolism. Thus, it has no interactions with inhibitors or inducers of cytochrome P450 enzymes. However, concerns have been raised about cases of misuse.

Tricyclic Antidepressants (TCAs)

Clomipramine and imipramine are shown to be effective for anxiety disorders. The main limitations of these medications include higher frequency and intensity of side effects compared to SSRIs and SNRIs, constituting them as the second line of treatment for anxiety disorders. It is important to mention the need for slow titration as well as precautions necessary in patients with high suicide risk, as TCSs are potentially fatal after an overdose.

Other Medication Options

Buspirone is an azapirone, acting as a 5-HT1A agonist and is shown to be effective in the treatment of GAD. However, there are also some negative studies not showing its effectiveness compared to standard drugs.

Monoamine Oxidase Inhibitors (MAOI)

Moclobemide is a drug that selectively and reversibly inhibits monoamine oxidase A (MAO-A). The use of these drugs is limited due to the presence of more side effects compared to first-line treatments, more interactions with other drugs metabolized through MAO-A and even some dietary limitations.

Phenelzine inhibits MAO in an irreversible way and is most commonly used for the treatment of panic disorder and social phobia. Like moclobemide, its use is currently limited due to side effects but also serious drug and dietary interactions.

Other antidepressants have been used for anxiety disorders with positive results in some randomized controlled trials but are not licensed for the treatment of anxiety disorders, and their use remains off-label. These drugs include *agomelatine* (melatonin MT1 and MT2 receptor agonist and serotonin 5-HT2C receptor antagonist) and *mirtazapine* (a noradrenergic and specific serotonergic drug) licensed for the treatment of depression with some positive results for GAD.

A second-generation antipsychotic, *quetiapine*, has also been used off-label in lower doses than schizophrenia, for generalized anxiety disorder with an earlier onset of efficacy but has significant side effects, including weight gain and sedation. Table 1 includes the most common medication used for the treatment of anxiety disorders.

Table 1 Pharmacological treatments for anxiety disorders

Drug	Drug class	Side effects	Clinical issues for certain drugs
Fluoxetine Sertraline Fluvoxamine Citalopram Escitalopram Paroxetine	SSRI	Jitteriness, nausea, restlessness, headache, fatigue, changes in appetite, weight loss or gain, tremor, sweating, sexual dysfunction, gastrointestinal side effects	Sedation, weight gain, sexual dysfunction, withdrawal symptoms after abrupt discontinuation (paroxetine)
			QTC interval prolongation, lower maximal dose for persons over age 65 (10 mg/day escitalopram, 2 mg/day citalopram)
Venlafaxine	SNRI	Jitteriness, nausea, restlessness, headache, fatigue, changes in appetite, weight loss or gain tremor, sweating, sexual dysfunction, gastrointestinal side effects	Withdrawal symptoms after abrupt discontinuation (venlafaxine)
Duloxetine			
Clomipramine	TCA	Anticholinergic effects, somnolence, dizziness, cardiovascular side effects, weight gain, nausea, headache, sexual dysfunction	Toxic when overdose, most effective for OCD
Pregabalin	Voltage-gated calcium channel modulator	Dizziness, somnolence, dry mouth, edema, blurred vision, weight gain, constipation, euphoric mood, imbalance, increased appetite, concentration difficulties	Renal clearance, suitable when hepatic insufficiency
Moclobemide	MAOI	Restlessness, insomnia, dry mouth, headache, dizziness, gastrointestinal symptoms, nausea, blurred vision	Drug interactions, possible dietary restrictions
Buspirone	Azapirone	Dizziness, nausea, headache, nervousness excitement, insomnia	

The Role of Benzodiazepines

Benzodiazepines are anxiolytic with high acute effect in most anxiety disorders (Gomez et al. 2018). No initial side effects in the form of increased anxiety and sleep disorder, as from the SSRIs/SNRIs, are presented. Due to their favorable direct effects, benzodiazepines are frequently used for anxiety disorders and are even described as long-term treatment (Balon and Starcevic 2020).

Nevertheless, benzodiazepines, after prolonged use, have a high dependency risk, especially in patients with alcohol or substance abuse, increasing the risk further due to synergic effects. In addition, there is a high risk for relapse after discontinuation. Other cautions associated with the use of benzodiazepines include fatigue, depression of the central nervous system, impaired reflexes, dizziness, and increased reaction time. They can lead to impairment of driving skills and are related to an increased number of traffic accidents. On the long term, they also cause impairment of cognitive functions, most severely in the elderly. The elderly patients are also more prone to falls and accidents due to balance impairment. For the reasons listed above, benzodiazepines are not considered as first-line treatments for anxiety disorders although they are considered key drugs for some patients (Balon and Starcevic 2020; Bandelow 2020).

Thus, the use of benzodiazepines is suggested for a limited period of time, in patients with more severe symptoms, in inpatient settings, and when other medications cannot be used or first-line treatments are not effective or tolerated. Benzodiazepines can also be used in combination with SSRIs/SNRIs at the initial titration of the drug, waiting for the onset of efficacy or to specifically target insomnia.

Duration of Treatment

Maintenance studies for 6–18 months following response to a drug have shown that the continuation of treatment is associated with favorable effects regarding relapse prevention. Study results and expert consensus suggest a continuation of treatment for at least 12 months after achieving remission and slow tapering of the medication to minimize discontinuation symptoms.

Treatment Resistance and Augmentation Strategies

In cases of treatment resistance, the first priority is reevaluation of the patient regarding diagnosis, compliance to the prescribed treatment, evaluation of the dose, and treatment duration. Comorbidity should be considered as well as other psychosocial factors. In general, non-response to an adequate dose for at least 4 weeks should lead to change of the treatment plan. The possibility for a late response is relatively low (around 20%) (Baldwin et al. 2009). In cases of partial response, the time period can be extended to another 4 weeks considering a higher dosage.

Although there is a need for further research and more evidence on treatment resistance, some strategies are often used in clinical praxis. Firstly, the combination of medication with psychotherapy might have better results than medication only. Regarding pharmacological interventions, a switch to a different class of antidepressants (from one SSRI to another, from an SSRI to an SNRI, or vice versa, to a TCA) can be applied. In GAD, a switch to pregabalin is also an option. Additionally, a switch to a second-line drug such as MAOI (phenelzine, moclobemide) and buspirone can be applied. Finally, augmentation with a benzodiazepine, in certain cases, is also an alternative. As a last resort, off-label medication can be used considering medicolegal issues.

Novel Pharmacological Targets

There have been a lot of difficulties in the last two decades in the development of novel compounds for the treatment of anxiety disorders. This was mainly due to lack of interest from pharmaceutical companies. However, there is a great expansion of knowledge regarding neurobiological mechanisms in anxiety disorders. Although the serotonergic system is a possible drug target, as evident from the established drugs for anxiety disorders, no new serotonergic drug was developed possibly due to the existence of cheap alternatives. In addition, the mechanisms of 5-HT that are related to anxiolytic actions are still unclear. Although there is a high diversity of 5-HT receptors, it is proposed that agonists of 5-HT2B and antagonists of 5-HT2A and 5-HT3 have anxiolytic effects. Other receptors such as 5-HT1A, 5-HT1B, 5-HT2C, 5-HT4, 5-HT6, and 5-HT7 have mixed results dependent of brain localization (Żmudzka et al. 2018). Likewise, different 5-HT receptors have a different contribution to the presence of side effects of SSRIs. Thus, strategies such as having partial agonists or selectively targeting specific receptors can be applied. Examples of medication already licensed for other indications include vilazodone, brexpiprazole, vortioxetine, agomelatine, and cyclobenzaprine.

γ-Aminobutyric Acid (GABA)

GABA is the main inhibitory neurotransmitter in the brain, and drugs acting at the γ-aminobutyric acid (GABA) binding site and reinforcing the effects of GABA hold a promise for the treatment of anxiety disorders. The aim is to target the GABA receptor without the effects of benzodiazepines, such as sedation and potential misuse. Examples of such medication include flavonoids, found in plants and fungi with the example of methoxyflavanone, and drugs targeting the translocator protein

(18 kDa), (Akbar et al. 2017; Wang et al. 2017). Neurosteroids bind to the α-intrasubunit, the β-intrasubunit, and the βα-intersubunit sites of the GABA-A receptors different than those bound by BDZs. Examples of compounds acting as neurosteroids or increasing neurosteroid levels include etifoxine already approved in some countries, as well as pregnenolone and fasedienol.

Glutamatergic Drugs

Glutamate is the major excitatory neurotransmitter in the brain. The suppression of the glutamate hyperexcitability was proposed to lead to anxiolytic effects. Although prospective glutamatergic drugs had severe side effects, recent drugs acting on metabotropic glutamate (mGlu) receptors exhibit anxiolytic effects (Ferraguti 2018).

Ketamine is an NMDA receptor antagonist by binding inside the open channel of the receptor resulting in brain-derived neurotrophic factor (BDNF) signaling. Most studied in depression with fast antidepressive effects, ketamine has shown promising results in the treatment of generalized anxiety disorder and social anxiety disorder in some recent studies (Glue et al. 2020). Questions remain to be answered regarding efficacy, safety, and durability of ketamine administration in anxiety disorders. Another example of a NMDA receptor antagonist is xenon gas currently under investigation. Riluzole and troriluzole act as voltage-sensitive sodium channel blockers, and by blocking NMDA receptors, they reduce glutamatergic neurotransmission. In addition, they stimulate the synthesis of neurotrophic factors and even affect GABA-A receptors. These are tested in treatment-refractory OCD and other anxiety disorders (Pittenger et al. 2015).

Endocannabinoid System

The endocannabinoid system modulates fear and anxiety with enhancing signaling and thus reducing stress and anxiety responses (Patel et al. 2017). Cannabis has long been used for recreational and medical reasons and is constituted by Δ9-tetrahydrocannabinol (THC) and cannabidiol (CBD) with THC mainly responsible for the psychotropic actions, while cannabidiol modulates the activity in anxiety-relevant brain areas. There are only a few studies investigating the effects of cannabinoids in patients with anxiety disorders, with Cannabidiol reducing anxiety (Bergamaschi et al. 2011). Other examples of compounds acting on the endocannabinoid system include nabilone (a synthetic CB1 and CB2 receptor agonist and THC analogue) tested in combination with other medications and psychotherapy for PTSD. Furthermore, different THC:CBD ratios are also under investigation (Kamal et al. 2018).

Drugs blocking the degrading enzymes of endogenous ligands (anandamide and 2-arachidonoylglycerol to the endocannabinoid system such as hydrolase fatty acid amide hydrolyze (FAAH) cause increased endocannabinoid signaling reducing anxiety. Thus, FAAH inhibitors are also proposed as possible treatments (Patel et al. 2017).

Neuropeptides

Neuropeptide S (NPS), neuropeptide Y (NPY), and oxytocin (OXT) have anxiety-reducing effects and are possible candidates for the treatment of anxiety disorders (Kupcova et al. 2022). Alternatively, blocking of molecules with anxiogenic effects such as corticotropin-releasing hormone (CRH), vasopressin, substance P, and cholecystokinin can lead to reduced anxiety. Molecules targeting vasopressin and oxytocin receptors are already tested. Likewise, drugs targeting the orexin system such as the orexin receptor antagonist suvorexant, prescribed for insomnia, are already tested for anxiety disorders. Unfortunately, CRHR1 receptor antagonists have not proven effective for anxiety disorders, although there were very promising results in rodents.

Natural Molecules

Different natural compounds are being studied such as extracts from *Piper methysticum* (kava), *Ginkgo biloba*, *Matricaria chamomilla*, and *Valeriana officinalis*. Even randomized clinical trials have been conducted with kava that has multiple actions such as positive allosteric modulation of GABA-A receptors and inhibition of voltage-gated sodium and calcium channels. Still, there is insufficient evidence to support its use in clinical praxis (Ooi et al. 2018).

Pharmacological Augmentation of Psychotherapy

Pharmacological strategies are proposed to enhance the effect of psychotherapy. The rational of these strategies is to facilitate the fear extinction. This can be done through manipulation of memory reconsolidation and fear extinction.

D-Cycloserine (partial NMDA receptor agonist) has been tested to facilitate fear extinction in patients with acrophobia and other anxiety disorders, with positive results (Hofmann et al. 2015). Likewise, MDMA (3,4-methylenedioxymetampheta mine, ecstasy) acts not only on monoamines, mainly serotonin, but also on other systems such as OXT, vasopressin, and cortisol. It has effects on the reconsolidation of fear memories, increasing tolerability of exposure therapy, and been studied as adjunct to psychotherapy for PTSD with positive preliminary results (Feduccia and Mithoefer 2018). Interestingly, ketamine, already mentioned previously, is proposed to interference with fear-memory reconsolidation in PTSD (Veen et al. 2018). *Oxytocin* can also be combined with psychotherapy, and it was reported to facilitate the extinction of conditioned fear with positive preliminary results in patients with PTSD (Flanagan et al. 2018). Other drugs targeting fear-memory (re) consolidation include propranolol (β-adrenoceptor blocker), doxazosin (α1-adrenoceptor blocker), mifepristone (glucocorticoid receptor antagonist), and rapamycin (mTOR inhibitor) that are tested in PTSD.

Finally, serotonergic psychedelics such as lysergic acid diethylamide (*LSD*) and *psilocybin* have long been used as adjunct to psychotherapy causing an altered state consciousness (Johnson et al. 2019). Research in these drugs has regained interest after a long period of restrictions in their use due to legislations, and clinical trials are now conducted.

Conclusions

Anxiety disorders are the most prevalent mental disorders, and psychopharmacology has a key role in the treatment. Effective treatments currently include SSRIs, SNRIs, and other licensed drugs mentioned above. However, there is a need for novel effective treatments, with fewer side effects and long-standing effects. As the knowledge on the pathophysiology of anxiety disorders is constantly expanding, novel pharmacological targets are identified helping drug development and clinical trials. Novel approaches include refined drugs targeting known systems such as monoamines, GABA, glutamate, and new targets including the endocannabinoid system and neuropeptides. Finally, new approaches with drugs interacting with psychotherapy are currently tested with promising results.

References

Akbar, S., Subhan, F., Karim, N., Aman, U., Ullah, S., Shahid, M., … Sewell, R. D. E. (2017). Characterization of 6-methoxyflavanone as a novel anxiolytic agent: A behavioral and pharmacokinetic approach. *European journal of pharmacology, 801*, 19–27. Retrieved from

Alonso, J., & Lépine, J. P. (2007). Overview of key data from the European Study of the Epidemiology of Mental Disorders (ESEMeD). *J Clin Psychiatry, 68 Suppl 2*, 3–9.

Alonso, J., Liu, Z., Evans-Lacko, S., Sadikova, E., Sampson, N., Chatterji, S., … Thornicroft, G. (2018). Treatment gap for anxiety disorders is global: Results of the World Mental Health Surveys in 21 countries. *Depress Anxiety, 35*(3), 195–208. https://doi.org/10.1002/da.22711

Baldwin, D. S., Ajel, K., Masdrakis, V. G., Nowak, M., & Rafiq, R. (2013). Pregabalin for the treatment of generalized anxiety disorder: an update. *Neuropsychiatr Dis Treat, 9*, 883–892. https://doi.org/10.2147/ndt.S36453

Baldwin, D. S., Anderson, I. M., Nutt, D. J., Allgulander, C., Bandelow, B., den Boer, J. A., … Wittchen, H. U. (2014). Evidence-based pharmacological treatment of anxiety disorders, post-traumatic stress disorder and obsessive-compulsive disorder: a revision of the 2005 guidelines from the British Association for Psychopharmacology. *J Psychopharmacol, 28*(5), 403–439. https://doi.org/10.1177/0269881114525674

Baldwin, D. S., Stein, D. J., Dolberg, O. T., & Bandelow, B. (2009). How long should a trial of escitalopram treatment be in patients with major depressive disorder, generalised anxiety disorder or social anxiety disorder? An exploration of the randomised controlled trial database. *Hum Psychopharmacol, 24*(4), 269–275. https://doi.org/10.1002/hup.1019

Balon, R., & Starcevic, V. (2020). Role of Benzodiazepines in Anxiety Disorders. In Y.-K. Kim (Ed.), *Anxiety Disorders: Rethinking and Understanding Recent Discoveries* (pp. 367–388). Singapore: Springer Singapore.

Bandelow, B. (2020). Current and Novel Psychopharmacological Drugs for Anxiety Disorders. In Y.-K. Kim (Ed.), *Anxiety Disorders: Rethinking and Understanding Recent Discoveries* (pp. 347–365). Singapore: Springer Singapore.

Bandelow, B., Baldwin, D., Abelli, M., Altamura, C., Dell'Osso, B., Domschke, K., … Riederer, P. (2016). Biological markers for anxiety disorders, OCD and PTSD – a consensus statement. Part I: Neuroimaging and genetics. *World J Biol Psychiatry, 17*(5), 321–365. https://doi.org/10.1080/15622975.2016.1181783

Bandelow, B., Baldwin, D., Abelli, M., Bolea-Alamanac, B., Bourin, M., Chamberlain, S. R., … Riederer, P. (2017). Biological markers for anxiety disorders, OCD and PTSD: A consensus statement. Part II: Neurochemistry, neurophysiology and neurocognition. *World J Biol Psychiatry, 18*(3), 162–214. https://doi.org/10.1080/15622975.2016.1190867

Bandelow, B., Reitt, M., Röver, C., Michaelis, S., Görlich, Y., & Wedekind, D. (2015). Efficacy of treatments for anxiety disorders: a meta-analysis. *Int Clin Psychopharmacol, 30*(4), 183–192. https://doi.org/10.1097/yic.0000000000000078

Bandelow, B., Sher, L., Bunevicius, R., Hollander, E., Kasper, S., Zohar, J., & Möller, H. J. (2012). Guidelines for the pharmacological treatment of anxiety disorders, obsessive-compulsive disorder and posttraumatic stress disorder in primary care. *Int J Psychiatry Clin Pract, 16*(2), 77–84. https://doi.org/10.3109/13651501.2012.667114

Bergamaschi, M. M., Queiroz, R. H. C., Chagas, M. H. N., de Oliveira, D. C. G., De Martinis, B. S., Kapczinski, F., … Crippa, J. A. S. (2011). Cannabidiol Reduces the Anxiety Induced by Simulated Public Speaking in Treatment-Naïve Social Phobia Patients. *Neuropsychopharmacology, 36*(6), 1219–1226. https://doi.org/10.1038/npp.2011.6

Bighelli, I., Castellazzi, M., Cipriani, A., Girlanda, F., Guaiana, G., Koesters, M., … Barbui, C. (2018). Antidepressants versus placebo for panic disorder in adults. *Cochrane Database Syst Rev, 4*(4), Cd010676. https://doi.org/10.1002/14651858.CD010676.pub2

Cipriani, A., Furukawa, T. A., Salanti, G., Geddes, J. R., Higgins, J. P., Churchill, R., … Barbui, C. (2009). Comparative efficacy and acceptability of 12 new-generation antidepressants: a multiple-treatments meta-analysis. *Lancet, 373*(9665), 746–758. https://doi.org/10.1016/s0140-6736(09)60046-5

Curtiss, J., Andrews, L., Davis, M., Smits, J., & Hofmann, S. G. (2017). A meta-analysis of pharmacotherapy for social anxiety disorder: an examination of efficacy, moderators, and mediators. *Expert Opin Pharmacother, 18*(3), 243–251. https://doi.org/10.1080/14656566.2017.1285907

de Vries, Y. A., Roest, A. M., Burgerhof, J. G. M., & de Jonge, P. (2018). Initial severity and antidepressant efficacy for anxiety disorders, obsessive-compulsive disorder, and posttraumatic stress disorder: An individual patient data meta-analysis. *Depress Anxiety, 35*(6), 515–522. https://doi.org/10.1002/da.22737

Diagnostic and statistical manual of mental disorders*: DSM-5*. (2013). Arlington, VA: American Psychiatric Association.

Duits, P., Cath, D. C., Lissek, S., Hox, J. J., Hamm, A. O., Engelhard, I. M., … Baas, J. M. (2015). Updated meta-analysis of classical fear conditioning in the anxiety disorders. *Depress Anxiety, 32*(4), 239–253. https://doi.org/10.1002/da.22353

Enck, P., Bingel, U., Schedlowski, M., & Rief, W. (2013). The placebo response in medicine: minimize, maximize or personalize? *Nat Rev Drug Discov, 12*(3), 191–204. https://doi.org/10.1038/nrd3923

Feduccia, A. A., & Mithoefer, M. C. (2018). MDMA-assisted psychotherapy for PTSD: Are memory reconsolidation and fear extinction underlying mechanisms? *Progress in Neuro-Psychopharmacology and Biological Psychiatry, 84*, 221–228. https://doi.org/10.1016/j.pnpbp.2018.03.003

Ferraguti, F. (2018). Metabotropic glutamate receptors as targets for novel anxiolytics. *Curr Opin Pharmacol, 38*, 37–42. https://doi.org/10.1016/j.coph.2018.02.004

Flanagan, J. C., Sippel, L. M., Wahlquist, A., Moran-Santa Maria, M. M., & Back, S. E. (2018). Augmenting Prolonged Exposure therapy for PTSD with intranasal oxytocin: A randomized, placebo-controlled pilot trial. *Journal of Psychiatric Research, 98*, 64–69. https://doi.org/10.1016/j.jpsychires.2017.12.014

Glue, P., Neehoff, S., Sabadel, A., Broughton, L., Le Nedelec, M., Shadli, S., … Medlicott, N. J. (2020). Effects of ketamine in patients with treatment-refractory generalized anxiety and social anxiety disorders: Exploratory double-blind psychoactive-controlled replication study. *J Psychopharmacol, 34*(3), 267–272. https://doi.org/10.1177/0269881119874457

Gomez, A. F., Barthel, A. L., & Hofmann, S. G. (2018). Comparing the efficacy of benzodiazepines and serotonergic anti-depressants for adults with generalized anxiety disorder: a meta-analytic review. *Expert Opin Pharmacother, 19*(8), 883–894. https://doi.org/10.1080/14656566.2018.1472767

Hofmann, S. G., Otto, M. W., Pollack, M. H., & Smits, J. A. (2015). D-cycloserine augmentation of cognitive behavioral therapy for anxiety disorders: an update. *Curr Psychiatry Rep, 17*(1), 532. https://doi.org/10.1007/s11920-014-0532-2

Johnson, M. W., Hendricks, P. S., Barrett, F. S., & Griffiths, R. R. (2019). Classic psychedelics: An integrative review of epidemiology, therapeutics, mystical experience, and brain network function. *Pharmacology & Therapeutics, 197*, 83–102. https://doi.org/10.1016/j.pharmthera.2018.11.010

Kalin, N. H. (2017). Mechanisms underlying the early risk to develop anxiety and depression: A translational approach. *European Neuropsychopharmacology, 27*(6), 543–553. https://doi.org/10.1016/j.euroneuro.2017.03.004

Kamal, B. S., Kamal, F., & Lantela, D. E. (2018). Cannabis and the Anxiety of Fragmentation-A Systems Approach for Finding an Anxiolytic Cannabis Chemotype. *Front Neurosci, 12*, 730. https://doi.org/10.3389/fnins.2018.00730

Kupcova, I., Danisovic, L., Grgac, I., & Harsanyi, S. (2022). Anxiety and Depression: What Do We Know of Neuropeptides? *Behav Sci (Basel), 12*(8). https://doi.org/10.3390/bs12080262

Lamers, F., van Oppen, P., Comijs, H. C., Smit, J. H., Spinhoven, P., van Balkom, A. J., … Penninx, B. W. (2011). Comorbidity patterns of anxiety and depressive disorders in a large cohort study: the Netherlands Study of Depression and Anxiety (NESDA). *J Clin Psychiatry, 72*(3), 341–348. https://doi.org/10.4088/JCP.10m06176blu

Melaragno, A. J. (2021). Pharmacotherapy for Anxiety Disorders: From First-Line Options to Treatment Resistance. *Focus (Am Psychiatr Publ), 19*(2), 145–160. https://doi.org/10.1176/appi.focus.20200048

Monfils, M. H., & Holmes, E. A. (2018). Memory boundaries: opening a window inspired by reconsolidation to treat anxiety, trauma-related, and addiction disorders. *Lancet Psychiatry, 5*(12), 1032–1042. https://doi.org/10.1016/s2215-0366(18)30270-0

Moreno-Peral, P., Conejo-Cerón, S., Rubio-Valera, M., Fernández, A., Navas-Campaña, D., Rodríguez-Morejón, A., … Bellón, J. (2017). Effectiveness of Psychological and/or Educational Interventions in the Prevention of Anxiety: A Systematic Review, Meta-analysis, and Meta-regression. *JAMA Psychiatry, 74*(10), 1021–1029. https://doi.org/10.1001/jamapsychiatry.2017.2509

Ooi, S. L., Henderson, P., & Pak, S. C. (2018). Kava for Generalized Anxiety Disorder: A Review of Current Evidence. *J Altern Complement Med, 24*(8), 770–780. https://doi.org/10.1089/acm.2018.0001

Patel, S., Hill, M. N., Cheer, J. F., Wotjak, C. T., & Holmes, A. (2017). The endocannabinoid system as a target for novel anxiolytic drugs. *Neuroscience & Biobehavioral Reviews, 76*, 56–66. https://doi.org/10.1016/j.neubiorev.2016.12.033

Penninx, B. W., Pine, D. S., Holmes, E. A., & Reif, A. (2021). Anxiety disorders. *Lancet, 397*(10277), 914–927. https://doi.org/10.1016/s0140-6736(21)00359-7

Pine, D. S., & Fox, N. A. (2015). Childhood antecedents and risk for adult mental disorders. *Annu Rev Psychol, 66*, 459–485. https://doi.org/10.1146/annurev-psych-010814-015038

Pittenger, C., Bloch, M. H., Wasylink, S., Billingslea, E., Simpson, R., Jakubovski, E., … Coric, V. (2015). Riluzole augmentation in treatment-refractory obsessive-compulsive disorder: a pilot randomized placebo-controlled trial. *J Clin Psychiatry, 76*(8), 1075–1084. https://doi.org/10.4088/JCP.14m09123

Sartori, S. B., & Singewald, N. (2019). Novel pharmacological targets in drug development for the treatment of anxiety and anxiety-related disorders. *Pharmacology & Therapeutics, 204*, 107402. https://doi.org/10.1016/j.pharmthera.2019.107402

Veen, C., Jacobs, G., Philippens, I., & Vermetten, E. (2018). Subanesthetic Dose Ketamine in Posttraumatic Stress Disorder: A Role for Reconsolidation During Trauma-Focused Psychotherapy? In E. Vermetten, D. G. Baker, & V. B. Risbrough (Eds.), *Behavioral Neurobiology of PTSD* (pp. 137–162). Cham: Springer International Publishing.

Wang, D.-S., Han, J., Li, S., Sun, T., Guo, Y.-Y., Kang, W.-B., … Zhao, M.-G. (2017). Antidepressant-Like and Anxiolytic-Like Effects of ZBD-2, a Novel Ligand for the Translocator Protein (18 kDa). *Neuromolecular medicine, 19*(1), 57–68. https://doi.org/10.1007/s12017-016-8425-7

WHO. (2019). ICD-11: International classification of diseases (11th revision).

Żmudzka, E., Sałaciak, K., Sapa, J., & Pytka, K. (2018). Serotonin receptors in depression and anxiety: Insights from animal studies. *Life Sciences, 210*, 106–124. https://doi.org/10.1016/j.lfs.2018.08.050

Social Anxiety Disorder, Public Speaking Anxiety and Virtual Reality Exposure Therapy

Thekla Konstantinou and Georgia Panayiotou

Introduction

Social Anxiety Disorder

Social anxiety disorder (SAD) or social phobia (SP) is a common psychological condition that is characterized by fear and/or anxiety of social situations in which a person expects unfavourable judgments from others or believes that their presence would make others uncomfortable (American Psychiatric Association 2022, p. 230; Heimberg et al. 2014). The anxiety/fear people experience in social circumstances is adaptive when it occurs at moderate levels, as this increases awareness of social interactions and behaviours. From an evolutionary point of view, this enables greater social integration, maintains social desirability and prevents rejection. However, in some cases, these symptoms exceed the normative experience, causing marked distress and dysfunction in daily life, hence meeting the criteria for the SAD disorder. It is important to note that SAD also exceeds in severity and dysfunction caused by the normative personality trait of shyness (American Psychiatric Association 2022, p. 234; Cox et al. 2005).

Comparative to people without SAD, individuals meeting the criteria tend to display fewer facial expressions, avert their gaze more frequently and exhibit greater difficulties starting and maintaining conversations. This can cause difficulties in daily functioning, such as fear of conducting everyday tasks like making phone calls or meeting new people. As a result, this may lead to having fewer social encounters or to avoiding social interactions completely. The symptoms such as shaking, blushing, sweating and appearing tense, uninterested or incompetent (Stein and Stein 2008) can arise during or in the anticipation of social encounters. The symptoms can

T. Konstantinou (✉) · G. Panayiotou
Department of Psychology, University of Cyprus, Nicosia, Cyprus
e-mail: constantinou.thekla@ucy.ac.cy

C. Charis, G. Panayiotou (eds.), *Anxiety Disorders and Related Conditions*,
https://doi.org/10.1007/978-3-031-56798-8_6

be triggered by a wide range of situations including formal or informal social interactions (e.g., meeting unfamiliar people), being observed while eating, drinking and performing in front of others (e.g., giving a speech, singing, acting) (American Psychiatric Association 2022, p. 230). SAD is typically identified more frequently among women compared to men (Asher and Aderka 2018). This difference in prevalence among genders peaks in adolescence and decreases throughout adulthood (American Psychiatric Association 2022, p. 232). SAD has almost always an onset in childhood or adolescence (Beidel 1998).

A study (Jefferies and Ungar 2020) with a large sample size ($n = 6825$) assessing the prevalence of SAD in young adults (aged 16–29 years) from seven different countries around the world (Brazil, China, Indonesia, Russia, Thailand, the United States and Vietnam) found that 36% of responders fitted the threshold criteria of SAD. Eighteen percent of the participants did not identify themselves as socially anxious individuals; however, their SAD scores showed that they were meeting the SAD criteria or even exceeding the minimum requirements for a diagnosis. The lifetime prevalence of SAD seems to fluctuate depending on the cultural context. Western societies tend to score higher lifetime prevalence compared to Easter societies. For instance, in the United States, the lifetime prevalence ranges between 7% and 13% (American Psychiatric Association 2022, p. 232; Kessler et al. 2005; Kessler et al. 2012) in Canada 8.1% (MacKenzie and Fowler 2013) and in New Zealand 9.4% (Oakley Browne et al. 2006). In Europe, there is an important level of variation regarding the prevalence estimates (e.g., Italy 3.7% (Faravelli et al. 2004), Switzerland 6% (Merikangas et al. 2002), France 7.3% (Pélissolo et al. 2000) and Norway 13.7% (Kringlen et al. 2001)), but still the scores are higher than those found in Eastern societies (e.g., China 0.5%, Lee et al. 2007; Iran 0.82%, Mohammadi et al. 2006). These percentages should be interpreted with caution as different methodological variables (e.g., diagnostic criteria and threshold, assessment methods) could have influenced the differences identified among the different countries (Furmark 2002).

Evidence suggests that SAD significantly impacts functioning in various life domains (work, academic and social life; Aderka et al. 2012). SAD has a bidirectional relationship with bullying in childhood and adolescence (Acquah et al. 2016; Pabian and Vandebosch 2016), higher possibilities of premature school withdrawal (Van Ameringen et al. 2003) and general poorer academic achievement (Leigh et al. 2021). The negative effect of SAD is apparent in young adults and especially university students with effects on their overall wellbeing (Hajure and Abdu 2020), including their satisfaction with romantic relationships (Montesi et al. 2013; Sparrevohn and Rapee 2009). A significant impact is caused on work performance and job satisfaction. It has been suggested that individuals meeting the SAD criteria, compared to normative samples, have three times higher rates of unemployment, missed working hours due to issues related to social anxiety and overall reduced work performance (Wittchen et al. 2000). SAD has also been associated with an increased risk for the development of depression (Beesdo et al. 2007; Ohayon and Schatzberg 2010) and substance abuse (Sareen et al. 2006). Lastly, clinical samples with SAD rate their overall quality of life as lower compared to normative samples (Safren et al. 1996). Others have found that patients with SAD exhibit attenuated executive functioning compared to healthy controls (Fujii et al. 2013).

Public Speaking Anxiety

Public speaking anxiety (PSA) or performance anxiety is a specific SAD subtype that is identified in individuals who experience significant distress while speaking or performing (including the anticipation phase) in public (American Psychiatric Association 2022, p. 231). Some anxiety during such conditions is to be expected and of course can be an adaptive response (Crozier and Alden 2005). Most people can deal with their anticipating or on-task anxiety without any significant effect on their performance. In some cases, however, the anxiety severity can be disabling (Powell 2004). This condition is highly prevalent in community samples (Pull 2012) and can be found in various contexts in which a person is expected to perform in front of others (e.g., public speaking or performance activities like dancing, acting or playing music). Anxiety in such cases can be manifested in the form of memory problems, vocal issues (e.g., pitched or quivering voice), rapid and shallow breathing, increased muscle tension (Sharp and Drawson 1992), physical discomfort, trembling (Beatty 1988) and a desire to avoid and withdraw from speaking (Powell 2004). Additionally, cognitively, individuals with high PSA experience concerns about doing or saying something embarrassing, are afraid that their mind will go blank, are unable to continue talking, say something foolish or are concerned about their anxiety being visible (e.g., showing to others that are anxious, trembling, sweating and blushing) (Stein et al. 1996).

Typically, PSA has an onset during teenage years or young adulthood (Stein et al. 1996) and can have a long-lasting impact on peoples' lives, such as interfering with their work (e.g., limiting careers or fewer promotion opportunities), social life and education (Stein et al. 1996). The prevalence of PSA varies significantly based on differences in measurements and assessments (Ruscio et al. 2008). Speaking in public is the most reported fear in the general population (Dwyer and Davidson 2012) and has a high prevalence among university students (Marinho et al. 2019). Additionally, PSA is frequently considered one of the most common fears experienced by individuals with SAD (Ruscio et al. 2008). However, evidence supports that the PSA-only condition is a distinct subtype and qualitatively and quantitatively different (Blöte et al. 2009) than generalized SAD with a predominant fear for public speaking. Specifically, it has been suggested that individuals with PSA (without experiencing other social interaction anxieties) have greater levels of autonomic arousal (elevated heart rate) than those with SAD, before and during social anxiety-induced tasks such as speech tasks (Heimberg et al. 1990; Hughes et al. 2006; Levin et al. 1993). Beyond these differences, PSA can be considered a subtype of SAD, as the two share similarities in key dimensions such as fear of evaluation, scrutiny by others (Heimberg et al. 1990), avoidance of the feared situations and marked distress. On a severity level, SAD groups tend to experience significantly more anxiety and disruption of functioning in their lives compared to those with PSA-only symptoms (Heimberg et al. 1990).

Virtual Reality Exposure Therapy (VRET)

Cognitive-behavioural therapy (CBT) is a frequently used treatment for various anxiety disorders (including SAD and PSA; Mayo-Wilson et al. 2014; Rodebaugh et al. 2004), and it is considered efficacious and effective (e.g., Hofmann and Smits 2008; Kaczkurkin and Foa 2022; Norton and Price 2007). CBT incorporates a class of interventions that support change through cognitive and behavioural techniques (Beck et al. 2005). Typically, CBT protocols include psychoeducation, cognitive restructuring, exposure (imaginal or in vivo), progressive muscle relaxation, social skills training and video feedback (Huppert et al. 2003). Regarding SAD and PSA, CBT protocols are adapted on the premises of cognitive models, emphasizing the relationship between dysfunctional belief systems and behavioural avoidance (Beck et al. 2005; Clark and Wells 1995; Heimberg et al. 2010; Rapee and Heimberg 1997).

Exposure is considered a core element of CBT in treating anxiety disorders (Kaczkurkin and Foa 2022). Such methods can be incorporated into the traditional CBT protocols (Stein and Stein 2008; Ebrahimi et al. 2019) or can stand independently as exposure therapy. Below we describe and evaluate exposure-based techniques with an emphasis on the modern application of this method, which involves virtual reality exposure methodologies.

The exposure method involves a client entering and remaining in a feared situation, with the expectation that exposure of sufficient length will produce new learning or habituation and therefore reduce anxiety in that situation (Foa and Kozak 1986). This methodology traditionally is applied in vivo (real life), in vitro (imaginal) and, more recently, in virtual. Evidence comparing the traditional methods supports the efficacy of in vivo exposure techniques (Rodebaugh et al. 2004) and their superiority to in vitro exposures (e.g., Safir et al. 2011). However, creating safe, controlled and easily accessible real-life exposure environments can be costly and, in some cases, impossible to recreate in therapy settings (for instance, to conduct exposure therapy for an individual with PSA, one would need to gather an audience and control their reactions). In in vivo exposures, there is the risk of encountering people the individual may know, thus affecting confidentiality (Bouchard et al. 2007; Safir et al. 2011). Furthermore, in some cases, patients may be reluctant to expose themselves to the real situation as they may be causing too much distress (Repetto et al. 2013).

Virtual reality (VR) technologies can now be effectively applied in exposure therapy (virtual reality exposure therapy, VRET) to treat phobias and anxiety disorders (Parsons and Rizzo 2008; Wechsler et al. 2019). There is cumulative evidence on the efficacy of VRET specifically for treating SAD Public speaking anxiety

(PSA). Systematic reviews and meta-analyses for SAD suggest that VRET is an appropriate treatment methodology, indicating no significant differences in effect sizes between VRET and traditional methods (e.g., in vivo and imaginal) (Chesham et al. 2018; Emmelkamp et al. 2020). However, others add that in long-term follow-ups, VRET efficacy lessens compared to in vivo exposure (e.g., Horigome et al. 2020). Regarding the specific SAD subtype, PSA, the evidence is similar; it has been suggested that VRET is effective for PSA reduction (Hinojo-Lucena et al. 2020; Lim et al. 2022). When compared to in vivo exposure techniques, VRET scores are marginally inferior but still equally effective (Reeves et al. 2022). Nevertheless, VRET is considered less invasive (Hinojo-Lucena et al. 2020) and less threatening than in vivo techniques (Garcia-Palacios et al. 2007), allowing for systematic exposure in controlled environments (Kampmann et al. 2016) in which immersion can be fully managed (level of challenge and context variety), thus securing confidentiality (Craske et al. 2014).

Assessing Mechanisms of Change in Exposure Therapy: New Directions

As per the review above, an amplitude of evidence exists supporting the efficacy of exposure for treating anxiety disorders. Irrespective of the mode of delivery (in vivo, in vitro or virtual), a missing piece still exists. We are still apprehensive about why and how exposure works (Tryon 2005). A series of mechanisms have been proposed as the agents leading to effective change during exposure. Some suggest behavioural/learning processes taking place (e.g., reciprocal inhibition, Wolpe 1968, 1995; counterconditioning, Wolpe 1968; habituation, Harris 1943; extinction, Waters et al. 1972; classical conditioning coupled with fear reduction behaviours, Mowrer 1960), whereas others advocate for more active cognitive/emotional processes (e.g., through cognitive changes such as enhancement of the perceptions of self-efficacy, Bandura 1977, 1982; bio-informational model, Lang 1977; Drobes and Lang 1995; emotional processing, Foa and Kozak 1986; learning-memory principles, Tryon 2005; inhibitory learning, Craske et al. 2008). The following review provides a critical analysis of the habituation model and the most recent approach in exposure mechanisms, the inhibitory learning approach (Craske et al. 2008; Craske et al. 2014).

Habituation Model

Until today, exposure-based protocols are conducted on the premise that the client should habituate to the anxiety and/or fear during exposure while eliminating any avoidance behaviours (e.g., emotion processing theory, Foa and Kozak 1986; Foa and McNally 1996). Specifically, an individual is repeatedly exposed to the feared stimuli (e.g., public speaking) until habituation takes place. Through repeated and graduated exposures, the severity of symptoms decreases (emotion processing theory; Foa and Kozak 1986; Foa and McNally 1996), and the client recognizes the inaccurate appraisal of feared outcomes; thus new learning incompatible with the existing knowledge develops and strengthens.

According to the habituation model, in order to be optimal, exposures should (1) be able to activate the related fear structure, (2) behaviours providing negative reinforcement via anxiety reduction need to be minimized (e.g., avoidance) and (3) anxiety (typically measured via subjective reports or physiological measures) should show a reduction within and across exposure tasks (Foa and Kozak 1986). In line with this model, the primary goal during exposure is anxiety reduction. Thus, when fear elicited by a stimulus has decreased, it is supposed that habituation has taken place.

The habituation model has been empirically assessed and received mixed evidence. Some evidence supports or partially supports the habituation mechanisms. In this direction, a meta-analysis conducted by Rupp et al. (2017) assessed the correlations between the habituation principles (initial fear activation, within-session habituation and between-session habituation) and treatment outcome. The results showed that indeed habituation within and between sessions correlated with treatment outcome, however, was not the case for the initial fear activation principle. The relationship between within-session habituation and clinical improvement received less empirical support compared to the relationship between improvement and between-session habituation or reductions across exposure trials (Benito et al. 2018; Essayli et al. 2023; Harned et al. 2015; Sripada and Rauch 2015). Others found no support for any of the three suggested habituation principles in relation to exposure outcome (Baker et al. 2010; Peterman et al. 2019) or found partial relationships being associated with treatment efficacy only in the short term (Baker et al. 2010).

Through this brief description of the model and the empirical evidence provided above, several questions arise in relation to habituation and exposure efficacy: (1) Is habituation (within and between sessions) a necessary ingredient in exposure? (2) Is habituation an accurate indicator of exposure efficacy? and (3) what may be the active mechanisms during exposure that lead to change? It has been suggested that habituation should not be considered as an actual mechanism of change during exposure as others are supporting (Maples-Keller and Rauch 2020; Foa and Kozak 1986). Habituation could be identified alternatively, as a practical marker of the initial extinction learning process or even a possible moderator of the relationship between fear activation and outcome (Benito et al. 2018). Additionally, along the same line, habituation could reflect an indication of processing during exposure, which may be a sign that other mechanisms of change have taken or are taking place (Benito and Walther 2015).

Inhibition Learning

Recently, a new approach aiming to maximize the efficacy of exposure has been proposed, and it's been receiving promising empirical support. This approach, known as the 'inhibitory learning theory' (Craske et al. 2008, 2014), not only offers an explanation of why exposure is effective but also delineates a series of factors that can increase the effects of exposure. According to this approach, the attention is directed to the mechanisms of change, i.e., the new learning, instead of the cessation of the aversive emotional responding (i.e., habituation).

Based on the aforementioned model (Craske et al. 2008), the reductions in emotional reactions during exposure should not be considered as indexes of corrective learning. Instead, the focus should be directed towards the toleration of distress within a structure that enhances inhibitory learning over context and time. The above arguments are based on evidence deriving from theories such as extinction learning, principles in learning and memory (Craske et al. 2008).

Research on fear conditioning and extinction learning provide useful insights into understanding the factors underlying the development and elimination of maladaptive fear responses (Craske et al. 2018). Fear conditioning involves the pairing of a neutral stimulus (e.g., audience) with an aversive unconditioned stimulus (US, e.g., scrutiny by others causing the unconditioned response, fear or anxiety). The neutral stimulus initially elicits no emotional reaction, but after repeated pairings with the US, the neutral stimulus becomes a conditioned stimulus (CS) signalling the US onset and inducing anxiety associated with the anticipation of the aversive US. Typically, fear conditioning is considered an adaptive form of learning; it can also be a source of pathology when anxious reactivity to a CS persists in the absence of a CS/US contingency (Lissek et al. 2005).

Fear extinction principles can explain the mechanisms taking place during exposure therapy. More specifically, a conditioned stimulus (CS, e.g., audience) that was previously paired with an aversive unconditioned stimulus (US, e.g., scrutiny by others) is repeatedly presented without the US, resulting in a decline in fear responses over time. Similarly, in exposure therapy, repeatedly approaching a feared stimulus (situation, object or memory, i.e., a CS) allows clients to learn that their feared consequences (the US, e.g., scrutiny by others) are unlikely to occur, leading to a similar decline in fear (Carpenter et al. 2019).

According to inhibitory learning theory, after a successful exposure, the stimulus possesses both the original meaning (conditioned-unconditioned association) and the new inhibitory association (conditioned-no unconditioned association). Through the process of exposure (i.e., extinction learning), the memory that underlies emotions is modified, allowing new non-threatening associations to be stored. This means that even if fear decreases after exposure, the original conditioned-unconditioned association can be recovered under certain conditions (i.e., *spontaneous recovery*; renewal (Craske et al. 2014).

Craske and colleagues (Craske et al. 2008, 2012, 2014) suggest that successful and an efficacious exposure should aim at maximizing inhibitory learning through

(a) developing new, non-threat associations and (b) enhancing the accessibility and retrieval of newly learned associations. A series of strategies aiming to optimize exposure therapy have been proposed, including expectancy violation, elimination of safety signals, deepened extinction, stimulus variability, attentional focus, occasional reinforced extinction and enhancing retrieval of inhibitory learning via multiple contexts and retrieval cues (Sewart and Craske 2020; Craske et al. 2014). For the purposes of this review, the strategy of expectancy violation will be critically examined (for a full explanation, see Craske et al. 2008, 2012, 2014).

Expectancy Violation

The expectancy violation strategy suggests designing exposures that allow the violation of expectancies regarding the frequency (Gallistel and Gibbon 2000; Rescorla 1972) or intensity (Davey 1992) of aversive outcomes. This strategy derives from the premise that the mismatch between expectancy and outcome is critical for new learning (Rescorla 1972) and for the development of inhibitory expectancies that will compete with the existing threatening expectancies. Therefore, the overall aim is to create conditions during exposure in which the individual can maximally disconfirm the threat expectancy. Studies (e.g., Baker et al. 2010, in a sample of acrophobic sample) showed that one trial of 'disconfirmation' exposure each day (staying in the situation for periods of time that exceeded the point at which they believed the aversive event was expected to occur) was as effective as multiple trials of 'non-disconfirmation' exposure each day. The exposure tasks in this approach target the increase of new learning, omitting the emphasis on fear reduction or instructions such as stay in the situation until fear declines (Craske 2015). It has been noted that traditional cognitive restructuring techniques (e.g., threat overestimation or decatastrophizing) can impede the expectancy violation process during extinction. For instance, such cognitive restructuring prior exposure can reduce the threat expectancy and jeopardize the extinction learning. According to Craske (2015), cognitive restructuring exercises are reserved post-exposure, as a tool to enhance the assimilation of learning.

The challenge now is to empirically assess the effectiveness of expectancy violation strategy and of course all the other strategies proposed by the inhibition learning theory. Specifically, for expectancy violation, the evidence is still scarce and mixed. When compared to habituation methods, in some cases, expectancy violation seems to produce higher reductions in symptomatology (Salkovskis et al. 2007; Schemer et al. 2020), whereas others find that both are equally important for an effective change in exposure therapy (Elsner et al. 2022; Schyns et al. 2018). Studies assessing specifically expectancy violation strategies are very limited in number, with some so far finding no relationship with symptom change (De Kleine et al. 2017), or even challenge the possibility to apply an expectancy violation technique in virtual methodologies such as in public speaking anxiety (Scheveneels et al. 2019). However, the overall inhibition learning theory approach has been tested empirically and (e.g., OCD, Arch and Abramowitz 2015; Obesity, van den Akker et al. 2016; Anorexia nervosa, Cardi et al. 2019), and it is being supported to be used in clinical settings for various psychological disorders with promising outcomes (Abramowitz and Arch 2014; Gropalis et al. 2018; Tolin 2019).

Conclusion

Public speaking anxiety, a subtype of social anxiety disorder, is a common phenomenon among the community that affects the function of vital domains in everyday life (e.g., Stein et al. 1996). Exposure therapy in such conditions is considered the gold standard (e.g., Hinojo-Lucena et al. 2020). Evidence supports the efficacy of exposure therapy irrespective of the mode of delivery (in vivo, in vitro or virtual). Modern approaches have incorporated virtual reality technology in exposure therapy (i.e., VRET) with promising results. However, the literature review provided above showed that virtual modes of exposure are slightly inferior to in vivo techniques (e.g., Horigome et al. 2020; Reeves et al. 2022). Despite the evidence suggesting the efficacy of exposure therapy, there are still a lot of gaps in relation to the exact mechanisms underlying exposure therapy that leads to effective treatment outcomes. The current text reviewed the traditional habituation model and the more recent approach in understanding exposure mechanisms as proposed by the inhibition learning theory (Craske et al. 2008). The inhibition learning theory lies on well-established theoretical premises such as extinction theory, learning and memory. A series of strategies have been suggested and tested empirically; however, the evidence is still inconclusive necessitating more RCTs comparing these strategies with more traditional approaches (e.g., habituation). A better understanding of how exposure works and the identification of underlying mechanisms of change are critical for enhancing clinical outcomes and advancing exposure therapy methodologies.

References

Abramowitz, J. S., & Arch, J. J. (2014). Strategies for improving long-term outcomes in cognitive behavioral therapy for obsessive-compulsive disorder: Insights from learning theory. *Cognitive and Behavioral Practice*, *21*(1), 20–31. https://doi.org/10.1016/j.cbpra.2013.06.004

Acquah, E. O., Topalli, P. Z., Wilson, M. L., Junttila, N., & Niemi, P. M. (2016). Adolescent loneliness and social anxiety as predictors of bullying victimisation. *International Journal of Adolescence and Youth*, *21*(3), 320–331. https://doi.org/10.1080/02673843.2015.1083449

Aderka, I. M., Hofmann, S. G., Nickerson, A., Hermesh, H., Gilboa-Schechtman, E., & Marom, S. (2012). Functional impairment in social anxiety disorder. *Journal of anxiety disorders*, *26*(3), 393–400. https://doi.org/10.1016/j.janxdis.2012.01.003

American Psychiatric Association. (2022). Anxiety disorders. In *Diagnostic and statistical manual of mental disorders* (5th ed.). https://doi.org/10.1176/appi.books.9780890425596.dsm05

Arch, J. J., & Abramowitz, J. S. (2015). Exposure therapy for obsessive–compulsive disorder: An optimizing inhibitory learning approach. *Journal of obsessive-compulsive and Related Disorders*, *6*, 174–182. https://doi.org/10.1016/j.jocrd.2014.12.002
Asher, M., & Aderka, I. M. (2018). Gender differences in social anxiety disorder. *Journal of clinical psychology,* 74(10), 1730–1741. https://doi.org/10.1002/jclp.22624
Baker, A., Mystkowski, J., Culver, N., Yi, R., Mortazavi, A., & Craske, M. G. (2010). Does habituation matter? Emotional processing theory and exposure therapy for acrophobia. *Behaviour research and therapy*, *48*(11), 1139–1143. https://doi.org/10.1016/j.brat.2010.07.009
Bandura, A. (1977). Self-efficacy: toward a unifying theory of behavioral change. *Psychological review*, *84*(2), 191. https://doi.org/10.1037/0033-295X.84.2.191
Bandura, A. (1982). Self-efficacy mechanism in human agency. *American Psychologist, 37*(2), 122–147. https://doi.org/10.1037/0003-066X.37.2.122
Beatty, M. J. (1988). Situational and predispositional correlates of public speaking anxiety. *Communication education*, *37*(1), 28–39. https://doi.org/10.1080/03634528809378701
Beck, A. T., Emery, G., & Greenberg, R. L. (2005). *Anxiety disorders and phobias: A cognitive perspective*. Basic books. https://psycnet.apa.org/record/2006-01301-000
Beesdo, K., Bittner, A., Pine, D. S., Stein, M. B., Höfler, M., Lieb, R., & Wittchen, H. U. (2007). Incidence of social anxiety disorder and the consistent risk for secondary depression in the first three decades of life. *Archives of general psychiatry*, *64*(8), 903–912. https://doi.org/10.1001/archpsyc.64.8.903
Beidel, D. C. (1998). Social anxiety disorder: Etiology and early clinical presentation. *Journal of Clinical Psychiatry*, *59*(17), 27–32. https://www.psychiatrist.com/read-pdf/33972/
Benito, K. G., & Walther, M. (2015). Therapeutic process during exposure: Habituation model. *Journal of obsessive-compulsive and related disorders*, *6*, 147–157. https://doi.org/10.1016/j.jocrd.2015.01.006
Benito, K. G., Machan, J., Freeman, J. B., Garcia, A. M., Walther, M., Frank, H., ... & Franklin, M. (2018). Measuring fear change within exposures: Functionally-defined habituation predicts outcome in three randomized controlled trials for pediatric OCD. *Journal of Consulting and Clinical Psychology*, *86*(7), 615. https://doi.org/10.1037/ccp0000315
Blöte, A. W., Kint, M. J., Miers, A. C., & Westenberg, P. M. (2009). The relation between public speaking anxiety and social anxiety: A review. *Journal of anxiety disorders*, *23*(3), 305–313. https://doi.org/10.1016/j.janxdis.2008.11.007
Bouchard, S., Côté, S., & Richard, D. C. (2007). Virtual reality applications for exposure. In Handbook of exposure therapies (pp. 347–388). Academic Press. https://doi.org/10.1016/B978-012587421-2/50017-X
Cardi, V., Leppanen, J., Mataix-Cols, D., Campbell, I. C., & Treasure, J. (2019). A case series to investigate food-related fear learning and extinction using in vivo food exposure in anorexia nervosa: A clinical application of the inhibitory learning framework. *European eating disorders review*, *27*(2), 173–181. https://doi.org/10.1002/erv.2639
Carpenter, J. K., Pinaire, M., & Hofmann, S. G. (2019). From extinction learning to anxiety treatment: Mind the gap. *Brain sciences*, *9*(7), 164. https://doi.org/10.3390/brainsci9070164
Chesham, R. K., Malouff, J. M., & Schutte, N. S. (2018). Meta-analysis of the efficacy of virtual reality exposure therapy for social anxiety. *Behaviour Change*, *35*(3), 152–166. https://doi.org/10.1017/bec.2018.15
Clark, D. M., & Wells, A. (1995). A cognitive model of social phobia. In R. G. Heimberg, M. R. Liebowitz, D. A. Hope, & F. R. Schneier (Eds.), *Social phobia: Diagnosis, assessment, and treatment* (pp. 69–93). The Guilford Press. https://psycnet.apa.org/record/1995-98887-004
Cox, B. J., MacPherson, P. S., & Enns, M. W. (2005). Psychiatric correlates of childhood shyness in a nationally representative sample. *Behaviour Research and Therapy*, *43*(8), 1019–1027. https://doi.org/10.1016/j.brat.2004.07.006
Craske, M. (2015). Optimizing exposure therapy for anxiety disorders: an inhibitory learning and inhibitory regulation approach. *Verhaltenstherapie*, *25*(2), 134–143. https://doi.org/10.1159/000381574

Craske, M. G., Hermans, D., & Vervliet, B. (2018). State-of-the-art and future directions for extinction as a translational model for fear and anxiety. *Philosophical Transactions of the Royal Society B: Biological Sciences*, *373*(1742), 20170025. https://doi.org/10.1098/rstb.2017.0025
Craske, M. G., Kircanski, K., Zelikowsky, M., Mystkowski, J., Chowdhury, N., & Baker, A. (2008). Optimizing inhibitory learning during exposure therapy. *Behaviour research and therapy*, 46, 5–27. https://doi.org/10.1016/j.brat.2007.10.003
Craske, M. G., Liao, B., Brown, L., & Vervliet, B. (2012). Role of inhibition in exposure therapy. *Journal of Experimental Psychopathology*, *3*(3), 322–345. https://doi.org/10.5127/jep.026511
Craske, M. G., Treanor, M., Conway, C. C., Zbozinek, T., & Vervliet, B. (2014). Maximizing exposure therapy: An inhibitory learning approach. *Behaviour research and therapy*, *58*, 10–23. https://doi.org/10.1016/j.brat.2014.04.006
Crozier, W. R., & Alden, L. E. (Eds.). (2005). *The essential handbook of social anxiety for clinicians*. John Wiley & Sons.
Davey, G. C. (1992). Classical conditioning and the acquisition of human fears and phobias: A review and synthesis of the literature. *Advances in Behaviour Research and Therapy*, *14*(1), 29–66. https://doi.org/10.1016/0146-6402(92)90010-L
De Kleine, R. A., Hendriks, L., Becker, E. S., Broekman, T. G., & van Minnen, A. (2017). Harm expectancy violation during exposure therapy for posttraumatic stress disorder. *Journal of Anxiety Disorders*, *49*, 48–52. https://doi.org/10.1016/j.janxdis.2017.03.008
Drobes, D. J., & Lang, P. J. (1995). Bioinformational theory and behavior therapy. In W. T. O'Donohue & L. Krasner (Eds.), *Theories of behavior therapy: Exploring behavior change* (pp. 229–257). American Psychological Association. https://doi.org/10.1037/10169-009
Dwyer, K. K., & Davidson, M. M. (2012). Is public speaking really more feared than death?. *Communication Research Reports*, *29*(2), 99–107. https://doi.org/10.1080/08824096.2012.667772
Ebrahimi, O. V., Pallesen, S., Kenter, R. M., & Nordgreen, T. (2019). Psychological interventions for the fear of public speaking: A meta-analysis. *Frontiers in psychology*, *10*, 488. https://doi.org/10.3389/fpsyg.2019.00488
Elsner, B., Jacobi, T., Kischkel, E., Schulze, D., & Reuter, B. (2022). Mechanisms of exposure and response prevention in obsessive-compulsive disorder: effects of habituation and expectancy violation on short-term outcome in cognitive behavioral therapy. *BMC psychiatry*, *22*(1), 66. https://doi.org/10.1186/s12888-022-03701-z
Emmelkamp, P. M., Meyerbröker, K., & Morina, N. (2020). Virtual reality therapy in social anxiety disorder. *Current psychiatry reports*, *22*, 1–9. https://doi.org/10.1007/s11920-020-01156-1
Essayli, J. H., Forrest, L. N., Zickgraf, H. F., Stefano, E. C., Keller, K. L., & Lane-Loney, S. E. (2023). The impact of between-session habituation, within-session habituation, and weight gain on response to food exposure for adolescents with eating disorders. *International Journal of Eating Disorders*. https://doi.org/10.1002/eat.23894
Faravelli, C., Abrardi, L., Bartolozzi, D., Cecchi, C., Cosci, F., D'Adamo, D., ... & Rosi, S. (2004). The Sesto Fiorentino study: point and one-year prevalences of psychiatric disorders in an Italian community sample using clinical interviewers. *Psychotherapy and Psychosomatics*, *73*(4), 226–234. https://doi.org/10.1159/000077741
Foa, E. B., & Kozak, M. J. (1986). Emotional processing of fear: Exposure to corrective information. Psychological Bulletin, 99, 20–35. https://doi.org/10.1037/0033-2909.99.1.20
Foa, E. B., & McNally, R. J. (1996). Mechanisms of change in exposure therapy. *Current controversies in the anxiety disorders*, 329–343.
Fujii, Y., Kitagawa, N., Shimizu, Y., Mitsui, N., Toyomaki, A., Hashimoto, N., ... & Kusumi, I. (2013). Severity of generalized social anxiety disorder correlates with low executive functioning. *Neuroscience letters*, *543*, 42–46. https://doi.org/10.1016/j.neulet.2013.02.059
Furmark, T. (2002). Social phobia: overview of community surveys. *Acta Psychiatrica Scandinavica*, *105*(2), 84–93. https://doi.org/10.1034/j.1600-0447.2002.1r103.x
Gallistel, C. R., & Gibbon, J. (2000). Time, rate, and conditioning. *Psychological review*, *107*(2), 289. https://doi.org/10.1037/0033-295X.107.2.289

Garcia-Palacios, A., Botella, C., Hoffman, H., & Fabregat, S. (2007). Comparing acceptance and refusal rates of virtual reality exposure vs. in vivo exposure by patients with specific phobias. *Cyberpsychology & behavior*, *10*(5), 722–724. https://doi.org/10.1089/cpb.2007.9962

Gropalis, M., Witthöft, M., Bailer, J., & Weck, F. (2018). Optimizing exposure therapy for pathological health anxiety: Considerations from the inhibitory learning approach. *Cognitive and Behavioral Practice*, *25*(2), 250–260. https://doi.org/10.1016/j.cbpra.2017.09.001

Hajure, M., & Abdu, Z. (2020). Social phobia and its impact on quality of life among regular undergraduate students of Mettu University, Mettu, Ethiopia. *Adolescent Health, Medicine and Therapeutics*, 79–87. https://doi.org/10.2147/AHMT.S254002

Harned, M. S., Ruork, A. K., Liu, J., & Tkachuck, M. A. (2015). Emotional activation and habituation during imaginal exposure for PTSD among women with borderline personality disorder. *Journal of Traumatic Stress*, *28*(3), 253–257. https://doi.org/10.1002/jts.22013

Harris, J. D. (1943). Habituatory response decrement in the intact organism. *Psychological bulletin*, *40*(6), 385. https://doi.org/10.1037/h0053918

Heimberg, R. G., Brozovich, F. A., & Rapee, R. M. (2010). A cognitive behavioral model of social anxiety disorder: Update and extension. In *Social anxiety* (pp. 395–422). Academic Press. https://doi.org/10.1016/B978-0-12-375096-9.00015-8

Heimberg, R. G., Hofmann, S. G., & Liebowitz, M. R. (2014). Social anxiety disorder in DSM-5. *Depress Anxiety*, *31*, 472–9. https://doi.org/10.1016/B978-0-12-394427-6.00024-8

Heimberg, R. G., Hope, D. A., Dodge, C. S., & Becker, R. E. (1990). DSM-III-R subtypes of social phobia: Comparison of generalized social phobics and public speaking phobics. https://doi.org/10.1097/00005053-199003000-00004

Hinojo-Lucena, F. J., Aznar-Díaz, I., Cáceres-Reche, M. P., Trujillo-Torres, J. M., & Romero-Rodríguez, J. M. (2020). Virtual reality treatment for public speaking anxiety in students. Advancements and results in personalized medicine. *Journal of personalized medicine*, *10*(1), 14. https://doi.org/10.3390/jpm10010014

Hofmann, S. G., & Smits, J. A. (2008). Cognitive-behavioral therapy for adult anxiety disorders: a meta-analysis of randomized placebo-controlled trials. *Journal of clinical psychiatry*, *69*(4), 621. https://doi.org/10.4088/jcp.v69n0415

Horigome, T., Kurokawa, S., Sawada, K., Kudo, S., Shiga, K., Mimura, M., & Kishimoto, T. (2020). Virtual reality exposure therapy for social anxiety disorder: a systematic review and meta-analysis. *Psychological medicine*, *50*(15), 2487–2497. https://doi.org/10.1017/S0033291720003785

Hughes, A. A., Heimberg, R. G., Coles, M. E., Gibb, B. E., Liebowitz, M. R., & Schneier, F. R. (2006). Relations of the factors of the tripartite model of anxiety and depression to types of social anxiety. *Behaviour Research and Therapy*, *44*(11), 1629–1641. https://doi.org/10.1016/j.brat.2005.10.015

Huppert, J. D., Roth, D. A., & Foa, E. B. (2003). Cognitive-behavioral treatment of social phobia: new advances. *Current psychiatry reports*, *5*(4), 289–296. https://doi.org/10.1007/s11920-003-0058-5

Jefferies, P., & Ungar, M. (2020). Social anxiety in young people: A prevalence study in seven countries. *PloS one*, *15*(9), e0239133. https://doi.org/10.1371/journal.pone.0239133

Kaczkurkin, A. N., & Foa, E. B. (2022). Cognitive-behavioral therapy for anxiety disorders: an update on the empirical evidence. *Dialogues in clinical neuroscience*. 10.31887/DCNS.2015.17.3/akaczkurkin

Kampmann, I. L., Emmelkamp, P. M., & Morina, N. (2016). Meta-analysis of technology-assisted interventions for social anxiety disorder. *Journal of anxiety disorders*, *42*, 71–84. https://doi.org/10.1017/S0033291721001690

Kessler, R. C., Berglund, P., Demler, O., Jin, R., Merikangas, K. R., & Walters, E. E. (2005). Lifetime prevalence and age-of-onset distributions of DSM-IV disorders in the National Comorbidity Survey Replication. *Archives of general psychiatry*, *62*(6), 593–602. https://doi.org/10.1001/archpsyc.62.6.593

Kessler, R. C., Petukhova, M., Sampson, N. A., Zaslavsky, A. M., & Wittchen, H. U. (2012). Twelve-month and lifetime prevalence and lifetime morbid risk of anxiety and mood disorders in the United States. *International journal of methods in psychiatric research*, *21*(3), 169–184. https://doi.org/10.1002/mpr.1359

Kringlen, E., Torgersen, S., & Cramer, V. (2001). A Norwegian psychiatric epidemiological study. *American journal of psychiatry*, *158*(7), 1091–1098. https://doi.org/10.1176/appi.ajp.158.7.1091

Lang, P. J. (1977). Imagery in therapy: An information processing analysis of fear. *Behavior therapy*, *8*(5), 862–886. https://doi.org/10.1016/S0005-7894(77)80157-3

Lee, S., Tsang, A., Zhang, M. Y., Huang, Y. Q., He, Y. L., Liu, Z. R., ... & Kessler, R. C. (2007). Lifetime prevalence and inter-cohort variation in DSM-IV disorders in metropolitan China. *Psychological medicine*, *37*(1), 61–71. https://doi.org/10.1017/S0033291706008993

Leigh, E., Chiu, K., & Clark, D. M. (2021). Is concentration an indirect link between social anxiety and educational achievement in adolescents?. PLoS One, 16(5), e0249952. https://doi.org/10.1371/journal.pone.0249952

Levin, A. P., Saoud, J. B., Strauman, T., Gorman, J. M., Fyer, A. J., Crawford, R., & Liebowitz, M. R. (1993). Responses of "generalized" and "discrete" social phobics during public speaking. *Journal of Anxiety Disorders*, *7*(3), 207–221. https://doi.org/10.1016/0887-6185(93)90003-4

Lim, M. H., Aryadoust, V., & Esposito, G. (2022). A meta-analysis of the effect of virtual reality on reducing public speaking anxiety. Current Psychology, 1–17. https://doi.org/10.1007/s12144-021-02684-6

Lissek, S., Powers, A. S., McClure, E. B., Phelps, E. A., Woldehawariat, G., Grillon, C., & Pine, D. S. (2005). Classical fear conditioning in the anxiety disorders: a meta-analysis. *Behaviour research and therapy*, *43*(11), 1391–1424. https://doi.org/10.1016/j.brat.2004.10.007

MacKenzie, M. B., & Fowler, K. F. (2013). Social anxiety disorder in the Canadian population: Exploring gender differences in sociodemographic profile. *Journal of anxiety disorders*, *27*(4), 427–434. https://doi.org/10.1016/j.janxdis.2013.05.006

Maples-Keller, J. L., & Rauch, S. A. M. (2020). Habituation. In J. S. Abramowitz & S. M. Blakey (Eds.), *Clinical handbook of fear and anxiety: Maintenance processes and treatment mechanisms* (pp. 249–263). American Psychological Association. https://doi.org/10.1037/0000150-014

Marinho, A. C. F., Medeiros, A. M. D., Lima, E. D. P., Pantuza, J. J., & Teixeira, L. C. (2019, October). Prevalence and factors associated with fear of public speaking. In *CoDAS* (Vol. 31). Sociedade Brasileira de Fonoaudiologia. https://doi.org/10.1590/2317-1782/20192018266

Mayo-Wilson, E., Dias, S., Mavranezouli, I., Kew, K., Clark, D. M., Ades, A. E., & Pilling, S. (2014). Psychological and pharmacological interventions for social anxiety disorder in adults: a systematic review and network meta-analysis. *The Lancet Psychiatry*, *1*(5), 368–376. https://doi.org/10.1016/S2215-0366(14)70329-3

Merikangas, K. R., Avenevoli, S., Acharyya, S., Zhang, H., & Angst, J. (2002). The spectrum of social phobia in the Zurich cohort study of young adults. *Biological psychiatry*, *51*(1), 81–91. https://doi.org/10.1016/S0006-3223(01)01309-9

Mohammadi, M. R., Ghanizadeh, A., Mohammadi, M., & Mesgarpour, B. (2006). Prevalence of social phobia and its comorbidity with psychiatric disorders in Iran. *Depression and anxiety*, *23*(7), 405–411. https://doi.org/10.1002/da.20129

Montesi, J. L., Conner, B. T., Gordon, E. A., Fauber, R. L., Kim, K. H., & Heimberg, R. G. (2013). On the relationship among social anxiety, intimacy, sexual communication, and sexual satisfaction in young couples. *Archives of sexual behavior*, *42*, 81–91. https://doi.org/10.1007/s10508-012-9929-3

Mowrer, O. H. (1960). *Learning theory and the symbolic processes*. John Wiley & Sons, Inc. https://doi.org/10.1037/10772-000

Norton, P. J., & Price, E. C. (2007). A meta-analytic review of adult cognitive-behavioral treatment outcome across the anxiety disorders. *The Journal of nervous and mental disease*, *195*(6), 521–531. https://doi.org/10.1097/01.nmd.0000253843.70149.9a

Oakley Browne, M. A., Elisabeth Wells, J., Scott, K. M., McGee, M. A., & New Zealand Mental Health Survey Research Team. (2006). Lifetime prevalence and projected lifetime risk of DSM-IV disorders in Te Rau Hinengaro: the New Zealand Mental Health Survey. *Australian & New Zealand Journal of Psychiatry*, *40*(10), 865–874. https://doi.org/10.1080/j.1440-1614.2006.01905.x

Ohayon, M. M., & Schatzberg, A. F. (2010). Social phobia and depression: prevalence and comorbidity. *Journal of psychosomatic research*, *68*(3), 235–243. https://doi.org/10.1016/j.jpsychores.2009.07.018

Pabian, S., & Vandebosch, H. (2016). An investigation of short-term longitudinal associations between social anxiety and victimization and perpetration of traditional bullying and cyberbullying. *Journal of youth and adolescence*, *45*, 328–339. https://doi.org/10.1007/s10964-015-0259-3

Parsons, T. D., & Rizzo, A. A. (2008). Affective outcomes of virtual reality exposure therapy for anxiety and specific phobias: A meta-analysis. *Journal of behavior therapy and experimental psychiatry*, *39*(3), 250–261. https://doi.org/10.1016/j.jbtep.2007.07.007

Pélissolo, A., André, C., Moutard-Martin, F., Wittchen, H. U., & Lépine, J. P. (2000). Social phobia in the community: relationship between diagnostic threshold and prevalence. *European psychiatry*, *15*(1), 25–28. https://doi.org/10.1016/S0924-9338(00)00214-5

Peterman, J. S., Carper, M. M., & Kendall, P. C. (2019). Testing the habituation-based model of exposures for child and adolescent anxiety. *Journal of Clinical Child & Adolescent Psychology*, *48*(sup1), S34-S44. https://doi.org/10.1080/15374416.2016.1163707

Powell, D. H. (2004). Treating individuals with debilitating performance anxiety: An introduction. *Journal of clinical psychology*, *60*(8), 801–808. https://doi.org/10.1002/jclp.20038

Pull, C. B. (2012). Current status of knowledge on public-speaking anxiety. *Current opinion in psychiatry*, *25*(1), 32–38. https://doi.org/10.1097/YCO.0b013e32834e06dc

Rapee, R. M., & Heimberg, R. G. (1997). A cognitive-behavioral model of anxiety in social phobia. *Behaviour research and therapy*, *35*(8), 741–756. https://doi.org/10.1016/S0005-7967(97)00022-3

Reeves, R., Curran, D., Gleeson, A., & Hanna, D. (2022). A meta-analysis of the efficacy of virtual reality and in vivo exposure therapy as psychological interventions for public speaking anxiety. *Behavior Modification*, *46*(4), 937–965. https://doi.org/10.1177/0145445521991102

Repetto, C., Gaggioli, A., Pallavicini, F., Cipresso, P., Raspelli, S., & Riva, G. (2013). Virtual reality and mobile phones in the treatment of generalized anxiety disorders: a phase-2 clinical trial. *Personal and Ubiquitous Computing*, *17*, 253–260. https://doi.org/10.1007/s00779-011-0467-0

Rescorla, R. A. (1972). A theory of Pavlovian conditioning: Variations in the effectiveness of reinforcement and non-reinforcement. *Classical conditioning, Current research and theory*, *2*, 64–69.

Rodebaugh, T. L., Holaway, R. M., & Heimberg, R. G. (2004). The treatment of social anxiety disorder. *Clinical Psychology Review*, *24*(7), 883–908. https://doi.org/10.1016/j.cpr.2004.07.007

Rupp, C., Doebler, P., Ehring, T., & Vossbeck-Elsebusch, A. N. (2017). Emotional processing theory put to test: A meta-analysis on the association between process and outcome measures in exposure therapy. *Clinical Psychology & Psychotherapy*, *24*(3), 697–711. https://doi.org/10.1002/cpp.2039

Ruscio, A. M., Brown, T. A., Chiu, W. T., Sareen, J., Stein, M. B., & Kessler, R. C. (2008). Social fears and social phobia in the USA: results from the National Comorbidity Survey Replication. *Psychological medicine*, *38*(1), 15–28. https://doi.org/10.1017/S0033291707001699

Safir, M. P., Wallach, H. S., & Bar-Zvi, M. (2011). Virtual Reality Cognitive-Behavior Therapy for Public Speaking Anxiety. *Behavior Modification,* 36, 235–246. https://doi.org/10.1177/0145445511429999.

Safren, S. A., Heimberg, R. G., Brown, E. J., & Holle, C. (1996). Quality of life in social phobia. *Depression and anxiety*, *4*(3), 126–133. https://doi.org/10.1002/(SICI)1520-6394(1996)4:3<126::AID-DA5>3.0.CO;2-E

Salkovskis, P. M., Hackmann, A., Wells, A., Gelder, M. G., & Clark, D. M. (2007). Belief disconfirmation versus habituation approaches to situational exposure in panic disorder with agoraphobia: A pilot study. *Behaviour research and therapy*, *45*(5), 877–885. https://doi.org/10.1016/j.brat.2006.02.008

Sareen, J., Chartier, M., Paulus, M. P., & Stein, M. B. (2006). Illicit drug use and anxiety disorders: findings from two community surveys. *Psychiatry research*, *142*(1), 11–17.

Schemer, L., Körfer, K., & Glombiewski, J. A. (2020). Evaluation of exposure instructions to pain: Should therapist focus on fear reduction or expectation violation? *Cognitive Therapy and Research*, *44*, 697–708. https://doi.org/10.1007/s10608-019-10070-7

Scheveneels, S., Boddez, Y., Van Daele, T., & Hermans, D. (2019). Virtually unexpected: No role for expectancy violation in virtual reality exposure for public speaking anxiety. *Frontiers in psychology*, *10*, 2849. https://doi.org/10.3389/fpsyg.2019.02849

Schyns, G., van den Akker, K., Roefs, A., Hilberath, R., & Jansen, A. (2018). What works better? Food cue exposure aiming at the habituation of eating desires or food cue exposure aiming at the violation of overeating expectancies?. *Behaviour Research and Therapy*, *102*, 1–7. https://doi.org/10.1016/j.brat.2017.12.001

Sewart, A. R., & Craske, M. G. (2020). Inhibitory learning. In J. S. Abramowitz & S. M. Blakey (Eds.), *Clinical handbook of fear and anxiety: Maintenance processes and treatment mechanisms* (pp. 265–285). American Psychological Association. https://doi.org/10.1037/0000150-015

Sharp, D., & Drawson, B. (1992). Send in the crowds. *Health*, *6*(2), 66–70.

Sparrevohn, R. M., & Rapee, R. M. (2009). Self-disclosure, emotional expression and intimacy within romantic relationships of people with social phobia. *Behaviour Research and Therapy*, *47*(12), 1074–1078. https://doi.org/10.1016/j.brat.2009.07.016

Sripada, R. K., & Rauch, S. A. (2015). Between-session and within-session habituation in Prolonged Exposure Therapy for posttraumatic stress disorder: A hierarchical linear modeling approach. *Journal of Anxiety Disorders*, *30*, 81–87. https://doi.org/10.1016/j.janxdis.2015.01.002

Stein, M. B., & Stein, D. J. (2008). Social anxiety disorder. *The lancet*, *371*(9618), 1115–1125. https://doi.org/10.1016/S0140-6736(08)60488-2

Stein, M. B., Walker, J. R., & Forde, D. R. (1996). Public-speaking fears in a community sample: Prevalence, impact on functioning, and diagnostic classification. *Archives of general psychiatry*, *53*, 169–174. https://doi.org/10.1001/archpsyc.1996.01830020087010

Tolin, D. F. (2019). Inhibitory learning for anxiety-related disorders. *Cognitive and Behavioral Practice*, *26*(1), 225–236. https://doi.org/10.1016/j.cbpra.2018.07.008

Tryon, W. W. (2005). Possible mechanisms for why desensitization and exposure therapy work. *Clinical psychology review*, *25*(1), 67–95. https://doi.org/10.1016/j.cpr.2004.08.005

Van Ameringen, M., Mancini, C., & Farvolden, P. (2003). The impact of anxiety disorders on educational achievement. *Journal of anxiety disorders*, *17*(5), 561–571. https://doi.org/10.1016/S0887-6185(02)00228-1

van den Akker, K., Schyns, G., & Jansen, A. (2016). Enhancing inhibitory learning to reduce overeating: Design and rationale of a cue exposure therapy trial in overweight and obese women. *Contemporary clinical trials*, *49*, 85–91. https://doi.org/10.1016/j.cct.2016.06.008

Waters, W. F., McDonald, D. G., & Koresko, R. L. (1972). Psychophysiological responses during analogue systematic desensitization and non-relaxation control procedures. *Behaviour Research and Therapy*, *10*(4), 381–393. https://doi.org/10.1016/0005-7967(72)90061-7

Wechsler, T. F., Kümpers, F., & Mühlberger, A. (2019). Inferiority or even superiority of virtual reality exposure therapy in phobias?—A systematic review and quantitative meta-analysis on randomized controlled trials specifically comparing the efficacy of virtual reality exposure to gold standard in vivo exposure in agoraphobia, specific phobia, and social phobia. *Frontiers in psychology*, *10*, 1758. https://doi.org/10.3389/fpsyg.2019.01758

Wittchen, H. U., Fuetsch, M., Sonntag, H., Müller, N., & Liebowitz, M. (2000). Disability and quality of life in pure and comorbid social phobia. Findings from a controlled study. *European Psychiatry*, *15*(1), 46–58. https://doi.org/10.1016/S0924-9338(00)00211-X

Wolpe, J. (1968). Psychotherapy by reciprocal inhibition. *Conditional reflex: a Pavlovian journal of research & therapy*, *3*, 234–240. https://doi.org/10.1007/BF03000093

Wolpe, J. (1995). Reciprocal inhibition: Major agent of behavior change. In W. T. O'Donohue & L. Krasner (Eds.), *Theories of behavior therapy: Exploring behavior change* (pp. 23–57). American Psychological Association. https://doi.org/10.1037/10169-002

Theoretical Digression

Christos Charis and Barbara Milrod

Panic-focused psychodynamic psychotherapy (PFPP) is a form of brief psychotherapy developed by Barbara Milrod, M.D. and her research group for treatment of panic disorder with or without agoraphobia. It has been adapted across anxiety disorders, for anxiety disorders of children and teens (Child and Adolescent Psychodynamic Psychotherapy [CAPP], Preter et al. 2018) and for posttraumatic stress disorder (Trauma Focused Psychodynamic Psychotherapy [TFPP], Busch et al. 2021). PFPP is a psychodynamic psychotherapy, meaning that it aims to reduce specific symptoms of anxiety by working psychodynamically on unconscious underpinnings to the symptoms. A brief introduction to the theoretical basis of this therapy can be found in this book in the chapter by Dr. Charis "Fear, Anxiety, and Their Meaning in Our Life" (more information about this can be found in Busch et al. 2011; or Subic-Wrana et al. 2012). This therapy has demonstrated efficacy, with independent replications, unusual in a psychodynamic psychotherapy, in a number of clinical trials over decades (Milrod et al. 2001, 2007a, b, 2016; Svensson et al. 2020). It is a brief therapy (24 sessions in 12 weeks) and consists of three phases: (a) the initial phase, which is the treatment of acute panic; (b) treatment of panic vulnerability; and (c) termination.

(a) In the initial phase, the symptoms and their underlying specific emotional meanings for the patient as well as the feelings associated with them are explored. By

C. Charis
Private Practice for Psychotherapy, Dillenburg, Hessen, Germany
e-mail: christos-charis@outlook.de

B. Milrod (✉)
Albert Einstein College of Medicine, New York, NY, USA

Psychotherapy Research at PRIME (Psychiatric Research Institute of Montefiore Einstein), New York, NY, USA
e-mail: bmilrod@montefiore.org

C. Charis, G. Panayiotou (eds.), *Anxiety Disorders and Related Conditions*,
https://doi.org/10.1007/978-3-031-56798-8_7

carefully tracking the conditions under which panic symptoms occur, the thoughts, the feelings, and the individual meanings of the symptoms, we get better access to underlying conflicts the patient is struggling with. It is important to understand these conflicts in context as this helps patients better understand why they are having panic. Panic attacks are often preceded by real or fantasized losses or separations from important, ambivalently held people in the patient's life. Patients fear being alone, feel small and weak, and worry they will not survive without the other person they feel unable to separate from. Against this background, treatment of such patients must focus on their intense fears of separation and of the greater agency that is necessary to function more autonomously (i.e., panic patients have trouble tolerating their own assertion and aggression). These patients are also frightened of their own anger, and whatever mixed feelings they may be aware of toward important people in their lives. Patients often experience conflicts in their wish to be more autonomous. In PFPP, the therapist actively explores panic attacks and associated anxiety if the patient does not do so on their own. (By definition, in DSM-described panic disorder, the panic attacks from the point of view of the patient come "out of the blue" or completely unexpectedly and patients often do not recognize any connection with their emotional lives.) Although intense fear is experienced at the forefront of a panic attack, a wide range of feelings arise during panic attacks (Fava et al. 1990). It is important to explore these and the issues associated with them. These feelings contribute to the development and maintenance of the symptoms that occur and their underlying meanings. To explain this better, CC gives a clinical example:

A 25-year-old man comes to therapy and reports panic attacks and abdominal discomfort. By exploring the circumstances in which he suffers the panic attacks, the patient succeeds in understanding the personal meaning of his panic attacks in therapy. One and a half years earlier, his mother died a dramatic death in front of his eyes. She had undressed in front of him due to sudden hot flushes and collapsed. Her death was due to a previously unrecognized abdominal aortic aneurysm which burst. On further inquiry, the patient reveals an extremely close relationship to his mother, as his father died in his early childhood. By exploring the symptoms, the patient begins to recognize their meaning for him personally. He becomes aware that he is filled with fear as soon as he feels physical discomfort in his abdomen, which specifically reminds him of losing his mother. In the further course of his therapy, he begins to recognize that he is firmly convinced that he is hereditarily burdened, i.e., that he also has an abdominal aortic aneurysm just like his mother (which is also an identification with his mother). Moreover, he also begins to recognize that he has the fantasy that his abdominal aortic aneurysm is about to rupture, which is why he now experiences the abdominal discomfort.

In further exploration of his thoughts and feelings, the patient realizes that he is grieving the death of his mother and that at the times that he experiences these symptoms he feels closer to her. He is also angry with her because she suddenly died and left him alone. He is ashamed of the loss of control he experiences during panic attacks. As can be seen from this example, it is obvious that by exploring the circumstances in which panic occurs, the thoughts, the feelings, and the individual meaning of the symptoms, we get better access to the underlying conflicts of the patient that lead him to experience panic in the first place.

Because of his terror of being alone without his mother, he moved in with his girlfriend after his mother's death, which enabled him to avoid his fear of being alone. Under these circumstances, he feels safer, although he does not feel well understood by his girlfriend. Panic patients can experience deficits in their tolerance of their affects (Busch et al. 1991, 2011). Panic disorders are afraid of their own anger and rage (Milrod et al. 1997; Shear et al. 1993; Subic-Wrana et al. 2012). This also corresponds to my personal experience with such patients. It is important to help these patients recognize that these dangers are in fantasy (Subic-Wrana et al. 2012).

(b) Treatment of panic vulnerability: In this phase of PFPP, work is done to reduce the patient's vulnerability to panic attacks and associated anxiety disorder symptoms and agoraphobic avoidance. This is done in part by working with the transference and working through, a psychoanalytic term meaning that the same underlying conflict emerges in a variety of different settings and capacities. Transference refers to the patient's feelings and fantasies toward the therapist that reflect a reliving of core emotional aspects of formative attachment relationships (Freud & Breuer 1966). The therapist must focus attention on the transference and explain its significance to the patient as it occurs, highlighting its relationship to panic symptoms. In this phase of therapy, panic attacks and associated anxiety continue to be the focus of therapy. Basic tenets of psychoanalytic therapy apply to PFPP, specifically: the therapy is not directed (despite its focus on panic), and the therapist follows the themes and associations that the patient brings up, and does not determine the focus of the session, but links what the patient brings up to themes and associations that have been determined to be associated with panic attacks and anxiety. It is important to give the transference room to unfold by the therapist not introducing their own agenda into the therapy and not being judgmental or actively intervening (such as by giving homework or telling patients what to do).

An example of this: A patient (Mr. W) of CC who is afraid of his anger immediately apologized because he was describing his own idea in the session and the therapist was of a different opinion. More precisely, the patient has set up a theory for himself how his panic attacks arise, and he explains his theory in the session. I answer him that it is good that he is dealing with the topic, but he will start to understand himself better if he concentrates more on his inner life. Mr. W does not feel appreciated by my intervention and he is angry, but because he is afraid of his anger, particularly in the context of his therapy—he worries I will be angry with him and refuse to treat him or somehow otherwise abandon him, he denies his anger. In the analysis of the transference, the patient was able to recognize his own underlying conflicts in dealing with anger. He was able to understand his fear of anger against the background of his experiences with anger in his family. His parents often fought viciously and bitterly throughout his childhood and adolescence and he had witnessed and survived child abuse. Mr. W's father had once injured his mother with an axe and yelled at him several times during the same incident so the patient was terrified that he might be attacked by his father too, so that he shivered all night and could not be calm down. For a patient like Mr. W, who had witnessed and survived severe interpersonal violence in childhood, it is unsurprising that trust of other people, and any experience of anger would be dysregulating.

If a patient experiences intense feelings in the transference and cannot express them, the therapist should help the patient recognize and acknowledge his feelings and express them in words. Working through means that the therapist notes ways in which the same conflicts occur in multiple aspects of the patients' lives in various settings and relationships in the patient's life, highlighting ways in which core conflicts underlying panic occur throughout their life. These understandings, and the emotional acknowledgement of key emotional conflicts and fantasies underlying panic, are what leads to symptomatic change. The aim of working through is that the patient becomes aware of the emotional significance of triggers of their panic attacks and begins to tolerate in verbal form some of the underlying emotional difficulties that have led to panic. The aim is to achieve more active attitudes through as a result of working through their fears and underlying fantasies, which leads to a reduction in anxiety. In working through this, the patient becomes more tolerant of their anger and rageful fantasies (Busch et al. 2011).

(c) Ending therapy: Panic patients often believe that becoming independent means separating from significant others and thus feeling abandoned. This is one reason that separations often trigger panic attacks, as the attacks can come to symbolize these losses. Panic patients are separation sensitive, and are prone to feeling abandoned, including in the context of their therapy. For these reasons, separations during the course of therapy provide access to this aspect of underlying panic-triggering conflicts. During separations from significant others, anger can arise toward people who the patient experiences as abandoning them. It is important to articulate and explore these conflicts of separation and the associated feelings and thoughts. Among other things, this means allowing, tolerating, and integrating anger that can arise from feeling abandoned. A typical goal in this process would be for the panic patient to feel more comfortable tolerating their anger and no longer to feel so threatened by it, facilitating smoother, less fraught and conflicted relationships and greater tolerance of autonomy. Experiences of separation in the course of therapy are thus carefully articulated and explored. The most important separation in treatment is the separation from the therapist at termination of this brief, time-limited psychotherapy. Termination gives the patient the opportunity to strengthen their sense of autonomy. This sense of greater mastery can be strengthened with the therapist carefully helping the patient to articulate in words their-inevitably- very mixed feelings about the treatment ending. This process gives the patient the important message: "I trust you to be able to manage your feelings better." Experience has shown that some patients quickly become symptom-free within the first several sessions of PFPP and begin the process of making sense of the feelings that lead to their panic. In PFPP, the therapist maintains a focus on ongoing conflicts underlying anxiety, even as patients improve symptomatically. PFPP has been well-tolerated in clinical trials, with a very low dropout rate (7–20% in RCTs).

Empirical evidence of effectiveness: Milrod et al.'s research group and others (Svensson et al. 2020) have conducted randomized controlled trials to test the efficacy of PFPP. All studies have used the Panic Disorder Severity Scale (PDSS; Shear 1997) as the primary outcome measure, as is standard in PD treatment research (Shear and Maser 1994). In the original open clinical trial, 21 patients with a diagnosis of panic disorder with or without agoraphobia were treated; psychopharmacotherapy was excluded. Four patients dropped out of the study, all had been forced to undergo benzodiazepine taper for study entry, which clearly was not tolerable. Sixteen patients successfully completed the treatment. (Milrod et al. 2001). In the initial RCT of PFPP, it was compared with an efficacious, exposure-based less-active but efficacious psychotherapy (Applied Relaxation Training (ART); Ost 1988) that includes in vivo exposure and relaxation exercises but lacks the interoceptive component of Panic Control Therapy (PCT; Craske et al. 2000) and has shown efficacy for PD. Applied Relaxation Training (ART) includes daily relaxation training and homework, and therapists were matched for experience and time with patients as in the PFPP condition. Forty-nine patients with PD ± Ag were randomly assigned, 26 to PFPP, and 23 to ART. The result of the study demonstrated the efficacy of PFPP with a between-group effect size of 0.95 on the PDSS, the primary outcome measure. Forty-nine percent of these subjects also met criteria for a personality disorder, 79% of whom had at least one cluster C disorder. PFPP imparted an advantage in this study for patients with comorbid cluster C disorders as compared with patients treated without cluster C disorder comorbidity (PFPP appeared still more advantageous than ART for subjects with an Axis II disorder (Cohen's $d = 1.19$) relative to those without an Axis II disorder (Cohen's $d = 0.55$). Cluster C disorders also appeared to moderate the treatment effect (cluster C, $d = 1.35$; no cluster C, $d = 0.69$). No moderating effect of cluster B was apparent (Cohen's $d = 1.10$ with cluster B vs. 0.91 without cluster B) (Milrod et al. 2007a, b). These personality disorder findings were not later replicated (Keefe et al. 2018).

The Cluster C findings were interpreted to mean that passivity of these patients, a hallmark of cluster C disorders, was specifically addressed in PFPP (Milrod et al. 2007a, b; Subic-Wrana et al. 2012). In a two-site RCT comparing 201 subjects with primary PD ± Ag in PFPP, CBT, and ART in a 2:2:1 ratio, overall attrition rates were ART 41%, CBT 25%, and PFPP 23%. The most severely ill patients dropped out of ART more than CBT or PFPP ($p = .013$). A site x treatment interaction ($p = .016$) for "response" (a priori 40% PDSS reduction) showed significant differences at Cornell (ART 30%, CBT 65%, PFPP 71% ($p = .003$)) but not at Penn (ART 63%, CBT 60%, PFPP 48% ($p = .37$)). Penn patients were more severe on PDSS, differed demographically from Cornell patients and had a 7.2-fold greater likelihood of taking medication and a 28-fold greater likelihood of taking p.r.n. benzodiazepines.

However, these differences did not explain site x treatment interactions. All treatments substantially improved PD ± Ag, but patients at both sites found ART less acceptable, particularly those who were the most severely ill. While CBT showed the most consistent performance across sites, the results for PFPP showed the promise of psychodynamic psychotherapy for this disorder (Milrod et al. 2016). In the 12-month follow-up of this study, McCarthy et al. (2018) examined the long-term effects of these three psychotherapies in this study. Of the 116 patients whose data were available at 12-month follow-up (largely responders), it was found that the improvements in all three forms of therapy were largely maintained in responders 1 year after the end of therapy; however ART was found to be less acceptable in the treatment for PD patients, as dropout rates were so much higher (McCarthy et al. 2018).

References

Busch, F. N., Milrod, B. L., Singer, M. B., Aronson, A. C. (2011): Manual of Panic focussed Psychodynamic Psychotherapy-eXtende Range. Routledge London.

Busch, F.N., Cooper, A.M., Klerman, G.L., Penzer, R.J., Shapiro, T., Shear, M.K. (1991): Neurophysiological, cognitive-behavioral and psychoanalytic approaches to panic disorder: Toward an integration. Psychoanalysis inquiry. 11, 316–332.

Busch F, Milrod B, Chen C, Singer M ((2021): Trauma-Focused Psychodynamic Psychotherapy. Bringing evidence-based psychodynamic treatment to patients with PTSD. Oxford University Press

Craske, M. G., Barlow, D. H., & Meadows, E. (2000). Master your own anxiety and panic: Therapist guide for anxiety, panic, and agoraphobia (MAP-3). San Antonio, TX: Graywind/ Psychological Corporation.

Fava M., Anderson K. & Rosenbaum J.F. (1990): "Anger attacks". Possible variant of panic and major depressive disorders. American Journal of Psychiatry. 147, 867–870.

Keefe JR, Milrod B, Barber JP et al: What is the effect on comorbid personality disorder of brief panic-focused psychotherapy in patients with panic disorder? Depression and Anxiety 2018 Mar;35(3):239–247

McCarthy, K. S., Chambless, D. L., Solomonoe, N., Milrod, B., Barber, J. P. (2018): Twelve-Month Outcomes Following Successful Panic-Focused Psychodynamic Psychotherapy, Cognitive-Behavioral Therapy, or Applied Relaxation Training for Panic Disorder. https://doi.org/10.4088/JCP.17m11807

Milrod B, Busch F, Cooper A, Shapiro T (1997): Manual of Panic - Focused Psychodynamic Psychotherapy APA Press, Washington, D.C..

Milrod B, Busch F, Leon AC, Aronson A, Roiphe J, Singer M, Shapiro T, Goldman H, Richter D, Shear MK (2001): A pilot open trial of brief psychodynamic psychotherapy for panic disorder Journal of Psychotherapy Practice and Research;10:239–245

Milrod B, Chambless DL, Gallop R et al (2016): Psychotherapies for panic disorder: a tale of two sites. Journal of Clinical Psychiatry; 77:927–935

Milrod B, Leon AC, Barber JP, Markowitz JC, Graf E (2007a): Do comorbid personality disorders moderate Panic-Focused Psychotherapy? An exploratory examination of the APA Practice Guideline Journal of Clinical Psychiatry;68:885–891

Milrod B, Leon, AC, Busch FN, Rudden M, Schwalberg M, Clarkin J, Aronson A, Singer M, Turchin W, Klass ET, Graf E, Teres JJ, Shear MK. (2007b): A randomized controlled clini-

cal trial of psychoanalytic psychotherapy for panic disorder. American Journal of Psychiatry; 164:265–272
Ost, L. G. (1988): Applied Relaxation in the treatment of panic disorder. Behavior Research and Therapy, 26, 13–22.
Preter S, Shapiro T, Milrod B (2018): Child and Adolescent Anxiety Psychodynamic Psychotherapy: A Manual Oxford University Press Print ISBN-13:9780190877712
Shear, M. K., Brown, T:A:, Barlow, D. H., Money, R., Sholomskas, D. E., Woods, S. W. et al. (1997): Multicenter collaborative panic disorder severity scale. American Journal of Psychiatry, 154, 1571–1575.
Shear M.K., Cooper, A.M., Klerman, G.L., Busch, F.N. & Shapiro, T (1993): A psychodynamic model of panic disorder. American Journal of Psychiatry. 150, 859–866.
Shear M.K., Maser JD. (1994). Standardized assessment for panic disorder research: a conference report. Archives of general psychiatry. Jamanetwork.com.
Svensson M, Nilsson T, Perrin S, Johansson H, Viborg G, Falkenström F, & Sandell R. (2020). Panic focused psychodynamic psychotherapy versus panic control treatment for panic disorder: A doubly randomised controlled preference trial. Psychotherapy & Psychosomatics.
C. Subic-Wrana, B, Milrod, M. Beutel, (2012): Panikfokussiete Psychdynamische Psychotherapie. Hogrefe, Göttingen.

Case Study of a 33-Year-Old Patient with a Panic Disorder, an Emetophobia (ICD-10 F 41.0/F 40.2) and a Moderate Depression on the Basis of a Recurrent Depressive Disorder (ICD-10 F 33.1) from Psychodynamic Point of View

Christos Charis

Introduction

I would like to present a case of a childless 33-year-old married administrative assistant who has been suffering from panic attacks since the age of 17 and at times becomes depressed, with panic disorder and emetophobia being at the forefront of the clinical picture. I treated the patient according to the concept of panic-focussed psychodynamic psychotherapy (PFPP) in a modified form. This means that the external transference was the subject of the therapy and not the transference, as recommended in PFPP. A total of 100 sessions took place. The aim of the therapy was not only to reduce the patient's symptoms but also to modify the patient's attitudes that contribute to their psychological destabilisation. In order for the reader to be able to follow me more easily, I will briefly explain the PFPP with the help of Professor Milrod in a theoretical digression (see above). The depth psychology-based therapy lasted for two and a half years. The patient came to therapy once a week. Mrs. X approached me on the recommendation of a patient who had completed her therapy with me some time before. She identified with the good results of her friend's therapy, which gave her encouragement and hope that her fervent wish to discontinue paroxetine would come true. Up until the time she presented to me, she had been taking the drug consistently every day for 11 years.

At the age of 17, she suffered her first panic attack and presented to a psychiatric outpatient clinic where she was prescribed paroxetine. Immediately before that, the patient, who was then an adolescent, had to reluctantly give up her second room to the children of her paternal uncle. This was because the parents of these children were both alcoholics and could not take care of their children. So the two children

C. Charis (✉)
Private Practice for Psychotherapy, Dillenburg, Hessen, Germany
e-mail: christos-charis@outlook.de

C. Charis, G. Panayiotou (eds.), *Anxiety Disorders and Related Conditions*,
https://doi.org/10.1007/978-3-031-56798-8_8

(about the same age as the patient) were taken in by the patient's family. Soon after, the patient's father suddenly collapsed unconscious one evening. The emergency doctor who rushed to help took her father to neurosurgery, where he had to be operated on due to a rupture of an aneurysm in the brain. A short time later, Mrs. X suffered her first panic attack after seeing her cousin vomiting in the room. From then on, Mrs. X suffered frequent panic attacks. At the beginning of 2018, Mrs. X vomited at home. The doctor on duty who came to her home recommended that the patient had to reduce paroxetine to 10 mg. As a result, she started suffering sudden panic attacks again that were accompanied by other symptoms (e.g. anticipated fear of future unexpected panic attacks, fear of going crazy, pronounced vegetative symptoms, etc.). Against this background, she came to me for therapy.

Biography

Mrs. X lives with her husband in their own home in a large city near the town where she grew up and where her parents are still settled today. Her husband (who is 12 years older than her) is a craftsman by profession. The patient was his "trophy wife!" He had seen her, and it went "bang" with him! He is matter-of-fact, and she experiences him as the "rock of their relationship". They got married in 2008, and they have had no children together so far partly because her husband does not want any more children and furthermore the patient is afraid that the children could vomit and that she herself could be infected by the vomit of her children. In addition, her husband has a 15-year-old daughter from a previous relationship, although he has no contact with her (see Table 1).

Mrs. X is tattooed on the right side of her body with the five names of her family of origin (her brother who is 8 years older and her sister who is 4 years older). When she told me this, I inferred a close family connection. Her sister fell ill with an infectious disease when she was 3 years old, in the course of which her sister also developed meningitis. The patient and her siblings were brought up by their parents in a very strict religious way (free evangelical). She says, "The other children were allowed everything. We had what we needed, but not what we wanted". She says her parents were very particular about hygiene: "Wash your hands! Don't put anything in your mouth!" Each family member had their own cutlery because her father had herpes. Moreover, the patient had herpes on her face when she was 6 months old, which was evidenced by a photo of her at that age. She emphasised how bad the herpes on her face was. In addition, the patient underwent an operation for appendicitis when she was 12 years old. A benign tumour was diagnosed in the

Table 1 Biographical data

33 years old. Occupation: administrative assistant. Married, childless
As for her own family now, her husband is a craftsman by profession and 12 years older than the patient. She is his "trophy wife!" He is the rock of their relationship
He has a 15-year-old daughter from a previous relationship

Table 2 Biographical data

Within her family there is a very close connection
The patient and her siblings (brother is 8 years and her sister is 4 years older than Mrs. X) were brought up by their parents in a very strict religious way (they belong to the free evangelical church)
Very strict hygiene rules within the family. For example, everybody had their own cutlery
Severe herpes on her face when she was 6 months old
When she was 12 years old, she developed a benign tumour, which is why the patient had to go to the clinic regularly for a few days for 5 years for check-ups

appendix that had been removed, which is why the patient had to go to the clinic regularly for a few days for 5 years for check-ups. The communication of Mrs. X's experiences triggered sympathy and understanding for the patient's pronounced hypochondriacal fears (see Table 2).

Her father who is 34 years older than her, receives disability benefit and is described by the patient as "the rock in the family" has been in a wheelchair since the patient was 17. He has always been quick-tempered. When he is wronged, he gets stomach ache and diarrhoea and yells, just like the patient. As a child, Mrs. X had witnessed several arguments between her father and her brother, during which her father had shouted so loudly at her brother that the patient had become afraid that her father would kill her brother. I think such experiences with aggression have left their mark on the patient or have shaped her ideas of aggression. She was a "daddy's girl" and had slept in her father's arms until she was 9 years old. He had done a lot with her. His word was law for the patient. She took on his fears. For example, he was afraid of flying. When she drives over a bridge, she looks at every screw of the bridge, and she asks herself "Will it hold?" These sequences testify to a particularly close bond with the father. I wondered during the first interview whether she has detached herself from him (Table 3). The patient was afraid of flying too.

Psychodynamics

There is an autonomy-dependence conflict and an oedipal conflict with structural deficits (self-(value)regulation, perceiving and differentiating affects) in the sense of Operationalised Psychodynamic Diagnostic 2 (OPD 2). According to her biography, Mrs. X was born and grew up in a climate of fear within her family of origin (the father's herpes, the patient's severe herpes in the face and later at the age of 12 a tumour, because of which the patient had to go to the clinic regularly for a few days for 5 years for check-ups. Her sister had meningitis). Such anxiety-provoking biographical factors certainly reduced her exploratory behaviour, which increased her dependence on her parents. In addition, her father's confrontations with her brother, which the patient experienced as life-threatening, increased the patient's

Table 3 Biographical data

Her father who is 34 years older than her, receives disability benefit and is described by the patient as "the rock in the family" has been in a wheelchair since the patient was 17
The patient can be described as a "daddy's girl". She took on his fears. For example, he was afraid of flying
As a child, Mrs. X had witnessed several arguments between her father and her brother. Therefore, the patient had become afraid that her father would kill her brother

Table 4 Psychodynamics

Pronounced dependence on her parents
She grew up in a climate of fear within her family of origin. Her father's herpes, the patient's severe herpes in the face and later at the age of 12 a tumour, because of which the patient had to go to the clinic regularly for a few days for 5 years for check-ups. Her sister had meningitis. The illness of her father when she was 17
Such anxiety-provoking biographical factors certainly reduced her exploratory behaviour, which increased her dependence on her parents. In addition, her father's confrontations with her brother, which the patient experienced as life-threatening, increased the patient's anxiety, weakening her willingness to detach from her parents

anxiety, weakening her autonomy in particular in her willingness to detach from her parents (see Table 4).

Mrs. X demonstrates her strong attachment to her parents and to her siblings, among other things, by the tattoo on her right leg. It is obvious that her pronounced dependence on her parents led to an increased intensity and frequency of negative affects (anger, fear). The patient was not able to cope with these affects because she was not able to form any supportive inner ideas of relationships against the background of her very ambivalent relationship with her parents. This means that against this background (structural deficits) she is not able to calm herself down or regulate her feelings. This is well illustrated by a scene with her husband, which Mrs. X describes as follows: When she suffers a panic attack, she puts her hand on her husband's chest and feels his heart, which calms her down. Or in other words, she went from one addiction to another. So she marries at the age of 22 and looks for a protective figure in her husband (father transference) just as she found a protective figure in her father, who paid a lot of attention to her, "daddy's girl". In this sense, it is better to understand when she says: The fact that she has not yet detached herself from her parental home to this day, it was noticed by her husband, who told the patient, "All three of you children have not managed to detach yourselves from home". She has remained the child, dependent on her husband, so that she does not trust herself to have children of her own. Thus her expression, she is his "trophy wife", is better understood. The experienced strong dependence on her parents and her husband triggers in Mrs. X a feeling of being weak herself, of being at the mercy of the significant others. She therefore adopts avoidance behaviour to protect herself from being flooded with negative feelings (anger, fear) (see Table 5).

Trigger of the patient's first panic attack: First, the children of her father's brother (he and his wife were alcoholics), who "stank", were taken into the patient's

Table 5 Psychodynamics

Negative affects
Her pronounced dependence on her parents led to an increased intensity and frequency of negative affects (anger, fear)
The patient was not able to cope with these affects. That means she is not able to calm herself down or regulate her feelings
Because of that she looks for a protective figure in her husband (father transference) just as she found a protective figure in her father ("daddy's girl"). Because of that she subordinates her desires and interests to the desires of her husband, whereby she hardly takes responsibility and remains the child. She does not trust herself to have children of her own

parental home. It stands to reason that the patient was very angry, not least because (in adolescence) she had to cede her living space to the two children. However, the patient could not express her anger against her father because of her dependence on him and fear of loss. She repressed her negative feelings and avoided confrontation with her parents. A few months after the children were admitted, their father had a sudden severe brain haemorrhage. It may be that the patient fantasised that she had made her father ill with her aggression. The fact that Mrs. X washed her hands often after a motorbike accident 2 years ago until the court case in which she was acquitted was over also speaks for the fact that she is dealing with her anger in and feelings of guilt. So it is conceivable, she thought, when children come, there are only disasters! They took away her living space, and her father almost died! When it came out a year later that her father also had *Salmonella* in his knees, which is why he could no longer walk, she blamed the children, as she told me the other day. The two children had originally brought the *Salmonella* into the house! In this way, she legitimises her anger at the two children who would have taken her space away from her, thereby exonerating herself. So today, when all her friends are having children (she is a godmother to two children) and she has turned 33, she finds herself in a dilemma. She wants to remain the child, does not want to be autonomous, does not take responsibility and wants to have her husband only for herself. On the other hand, she wants children, i.e. to be an autonomous mother. This potentiates the patient's feelings of helplessness and weakness and depression. There is a flooding of the ego with negative affects (anger, fear) (see Table 6).

Diagnoses

Case Study of a 33-Year-Old Patient with a Panic Disorder, an Emetophobia (ICD-10 F 41.0/F 40.2) and a Moderate Depression on the Basis of a Recurrent Depressive Disorder (ICD-10 F 33.1) from Psychodynamic Point of View.

Table 6 Psychodynamics

Trigger of the patient's first panic attack
The patient was very angry, not least because (in adolescence) she had to cede her living space to the two children
However, the patient could not express her anger against her father because of her dependence on him and fear of loss
A few months later, their father had a sudden severe brain haemorrhage. It may be that the patient fantasised that she had made her father ill with her aggression. So it is conceivable, she thought, when children come, there are only disasters! They took away her living space, and her father almost died!
So today, when all her friends are having children (she is a godmother to two children) and she has turned 33, she finds herself in a dilemma
She wants to remain the child, does not want to be autonomous, does not take responsibility and wants to have her husband only for herself. On the other hand, she wants children, i.e. to be an autonomous mother
This potentiates the patient's feelings of helplessness and weakness and depression. There is a flooding of the ego with negative affects (anger, fear)

Table 7 Therapy

Transference: the patient is looking for a paternal companion in me, whom she idealises and tries to find answers to her agonising life questions with me, just as she idealised her father and leaned on him
Countertransference: I felt invited to start the therapy because I identify with the patient's therapy goal
Motivation: To strengthen the patient's motivation and better prepare her for the upcoming therapy, I gave her the Greek poem by Kavafis "Ithaka" to read

Therapy

The therapy started on the patient's initiative in June 18. With regard to the transference, the patient is looking for a paternal companion in me, whom she idealises and tries to find answers to her agonising life question with me, just as she idealised her father and leaned on him. I felt invited to start the therapy because I identify with the patient's therapy goal. She wants to slowly wean herself off the medication while having her panic disorder treated psychotherapeutically. This idea of the patient corresponds exactly to how I envision the therapy, namely, to use as little medication as possible so that the underlying conflicts and deficits become more recognisable and thus get the opportunity to understand and work on the conflicts more comprehensively. To strengthen the patient's motivation and better prepare her for the upcoming therapy, I gave her the Greek poem by Kavafis "Ithaka" to read (see Table 7).

The poem reads:If you set out for Ithaca,
I wish you a long journey,
full of adventure and knowledge.
The blasphemers and the Cyclops,
The angry Poseidon fear not,

You will never find such things on your journey,
when your mind is high, when noble
When noble emotion stirs your mind and body.
To the blasphemers and cyclops,
...the furious Poseidon you shall not meet...,
if you do not carry them in your soul,
unless your soul builds them up before you.

After she read it, we discussed it. With the help of this poem, I wanted to tell the patient that (a) she should engage in a deeper therapy. (If you set out for Ithaca, wish yourself a long journey, full of adventure and knowledge.) (b) Moreover, we cause ourselves many conflicts with our view of things. In the poem it says: "You will not meet the blasphemers and cyclops, the angry Poseidon, if you do not carry them with you in your soul, if your soul does not build them up before you" (see Table 8).

After that I explained to her about the therapeutic work, and it is important to grasp the conditions of origin of her panic attacks: "She should pay attention to the feelings and fantasies associated with them, because they give us access to her conflicts. We will look at these conflicts together and solve them". In this sense, Mrs. X is sensitised to the conditions that lead to her panic attacks. The patient wants to understand which factors contributed to the development of her anxiety disorder and which factors maintain her anxiety disorder and how she can free herself from it (see Table 9).

With this in mind, Mrs. X realises that one day she suffers a panic attack while eating spicy food and therefore has to go to the toilet twice. She can observe she gets panic attacks when she believes that "I will vomit". This is the first thought that scares her. The second time the thought: "I have to vomit, and if I vomit, the panic attack won't stop!" The meaning of this fear remains unclear for the time being. What is the patient's real fear? We can't tell from this panic attack what she is really

Table 8 Therapy

The goal of the therapy is to help the patient become more autonomous with both her parents and her husband
In order to accomplish this step, the patient needs to admit to more healthy aggression
To achieve this it is important to grasp the conditions of origin of her panic attacks as suggested by the "panic-focussed psychodynamic psychotherapy": "She should pay attention to the feelings and fantasies on the verge of a panic attack, because they give us access to her conflicts"

Table 9 Therapy

With this in mind, Mrs. X realises that one day she suffers a panic attack while eating spicy food and therefore has to go to the toilet twice. The second time she is going to the toilet she is thinking: "I will vomit, and if I vomit, the panic attack won't stop!"
The meaning of this fear remains unclear for the time being, and we can't tell what she is really afraid of
Another important point in therapy is somatisation. I try to help the patient to become aware of the feelings associated with somatisation so that she can understand herself better

afraid of. Moreover, she came with a clear goal in mind, as mentioned earlier, to stop taking paroxetine. This is because she feels she has lived many years of her life "on crutches" under the influence of the drug. I understood this as an expression of the patient's wish to live or be independent of medication, i.e. as an expression of her anger because she has been dependent on the paroxetine for all these years. In order to strengthen the patient's self-confidence or her sense of autonomy and to reduce the extent of her anxiety, I leave the execution of the reduction of the paroxetine in the patient's hands, which is done in very small steps, but which, from a psychopharmacological point of view, do not make sense. It is important for Mrs. X to determine the dosage herself according to her feelings. She tells me about the individual reduction steps. I confirm her in this. In this first phase of the therapy, Mrs. X discusses her most important relationships in life. Her husband is very patient and calm, and she calms down with him by putting her hand on his chest. She is disappointed in herself because she puts too much strain on her husband because of her panic attacks and because she is horrible to him. She wonders how her husband can love her when she behaves like this! She admits to herself that her husband might even leave her against this background. Once again she realises how close the bond is within her family circle. She tells me, "There are no secrets in our family! If we get on each other's nerves, you say it and it's done!" Based on her life experiences, she says she has learnt that they can only get through life "as a family" that blood is thicker than water. In the episode, she recalls again when her father had brain haemorrhage, and she remembers many details from that time and mourns her father's fate and the fact that he is now in a wheelchair. "It tears my heart out to see how he is today!" I share in the patient's grief and show understanding for the blows of fate she has experienced in her life. I acknowledge their achievement as a family in getting through all that has happened to them. At the same time, I point out to the patient that the roots of her fears of infection by germs are to be found in these early life experiences with the herpes viruses. The patient feels understood to a certain extent, and her motivation for therapy increases. I ask myself, what is the deeper meaning of her explanations? Does she want to tell me at the beginning of the therapy what this therapy is about? That is, she wants to introduce me to all the important others in her life and already now partly unconsciously tells me how difficult it will be for her to detach herself from these important people with the help of therapy. But it can also be understood as an expression of her ambivalence about detachment from all these important others, because she is afraid of the consequent independence. In this phase of the therapy, Mrs. X introduces another important theme in her life, namely, her great ambivalence about having children of her own or not. In this context, she often reports about her contacts with the family of her godchild. She repeatedly describes her experiences with the two small children of the family, whom the patient often cares for. She is also concerned about the relationship between the children's parents. She finally admits to herself that her fear of vomiting is her specific problem, which does not generally burdened others, something she previously denied. In this context, it is noticeable that Mrs. X has problems recognising her feelings. I help her formulate her defensive feelings in therapy. For example, with interpretations like "Your fear of vomiting has to do with repressed feelings!" or if the patient is angry and she herself feels a lump in her throat, the interpretation: "Could it be that the lump in your throat is protection for you so that the anger does not erupt because you have learnt that you must not be angry?" This is because the patient is not aware that the lump in her throat is curbing her anger. Later on, the patient's father falls ill with an inoperable colon tumour, which, however, does not seem to have metastasised so far. In this sense, Mrs. X seeks to draw strength from the therapy to deal with her father's life-threatening illness. She reports in detail about her father's condition during the ongoing chemotherapy and radiation. She feels seen and accepted and is grateful that her concerns are being heard (see Table 10).

Now, despite her fear of losing her mother, she begins to distance herself more consistently after analysing her interactions with her mother through the therapy. Here is an example of this. In therapy she realises that her mother sees herself as "a saint". Because on the basis of a sequence of a telephone conversation with her mother, in which her mother demands of the patient that the patient goes out of her way after work to pick up her mother and take her to the hospital where the patient's father is being treated, the patient becomes aware that her mother is also comfortable taking her for granted. In becoming so, Mrs. X allows her anger towards her mother to show. She admits to herself, "My mother didn't ask me how I was, she wants me to pick her up!" The patient then hangs up on her. She adds, "I thought for 2 minutes", "Why is my mother so selfish? The main thing is that she comes to see my father!" As the patient's capacity for introspection has grown during the course of therapy, it occurs to her during this sequence, "Now comes the guilty conscience because I thought badly about my mother! Everything mum says is right! Says the little Nicole in me! Adult Nicole, however, says it can't be that everything Mama says is right!" The patient recalls, "Momma says with the panic attacks is the devil taking you away from God!" In the free church evangelical congregation, where she had been regularly as a child and teenager, she had learnt that illness was God's punishment! As a result, Mrs. X admits to herself that the perfect image of her mum is falling apart! Her upbringing was not as ideal as she had previously thought! She is angry at herself right now because she is already 33 years old and yet she is not able to distance herself from her mother. She could not say, "That's my mum and that's me!" In this context, Mrs. X expresses her disappointment rage against her parents, who had not protected the patient from the influence of their radical religious community (see Table 11).

Table 10 Therapy

Now, despite her fear of losing her mother, she allows her anger towards her mother to show
As the patient's capacity for introspection has grown during the course of therapy, it occurs to her during this sequence, "Now comes the guilty conscience because I thought badly about my mother!..." As a result, Mrs. X admits to herself that the perfect image of her mum is falling apart!
She is angry at herself right now because she is already 33 years old and yet she is not able to distance herself from her mother

Table 11 Therapy

The patient notices that the more she is upset about this, the greater her fears of vomiting become. She succeeds in becoming aware that her thoughts of vomiting are connected to her need to free herself from her mother
As a result of the therapy, she was able to better distance herself from her parents and became more autonomous
At the end of the therapy, Mrs. X is no longer depressed, and she has an occasional mild panic attack, which she manages herself. Her panic attacks could be successfully treated because Mrs. X's fear of her own anger has clearly diminished

The patient notices that the more she is upset about this, the greater her fears of vomiting become. Nevertheless, she does not succeed in expressing her anger directly against her father. This can be seen in a sequence with her father. Her father is scolding and yelling about the emergency doctor who is late for an accident in the village. The patient hears her father's scolding because she is standing next to him. However, she cannot reprimand her father, although she is very angry with him. For she perceives a voice within herself in the situation: "That's enough! It can't be that he talks like that!" On the other hand, Mrs. X had felt in the situation, "As if my father was grabbing me by throat!" She admits to herself, "I am helpless against this!" For she had learnt, "You shall honour your father and mother!" In this context, Mrs. X recalls once more that her father used to yell at her brother when she herself was a little girl. In that situation she had thought, "Stop it, you're scaring me!" However, she had said nothing to them. So the implication for therapy is that the patient should come to admit and express her anger against significant others, such as her father, despite her fears, even if she develops feelings of guilt in the process. At a later point in the therapy, it also becomes apparent how much the patient, who is trying to detach herself from her parents, is being held tightly by her mother. During a telephone conversation, the patient explained to her mother that the patient now had her own family, whereupon her mother cried and told the patient that her mother only had the patient's father and the neighbour. The patient then develops feelings of guilt, thinking that she is selfish if she wants to lead her own life and is not at the disposal of her family of origin. The patient makes herself aware that after this confrontation with her mother she had the feeling all the time that something bad was about to happen! Mrs. X remembers that when she drank a lot of alcohol with the others as a teenager, her mother always criticised the patient, saying that she had to answer for it herself before God. She then added that the patient had greatly disappointed her mother with her alcohol consumption. This moral reproach had been much worse for the patient than a thousand punishments! Because Mrs. X had been seeking her mother's approval all the time, which she had not received because of her sinful behaviour! In therapy, Mrs. X recognises that she is still courting the approval of important others in her life, e.g. the approval of her husband. She admits to herself that during sex with her husband she fantasises that her mother makes the comment "in the original language": "It's not right!" In this way, the patient succeeds in becoming aware that her thoughts of vomiting are connected to her need to free herself from her mother (see Table 12).

Table 12 Therapy

The patient's conflicts with her husband are revealed, including the issue of having her own children. Mrs. X has come closer to her thoughts regarding this topic. The patient partly admits her anger towards her husband. She begins to defend herself against him

Subsequently, she addresses one of her main issues, namely, "having children". She admits to herself that she does not want to take on the responsibility of having children, not least because this would mean a significant reduction in her quality of life. For example, she and her husband would like to stay in bed late on weekends, which would not be possible if she had small children. I show understanding for her fear, which encourages her to talk more about them. She could not keep the child from the grandparents. Besides, she would make herself dependent on her husband again if she no longer earned any money herself. Finally, she asks herself, "And what if I can't make it any more? What if I get depressed or have panic attacks and can no longer look after the child?" The child would then have to suffer, and it would be the patient's fault. Mrs. X admits to herself that the thought of having children is there, but it is associated with many fears. Furthermore, Mrs. X reports that she now dreams more often. Here is a dream as an example: Her husband had come home from work. He told the patient that everyone at work had stomach flu. He wanted to hug the patient. She rejected him. My interpretation: the deeper meaning of the dream had something to do with sex and getting pregnant, which she was probably afraid of in this scenario too. However, she did not accept my interpretation. According to the patient, this was a manifestation of her hypochondria, which means in this case a fear of infection from close contact with him. She sees in this dream more the restrictions in her life resulting from her hypochondriacal fears. In the further course, the patient realises that her panic attacks are mainly her fear of her own anger against the background of her experiences with her father's outbursts of anger at home. The patient remembers that she had often experienced, for example, that her father had acted out against her older brother in anger and how helpless she had felt in this context and had been afraid for both her father and her brother without being able to do anything about it herself. Similarly, her first panic attack (patient 17) is to be understood as she got angry with her parents because they took away one of her rooms and gave it to her cousin. As a result, her father collapsed with a brain haemorrhage. In the course of therapy, the patient has new experiences with her anger in interactions with other people, and she gradually and increasingly learns to recognise and admit her anger. Moreover, she recognises her tendency to somatise her anger (feeling of a lump in her throat), especially in connection with the clinging attitude of her mother, who, due to self-development of the patient, distances herself from her family of origin in favour of her own family and holds on to the patient more and more. As a result of this recognisable dynamic in the patient's relationship with her own parents, the patient is criticised by her two siblings for breaking away from the family unit, which frightens them because they themselves have not previously taken such steps towards autonomy. She also recognises her tendency to feel guilty readily, which she later relates to her experiences in her extremely religious community. Over time, the patient manages to distance herself to some extent from her decidedly strict conscience. In this way, Mrs. X succeeds in gradually discontinuing the antidepressant she had been taking for so many years and has been able to do without it until today. The patient was definitely able to overcome her inability to work for several days (due to an increase in her symptoms) after stopping paroxetine. Another important issue for the patient, as already mentioned, is having children. This topic preoccupies the patient in the final phase of therapy, which has not yet found a definite answer. The patient's fear in the end of the therapy becomes recognisable on the basis of a conversation with a colleague who talked about the fact that this colleague's sister had wet her pants. From this point of view, the patient's statement becomes more understandable: she was also "terrified" of wetting her pants herself. In this sense, I decide to carefully clarify: "I understand your fear of wetting your pants as fear of the end of the therapy, which is triggered by your colleague's report". Mrs. X feels understood by this intervention, so she speaks of her doubts about whether she can do it alone. She adds, "A back and forth!" In order to boost the patient's ego, I confront her about her successes in therapy so far. She admits to herself that she is happy to be able to deal with things on her own. She reflects on this and realises that she is angry about her dependence on her husband. If he were to leave, she would not be able to cope with life. I gently confront the patient with the thought that perhaps she herself wants to leave and projects her wish onto her husband. She laughs and denies it. However, it stands to reason that Mrs. X must be very angry with her husband, which she admits to herself in a very limited way. For he offends her with his remarks. For example, he tells her, "Knowing what I know today, I wouldn't have married you again today!" In this context, she allows her anger towards her husband: "Then you can go too!" I pick up on this response from the patient and address the conflict with her husband: "I think what is getting at you is the tension with your husband and not your colleague's telling you about her sister!" With this in mind, she admits her anger, "Yesterday when I was walking, I thought I was suffocating in my hatred towards myself!" So once again she realises, "It's hard for me to be angry! Because I think it is not proper to be angry as a woman!" Furthermore, she recognises she feels a strong moral bond towards her husband because he has done so much for her. That is why she does not allow herself to be angry with her husband. In summary, in the final phase of therapy, the patient's conflicts with her husband are revealed, including the issue of having her own children. Mrs. X has come closer to her thoughts regarding this topic, and her husband has not. The patient partly admits her anger towards her husband. This anger is not only the result of her dependence on her husband and her insufficiency to free herself from it but also because her husband repeatedly offends her. The therapy has shown that the patient somatises some of her anger ("lump in the throat", diarrhoea) and directs some of it against herself. However, since Mrs. X has partly succeeded in admitting her anger towards her husband, she begins to defend herself against him. At the end of the therapy, Mrs. X is no longer depressed; she has an occasional mild panic attack, which she manages to control herself. Her panic attacks could be successfully treated because Mrs. X's fear of her own anger has clearly diminished. In this way, she was able to express her pent-up anger, which is related to her previous disappointments through her experiences with her parents, including feeling her dependence on them. This development promoted the detachment from her parents, which the patient achieved. In the foreground of their experience was anger, less grief. (Usually, grief plays a central role in detachment processes.) Her permitted anger became a catalyst so that the patient could overcome her fear of independence to a certain extent, which allowed her to better differentiate herself from her parents and become more autonomous. She became more and more focused on her life with her husband, and their relationship became closer. Nevertheless, she has now become partly more independent in her married life, as I have described above. In the course of the therapy, the patient succeeded in partially loosening her strict conscience, which stems not least from the extremely strict religious education, and she has felt increasingly free in her everyday life. In a catamnesis of 1 and 2 years after the end of therapy, these results were stable.

Psychodynamic Approaches to Social Anxiety Disorder

Fredric N. Busch

Introduction

According to DSM-V (American Psychiatric Association 2013), criteria for social anxiety disorder include the following: (a) marked fear or anxiety about social situations in which the individual is exposed to possible scrutiny by others; (b) the individual fears that he or she will act in a way or show anxiety symptoms in a way that will be negatively evaluated; (c) the social situations almost always provoke fear and anxiety; (d) the social situations are avoided or endured with intense fear or anxiety.; and (e) the fear or anxiety is out of proportion to the actual threat posed by the social situation and to the sociocultural context, amongst other criteria. This disorder can have a significant adverse impact on interpersonal and work relationships.

Social anxiety disorder is associated with temperamental fearfulness, a probable precursor to the disorder. A link has been found between social anxiety disorder and behavioral inhibition in children (Rosenbaum et al. 1991; Biederman et al. 2001), considered a measure of temperamental fearfulness. Inhibited infants and children "…manifested long latencies to interact when exposed to novelty, retreated from the unfamiliar, and ceased play and vocalizations while clinging to their mothers" (Biederman et al. 1990, p. 21). According to DSM-V, childhood maltreatment and adversity are risk factors for social anxiety disorder, though not considered to play a causative role. A study that systematically assessed perceptions of parents found that those with social anxiety perceived their parents as less caring, more rejecting, and more overprotective compared to control subjects (Arrindell et al. 1983), further indicating developmental backgrounds with adverse events or trauma. It is not

F. N. Busch (✉)
Faculty, Weill Cornell Medical College, Columbia University Center for Psychoanalytic Training and Research, New York, NY, USA
e-mail: fnb2001@med.cornell.edu

C. Charis, G. Panayiotou (eds.), *Anxiety Disorders and Related Conditions*,
https://doi.org/10.1007/978-3-031-56798-8_9

clear on what basis the DSM-V concludes that these factors are not causative, as they likely predispose to fearfulness of others.

Temperamental fearfulness and early life stressors have a significant impact on the psychological development and dynamics of these patients. It can lead them to a view of themselves as inadequate, shameful, and unworthy, while they tend to experience others as judgmental and threatening. These self and other representations contribute to feelings of low self-esteem and an expectation of humiliation and rejection. Feelings of inadequacy can heighten attachment fears, creating a sense of incapability, threats surrounding autonomy, and difficulty tolerating angry feelings. Exhibitionistic and grandiose fantasies and wishes, which are often conflicted (Fenichel 1945), can develop in an unconscious effort to compensate for feelings of low self-esteem and inadequacy. Clarification of these dynamisms, which are described in greater depth below, can aid in treating patients who suffer from social anxiety disorder.

A Psychodynamic Formulation for Social Anxiety Disorder

A psychodynamic formulation identifies the contexts and emotions surrounding the triggering of symptoms, associated self and other representations, developmental history, relevant intrapsychic conflicts, defenses, and mentalization impairments involved with a particular disorder or problem (Busch 2021; Perry et al. 1987). A formulation for social anxiety disorder, described below, identifies several dynamic contributing factors, which can then be used as a basis for targeting interventions (Busch et al. 2012). In an individual case, some or all of the various dynamics may contribute to symptoms, and the therapist works to determine the formulation for that particular patient.

Emotions and Contexts Surrounding Symptoms

By definition patients with social anxiety disorder have symptoms triggered by social contexts. Overall, these consist of circumstances in which the patient's fears of being inadequate, humiliated, or rejected are triggered. However, the therapist works to identify for each patient what kinds of events are considered threatening and are avoided, which vary according to their particular history and dynamics. Furthermore, patients may have other emotional reactions to social situations, such as anger or feelings of superiority, that intermix with their social fears.

Self and Other Representations

Patients with social anxiety disorder typically have feelings of low self-esteem and anticipate being rejected or humiliated by others. These fears contribute to representations of themselves as inadequate and shameful and others as rejecting and judgmental. Thus, typical social situations become suffused with the risks of humiliation and criticism, contributing to intense anxiety and often avoidance. Patients may also see themselves as incapable and in need of others for a sense of safety and view others as anxious and overprotective. Finally, patients may have representations of themselves as special and others as admiring or submitting to them in the form of grandiose fantasies.

Developmental History

Identifying the origins of social fears helps patients understand how they developed low self-esteem, conflicted angry feelings, and compensatory grandiose and exhibitionistic fantasies. Patients often report adverse developmental events in which caregivers behaved in rejecting or critical ways, with little tolerance of the child's anger (Arrindell et al. 1983). Clarification of how patients have internalized these negative self and other representations can help determine how patients misperceive the danger of current social situations. They can also help identify the origins of compensatory grandiose and exhibitionistic fantasies, which often develop in childhood, and recognize the guilt they trigger.

Intrapsychic Conflicts

The identification of conflicts patients have about wishes and fantasies is a crucial component of psychodynamic psychotherapy (Freud 1926). Wishes for autonomy can become a source of conflict for patients with social anxiety disorder. Feelings of inadequacy and expectations of social rejection can create fears of being unable to function independently. Overprotective behavior by caregivers can create a sense that attachment figures are essential for effective functioning. These perceptions can add to a feeling that caregivers are unable to tolerate their independence. Socializing can therefore be experienced, often unconsciously, as betraying or disrupting relationships with important people in patients' lives. Regressive fantasies of helplessness are triggered, which further increase social anxiety and avoidance.

Patients can develop intensely angry feelings and fantasies toward others they perceive as rejecting and humiliating and fear that their anger will pose a threat to essential attachment figures (Busch et al. 2012). A sense of helplessness and incompetence, associated with low self-esteem, can further intensify anger at caregivers perceived as contributing to these feelings. Self-representations of incompetence and inadequacy can function defensively to ease threats from aggressive feelings and fantasies and diminish others' perceptions of the individual as being hostile and threatening.

When social fears are explored in greater depth, grandiose fantasies often emerge as a source of conflict, sometimes associated with sexually exhibitionistic wishes (Fenichel 1945; Gabbard 1992, 2000; Kaplan 1972; Zerbe 1994; Lipsitz and Marshall 2001). These fantasies often represent efforts to compensate for feelings of inadequacy and fears of humiliation. When these fantasies emerge, they typically trigger guilt and further expectations of punishment, increasing social anxiety and avoidance. However, grandiose fantasies, along with wishes to be treated as special or important, often cause disappointment and anger in actual social situations, increasing feelings of inadequacy and rejection.

Defenses

Patients with social anxiety disorder are prone to particular defenses (Freud 1946), including denial, projection, and identification with the aggressor, particularly in response to conflicted angry feelings and fantasies. Patients may deny angry feelings in an unconscious effort to protect against the dangers they associate with them. Anger that is denied may be projected and experienced as coming from others, leading others to be perceived as more judgmental or threatening, increasing fears of rejection and criticism. Socially anxious patients with grandiose compensatory fantasies may also demonstrate identification with the aggressor. In this defense patients may fantasize about being in control and possibly critical of others in the ways they experienced with caregivers and/or other authority figures. These wishes to dominate others may contribute to guilt about grandiose fantasies.

Mentalization Impairments

Mentalization refers to patients' capacities to understand their own mind and the mind of others (Fonagy and Target 1997). In social anxiety disorder, patients' mentalization skills are impaired by their convictions that they are inadequate and that others will view them critically or judgmentally. Therefore they find it difficult to consider that they may be misperceiving what others are experiencing, making it difficult to reevaluate these perceptions.

Thus several dynamic factors contribute to social anxiety and avoidance. Social avoidance can function to manage feelings of inadequacy, low self-esteem, and fears of rejection and humiliation associated with social anxiety. Patients also fear that social activity will lead to a disruption of their relationships with significant attachment figures. Social avoidance can ease the threats associated with the experience and expression of anger while partially expressing unconscious contempt. Compensatory grandiose and exhibitionistic wishes may relieve aspects of social inadequacy but can lead to a drop in self-esteem in social settings. Social avoidance can function as a defense against conflicted aggressive, sexually exhibitionistic, and grandiose wishes, and expectations of rejection and humiliation can represent a punishment for these wishes.

Social Anxiety and Avoidance Focused Psychodynamic Psychotherapy

Psychodynamic psychotherapy that addresses social anxiety and avoidance can be viewed as operating within the principles of problem-focused psychodynamic psychotherapy (Busch 2021). In this approach the therapist works to elaborate a psychodynamic formulation, including contexts and emotions surrounding symptoms, self and other representations, developmental contributors, conflicts and defenses, and mentalization skills. In the course of therapy, patients become aware that their fears derive from feelings of inadequacy, low self-esteem, conflicted anger, attachment threats, and guilt-ridden grandiose fantasies. Social anxiety is diminished as patients become able to identify contributory representations and conflicts and as their feelings and fantasies become detoxified. Therapists do not directly instruct patients to confront feared social situations but do explore contributors to avoidance, including what patients anticipate will happen if they attempt to do so. As psychodynamic exploration leads to reduced fears, patients become more willing to confront situations they have been avoiding. The therapist can explore persistent dangers patients experience in taking a more active role in their lives.

Identifying Contexts and Emotions Surrounding Symptoms

Initial therapeutic efforts are focused on elaborating the specific nature of the patient's symptoms and the contexts and emotional states that trigger or exacerbate them. Although patients with social anxiety disorder routinely experience feelings of social inadequacy and expectations of humiliation and rejection, the therapist works to identify specific symptoms and situations that trigger anxiety. For example, some individuals may feel safer in larger groups but fearful in more intimate situations or vice versa. Obtaining this information will help identify the emotional meanings of these symptoms, helping to ease the specific dangers patients feel in social contexts.

Clarifying and Addressing Self and Other Representations

The therapist works to elaborate the representations patients have of themselves and others, particularly as it relates to social contexts. Typically, these perceptions involve viewing themselves as inadequate and shameful and others as rejecting and critical. Therapists work to address feelings of low self-esteem and inadequacy that stem from patients' overly negative view of themselves and their anticipation of severe and harsh reactions of others. Therapists can identify how these views of self and others are harsh and excessive and the importance of understanding the meanings and origins of these conceptions in order to combat them. The experience of therapy, with the nonjudgmental and empathic support of the therapist, can aid patients in the development of more benign or supportive representations of themselves and others.

Developmental Interpretations

Therapists work to link symptoms and self/other representations to their developmental origins, helping patients identify the sources of their social fears. The therapist explores adverse developmental events, including patients' descriptions of their experiences with caretakers, that may have contributed to feelings of inadequacy and anxiety. These interventions help identify how patients overestimate the danger of current social situations based on their prior experiences. Therapists also work to determine contributors to compensatory grandiose and exhibitionistic fantasies, helping to reduce the guilt and disappointment they trigger.

Addressing Conflicted Feelings and Fantasies

The therapist works to elaborate and address conflicts involving autonomous, angry, and grandiose fantasies. Therapists identify the dangers that autonomy can present, including the threat of rejection by and loss of significant attachment figures and how social avoidance helps protect against these threats. An additional component of psychodynamic treatment is helping patients to become aware of, more tolerant of, and more able to express their various angry feelings and fantasies. Patients may associate self-assertion with anger, causing it to feel disorganizing, threatening, and sometimes intolerable. Therapists work to identify that patients' angry feelings and fantasies are understandable and less dangerous and toxic than they believe. As this work progresses, patients feel safer expressing anger and disappointment with others, including the therapist, allowing them to test out their fears of disruption.

Fantasies of grand power and being the center of attention often emerge in therapy. Patients tend to minimize the importance of these fantasies, given their manifest preoccupation with feelings of inadequacy. Therapists work to identify that these fantasies typically have an adverse impact on patients, causing guilt and disappointment, and work to connect them with the origins of their social anxiety. The therapist can explore these wishes and conflicts about them as they emerge in treatment and highlight their functions, including efforts to compensate for feelings of inadequacy. The patient comes to recognize that grandiose fantasies also represent high expectations that trigger anxiety and disappointment in social situations.

Addressing Defenses

In order to help gain access to areas of conflict, including angry feelings and fantasies, therapists point out that patients may *deny* these feelings because of their fear of disrupting relationships. In addition to this denial, therapists identify how angry feelings can become *projected* onto others, leading the patient to perceive an even more critical response. Therapists will assess and communicate to patients if they demonstrate *identification with the aggressor*, in which patients fantasize or act out wishes to control and dominate others, often triggering intense guilty reactions. These interpretations of defenses help patients better gain access to unconscious feelings and fantasies and detoxify them by reevaluating the perceived danger.

Addressing Mentalization Deficits

As noted above, patients' mentalization capacities are disrupted by their conviction that others will view them critically or judgmentally. The therapist helps patients identify this rigidity in their expectations and consider that they may be incorrect in their assumptions. They can point out that patients cannot be sure how others feel about them and that it is important to consider other possibilities other than negative reactions, working to expand their mentalization capacities. The transference represents another area where these notions can be examined, as patients often anticipate that therapists will be similarly judgmental.

Addressing the Transference

People with social phobia often anticipate they will be criticized or rejected by the therapist in a similar way that they expect will occur in other social situations. The transference (Freud 1905) provides a direct means of exploration of these fantasies as they emerge with the therapist. Fears of humiliation or ridicule projected on to their therapist may cause patients to avoid or skip sessions or even to leave treatment. They also anticipate criticism or punishment for their often secret grand and exhibitionistic fantasies, which they can be reluctant to reveal. Patients worry that they will be attacked for critical feelings and fantasies they have about the therapist. The therapist helps patients feel safe expressing these angry feelings and fantasies, working to reduce conflicts about them. The exploration of the transference allows for more direct identification of these fears and helps patients recognize ways in which their expectations of humiliation and criticism color other relationships.

Countertransference

Therapists must be alert to feelings of criticism or frustration that may occur in working with patients with social anxiety disorder. Frustration can be triggered by the pervasiveness of their feelings of inadequacy and incompetence and by the difficulty they have addressing these symptoms. Covert expression of angry feelings can lead to subtle criticisms by the therapist that can intensify patients' feelings of inadequacy. In addition, therapists should remain alert to their reaction to patients' anger toward them, to help them better address these conflicts. The therapist can use their reactions to understand what patients may be unconsciously provoking in others. Monitoring these reactions can also help maintain the therapist's nonjudgmental stance, which plays an important role in modifying negative, tormenting self and other representations.

Termination

In psychodynamic psychotherapy termination presents an opportunity to address persistent dynamic factors and further the gains of treatment (Gabbard 2009). Patients' feelings about separation from the therapist can be explored and addressed in the transference. In treatment of social phobic patients, angry reactions to termination and its meaning in terms of greater autonomy and independence can emerge, providing an opportunity to further detoxify these feelings and fantasies. In a problem-focused psychodynamic psychotherapy, therapists also work with patients to assess the extent of relief of symptoms and address remaining areas of difficulty. The goal is to leave treatment with a reduction and detoxification of negative feelings and fantasies, a greater awareness of contributing dynamics, and the use of skills to manage contributors to anxiety and avoidance.

Case Example

Mr. P, a 48-year-old lawyer, experienced intense anxiety in social settings and at work, fearing he would be judged or criticized for being inadequate or ineffective. He felt he was being pressured by others to perform and that he could not meet their expectations. He avoided others for fear of being reprimanded by them for some shortcoming. Stomach pains often accompanied his anxiety, and it emerged that he feared vomiting, which he would find terribly humiliating. He worried that something would disrupt the relationship with his boss or that a view of him as incompetent would lead to his being fired, threatening his financial security. His anxiety had even increased with his wife; she became more critical of him after their second child finished college and left home, leaving an empty nest. At the same time that he felt inadequate, he had fantasies of being the lead partner at the firm, in charge and in control of others. He would imagine himself giving orders to others, who might be fearful of him. He was evaluated, and the therapist recommended a weekly problem-focused psychodynamic psychotherapy that targeted his anxiety socially and at work.

The therapist explored Mr. P's background to gain a better sense of the origins of his anxiety. He recalled his parents having intense fights, often about his father's frequent absences from the home, and they divorced when he was age 8. He lived for the most part with his mother, and they struggled to make ends meet, in part because his father did not keep up his child support payments. He described his mother as a worrier, often warning him about going out, indicating he was safest being at home. In addition, she expressed anxiety and frustration about their financial situation. When he visited his father's house, it was evident that his father led a much more comfortable lifestyle. His mother remarried when he was 15, and he came to hate his stepfather. He saw him as inadequate because he was chronically unemployed and spent hours watching television and drinking beer, leading his mother to complain about being "alone." The patient felt some pressure to be at home to keep his mother company, though he did spend time with friends.

His relationship with his father alternated between severe criticism and neglect. When his father occasionally visited him at his mother's home, he would walk in unexpectedly and often reprimand the patient for being lazy, saying, "Why aren't you doing homework?" He chronically worried his father would catch him resting on the couch or playing games, despite the infrequency of his visits. His father even lambasted him for playing a complex strategy game, which Mr. P believed nurtured the development of his legal strategy skills. He would feel both humiliated and enraged by his father. He also worried about being financially dependent on him and believed that if he expressed too much irritation his father would withdraw support. His father was otherwise preoccupied with his business ventures and was involved in a series of relationships with women.

Mr. P's only persistently positive relationships growing up were with a close friend and his friend's family, whom he considered more "normal." Mr. P began to rebel in high school by smoking pot, avoiding schoolwork, and playing in a band. Although he still feared his father's reprimands, these worries were mitigated by his father's increasing absences. Looking back, he saw it as a way of expressing his anger and attempting to engage his father's attention in a provocative manner. However, he also felt badly about "screwing up" in school. Despite his rebellion, which he hoped would make him look "cool," he felt intense insecurity and social anxiety in groups and with girls, heightening his feelings of inadequacy.

The therapist identified how Mr. P's current fears and their triggers paralleled his experience of attacks by his father. He expected to be viewed as lazy and ineffective and worried his boss would walk into his office and reprimand him just as his father did. He feared being intruded upon or pressured, particularly from demands made by his boss and his wife. His fears of being fired linked to financial fears and his dependency on his father. The therapist pointed out how his actual performance at the job and promotion made this outcome unlikely: He had received strong reviews and had a recent promotion.

His self and other representations primarily consisted of viewing himself as inadequate and lazy and others as critical and attacking. At the same time, he muted his anger at others for what he experienced or anticipated to be unfair criticism, fearing he would be attacked for expressing it, an indication of significant conflict about these feelings. Therapist and patient identified he would become anxious in situations where he felt frustrated with others, such as when employees he managed did not complete their tasks, as he feared losing his temper and causing a disruption. The therapist linked this conflict to anger at his father, which was expressed indirectly via rebelliousness against "the establishment." In addition, he feared expressing anger in the same hurtful way his father did. It emerged that he felt guilty about his grandiose fantasies of being in control of others and their being frightened of him, a form of identification with the aggressor. The therapist worked with Mr. P in reevaluating the actual risks of his getting angry, particularly given that he was careful about how he expressed it.

In examining Mr. P's gastrointestinal symptoms, the therapist indicated that these somatic states were psychologically meaningful. In fact, several physical gastrointestinal evaluations found no evidence of medical issues. These symptoms represented his fears of being out of control and humiliated, paralleling his fears regarding his father. In addition, there was an aspect of fears of lack of control of his aggression, regarding a wish to "vomit on" others. Recognition of the origins of these symptoms helped him feel less threatened by these risks. Indeed, actual vomiting turned out to be a rare event.

The therapist identified how Mr. P's anxiety about others attacking him interfered with his capacity to consider their motives, increasing his anticipation of negative judgments. For example, he would fear that his associates working for him might be looking to criticize his behavior, projecting his own anger, not recognizing that they often were fearful of him or hoped to impress him. These fears also emerged in the transference, as Mr. P anticipated that the therapist would reject him as well. Exploration revealed that he worried the therapist would see him as incapable of being able to make progress in therapy. Indeed, he anticipated that the therapist might end his therapy or send him to a new therapist for not addressing his difficulties more assertively. The therapist pointed out that these beliefs demonstrated the pervasiveness of his fears, as the therapist was there to help the patient, not evaluate his progress and fire him if necessary like a boss at a job.

The therapist also interpreted that Mr. P's grandiose fantasies compensated for his feelings of insecurity by engaging in long-standing wishes to be in charge of others. Although he did manage a group of people, he was disappointed he was not the "big boss," adding to his feelings of inadequacy. The therapist identified how these fantasies, while in some way providing relief, continued to drive unrealistic expectations and recurrent disappointment in his accomplishments.

As this work progressed, Mr. P's social fears began to decrease, as he recognized that others were less judgmental than he believed, particularly given his success at work. In addition, he understood that his frustration with others was less likely to disrupt his relationships than he thought. At this point he developed the belief that the therapist was threatened by his increasing capability and autonomy and would warn him about potential dangers of being competent. The therapist linked this to the patient's struggle with his mother's warnings about leaving the house and the sense that she needed him to be at home. This understanding further aided in moving toward greater feelings of safety and social competence.

The patient's feelings of increased competence and reduced social anxiety and avoidance led to a discussion of termination. This phase allowed for additional working through of the patient's self and other representations, conflicts, and defenses. Mr. P had a resurgence of fears that he would be unable to manage without the therapist and his gains would fall apart. This related to early feelings of insecure attachment and the difficulty developing an internal sense of safety, as his mother often labeled the world as dangerous. However, identifying that the patient had been effectively managing multiple social and work situations helped ease these fears. Mr. P then had the onset of worries that the therapist was terminating treatment as a rejection of him, even though termination was mutually agreed upon, which the therapist linked to the feelings of rejection by his father. Additional anger and sadness about the increasing distance from his father as he grew older emerged, with the patient able to recognize that he was misattributing this to the therapist. Indeed, the pervasive threat of rejection he was anticipating throughout his life was not occurring in his actual life, as he increasingly recognized that this fear derived from experiences in his past and conflicts that developed about them. Indeed, tensions with his wife eased as well, as he more directly addressed her concerns and frustrations.

Research on Psychodynamic Treatment of Social Anxiety Disorder

Short-term, manualized, psychodynamic therapy has been found to be effective for the treatment of social anxiety disorder in randomized controlled trials, with superior response rates compared to wait-list or placebo groups (Knijnik et al. 2004; Leichsenring et al. 2013, 2014; Bogels et al. 2014; Leichsenring and Lewek 2017) and similar to those treated with CBT (Bogels et al. 2014; Leichsenring et al. 2013, 2014). Leichsenring et al. (2013) compared patients with social anxiety disorder (SAD), treated with either manualized CBT, supportive expressive therapy (SET), or a wait-list control. In supportive-expressive therapy (Luborsky 1984), the therapist formulates and targets a "core conflictual relationship theme," (CCRT) which identifies the patient's wish, the other's response, and the self's response. CBT and dynamic therapy response and remission rates were superior to that of the wait-list control. CBT was superior to SET in remission rates, but the difference was no longer significant at follow-ups of 6, 12, and 24 months. Bogels et al. (2014) compared patients with SAD treated with psychodynamic psychotherapy (PDT) or CBT. Treatments were effective (over 50% remission rates), with no differences found between PDT and CBT. A recent meta-analysis of studies by Zhang et al. (2022) further indicated that psychodynamic therapy was effective in treating social anxiety disorder.

Discussion

Thus psychodynamic psychotherapy is an approach that has demonstrated efficacy in the treatment of social anxiety disorder. Although not systematically studied, we have found in treatment of panic disorder that a problem-focused approach contributes to this efficacy, as it highlights and addresses the dynamics of the particular disorder (Keefe et al. 2018). In a problem-focused approach, the core dynamics surrounding social anxiety disorder, involving representations of oneself as inadequate and others as critical, conflicts surrounding anger, autonomy and grandiose wishes, the defenses of denial and projection, and mentalization disruptions, are defined and addressed as contributors to symptoms. Termination provides an additional opportunity to address these dynamics, particularly surrounding conflicts with anger and autonomy as they emerge in the transference. The treatment targets both relief of symptoms, addressing potential reemergence of symptoms and conflicts.

References

American Psychiatric Association: Diagnostic and Statistical Manual of Mental Disorders, 5th Edition. Washington, DC, American Psychiatric Association, 2013

Arrindell, W., Emmelkamp. P.M.G., Monsma, A., & Brilman, E. (1983). The role of perceived parental rearing practices in the etiology of phobic disorders: a controlled study. *British Journal of Psychiatry,* 143, 183–187.

Biederman, J., Hirshfeld-Becker, D.R., Rosenbaum, J.F., Hérot, C., Friedman, D., Snidman, N., Kagan, J., & Faraone, S.V. (2001). Further evidence of association between behavioral inhibition and social anxiety in children. *American Journal of Psychiatry*. 158(10),1673–1679

Biederman, J., Rosenbaum, J.F., Hirshfeld, D.R., Faraone, S.V., Bolduc, E.A., Gersten, M., Meminger, S.R., Kagan, J., Snidman, N., & Reznick, J.S. (1990). Psychiatric correlates of behavioral inhibition in young children of parents with and without psychiatric disorders *Archives of General Psychiatry* 47, 21–26

Bögels SM, Wijts P, Oort FJ, et al: Psychodynamic psychotherapy versus cognitive behavior therapy for social anxiety disorder: an efficacy and partial effectiveness trial. Depress Anxiety 2014; 31: 363–373

Busch, F.N. Problem Focused Psychodynamic Psychotherapy. Arlington, VA, American Psychiatric Press, 2021.
Busch, F.N., Milrod, B.L., Singer, M. and Aronson, A. Panic-Focused Psychodynamic Psychotherapy, eXtended Range. New York, NY: Routledge, 2012
Fenichel, O. (1945). *The psychoanalytic theory of neurosis*. New York, WW Norton
Fonagy P, Target M: Attachment and reflective function: their role in self-organization. Dev Psychopathol 1997; 9: 679–700
Freud, A. The Ego and the Mechanisms of Defense. New York, International Universities Press, 1946
Freud S: Fragment of an analysis of a case of hysteria (1905), in Standard Edition of the Complete Psychological Works of Sigmund Freud, Vol 7. Translated and edited by Strachey J. London, Hogarth Press, 1953, pp 3–122
Freud S: Inhibitions, symptoms and anxiety (1926), in Standard Edition of the Complete Psychological Works of Sigmund Freud, Vol 20. Translated and edited by Strachey J. London, Hogarth Press, 1959, pp 77–175
Gabbard, G.O. (1992). Psychodynamics of panic disorder and social phobia. *Bulletin of the Menninger Clinic,* 56 (2, supplement A), A3–A13
Gabbard, G.O. (2000). *Psychodynamic psychiatry in clinical practice, third edition*. Washington, DC, American Psychiatric Press.
Gabbard GO: What is a "good enough" termination? J Am Psychoanal Assoc 57(3):575–594, 2009
Kaplan, D.M. (1972). On shyness. *International Journal of Psychoanalysis*, 53, 439–454.
Keefe JR, Solomonov N, Derubeis RJ, Phillips AC, Busch FN, Barber JP, Chambless DL, Milrod BL. (2018) Focus is key: Panic-focused interpretations are associated with symptomatic improvement in panic-focused psychodynamic psychotherapy. Psychother Res. 18: 1–12
Knijnik DZ, Kapczinski F, Chachamovich E, Margis R, Eizirik CL. Psychodynamic group treatment for generalized social phobia. Rev Bras Psiquiatr 2004; 26:77–81. (In Portuguese).
Leichsenring F, Leweke F.N Social anxiety disorder. Engl J Med. 2017 Jun 8;376(23):2255–2264.
Leichsenring F, Salzer S, Beutel ME, et al. Long-term outcome of psychodynamic therapy and cognitive-behavioral therapy in social anxiety disorder. Am J Psychiatry 2014; 171: 1074–82.
Leichsenring F, Salzer S, Beutel ME, et al: Psychodynamic therapy and cognitive-behavioral therapy in social anxiety disorder: a multicenter randomized controlled trial. Am J Psychiatry 2013; 170: 759–767
Lipsitz, J.D., & Marshall, R.D. (2001), Alternative psychotherapy approaches for social anxiety disorder. *Psychiatric Clinics of North America,* 24, 817–829.
Luborsky L: Principles of Psychoanalytic Psychotherapy: A Manual for Supportive-Expressive Treatment. New York, Basic Books, 1984
Perry S, Cooper AM & Michels R. The psychodynamic formulation: its purpose, structure, and clinical application. Am J Psychiatry, 144, 543–550, 1987
Rosenbaum, J.F., Biederman, J., Hirshfeld, D.R., Bolduc, E.A., Faraone, S.J., Kagan, J., Snidman, N., & Reznick, J.S. (1991). Further evidence of an association between behavioral inhibition and anxiety disorders: results from a family study of children from a non-clinical sample. *Journal of Psychiatric Research*, 25, 49–65
Zerbe, K.J. (1994). Uncharted waters: Psychodynamic considerations in the diagnosis and treatment of social phobia. *Bulletin of the Menninger Clinic*; 58: (2, supplement A), A3–20.
Zhang Q, Yi, P, Song, G, Kangkang, X, Wang, Y, Liu, J, Chen, Z, Zhang, H, Ma, L, Liu, W, Li, X. The efficacy of psychodynamic therapy for social anxiety disorder—A comprehensive meta-analysis. Psychiatry Research, 2022-03-01, Volume 309

A Conceptual Review of Models and Findings Regarding Attention Bias for Social Anxiety

Klavdia Neophytou and Georgia Panayiotou

Social anxiety disorder (SAD) is a prevalent psychological disorder that affects approximately 13.3% of individuals (Barlow and Durand 2000). It is characterized by an intense fear of negative evaluation by others in social situations (APA 2013). SAD is the second most common psychological disorder in the general US population and the second most common anxiety disorder in Europe (Kessler et al. 2005; Wittchen et al. 2011). The disorder is associated with low quality of life, an increased risk for the development of additional psychopathology and economic costs stemming from disorder effects such as work absenteeism and healthcare utilization (Stein and Kean 2000; Schneier et al. 1992; Stuhldreher et al. 2014). DSM-5 distinguishes two main groups of individuals with SAD: those with primarily public performance or public speaking fears and those with general social fears (Kessler et al. 2014). However, most individuals with SAD experience both types of fears. General social fears are more persistent, have a greater impact on individuals' lives and have higher comorbidity with other disorders (Kessler et al. 2014). If left untreated, SAD can have a chronic and disabling course (Dewit et al. 1999).

Cognitive-behavioural therapy (CBT) is an evidence-based treatment for SAD and is considered the most effective for adults (Albano and DiBartolo 2007). However, a high percentage of individuals do not seek treatment due to reasons that include perceived stigmatization, biased beliefs about therapists, lack of willingness to discuss personal issues with strangers, concerns about confidentiality, lack of knowledge about appropriate services and their effectiveness and practical obstacles (Brown et al. 2006; Griffiths and Christensen 2007; Taylor and Luce 2003; Titov et al. 2008). In addition, the characteristics of SAD, such as avoidance and fear of

K. Neophytou (✉) · G. Panayiotou
Department of Psychology and Center for Applied Neuroscience, University of Cyprus, Nicosia, Cyprus
e-mail: neophytou.klavdia@ucy.ac.cy

C. Charis, G. Panayiotou (eds.), *Anxiety Disorders and Related Conditions*,
https://doi.org/10.1007/978-3-031-56798-8_10

negative evaluation, further deter individuals from seeking treatment (Cuijpers and Schuurmans 2007).

Attention bias modification therapy (ABMT) is a new treatment that showed promise in early investigations, as it has been proposed to overcome many of the above-mentioned obstacles. ABMT is a computerized intervention that aims to reduce anxiety by changing attentional processes, specifically by redirecting the attention of socially anxious individuals away from negative faces. SAD, like other anxiety disorders, involves attention biases, which refer to the preferential allocation of attention to disorder-congruent stimuli (i.e. threatening faces) compared to disorder- incongruent stimuli (Pergamin-Hight et al. 2015). Attention, the process that ABMT targets, refers to a cognitive process, which allows the brain to prioritize specific stimuli for elaboration (Shechner et al. 2012).

Attention biases (AB) in anxiety more generally interfere with normal stimulus processing and play a role in maintaining the disorder. They can include hypervigilance to threat, attentional avoidance and difficulty in disengagement from threat. *Hypervigilance* is the 'preference' of allocation of attention to threat relative to neutral stimuli (Bögels and Mansell 2004; Cisler and Koster 2010). This means that the threatening stimuli can be identified easier and quicker than neutral (Cisler et al. 2009). *Attentional avoidance* of threatening stimuli is considered to happen when attention is directed away from threatening stimuli (Cisler and Koster 2010). Finally, *difficulty in disengagement* refers to a delayed withdrawal of attention from a threatening stimulus towards a different task, because of the former's ability to hold attention (Clarke et al. 2013), although it has been considered as an adaptive and normal process by some theorists (Moriya and Tanno 2011).

Theoretical models of anxiety all emphasize the importance of AB as key processes in maintaining anxiety (see Table 1), and numerous studies have provided evidence in support of this assertion (Bar-Haim et al. 2007). However, existing models vary in their emphasis on specific types of attentional biases and their interaction with anxiety levels. Most models on the role of AB in anxiety focus on the facilitated attention to threat that characterizes anxious individuals, i.e. on

Table 1 Theoretical models of attention biases in anxiety

Attention processes included in model	Models
Facilitated attention to threat and difficulty in disengagement	Bar-Haim et al. (2007) Beck and Clark (1997) Eysenck et al. (2007) Rapee and Heimberg (1997)
Facilitated attention to threat	Matthews and Mackintosh (1998) Mogg and Bradley (1998) Ohman (1996) Wells and Matthews (1994) Clark and Wells (1995) (self-focused attention)
Facilitated attention to threat in HTA and attention avoidance in LTA	Williams et al. (1988)

Note: *HTA* highly trait-anxious individuals, *LTA* low trait-anxious individuals hypervigilance. This facilitated attention is based on the perceived importance or threatening value of the stimulus that occurs in interaction with state and trait anxiety levels (Bar-Haim et al. 2007; Eysenck et al. 2007; Matthews and Mackintosh 1998; Mogg and Bradley 1998; Ohman 1996; Williams et al. 1988).

Theoretical Models of Attention Biases in Anxiety

Attentional control theory by Eysenck et al. (2007) suggests that anxiety in normal populations affects central executive functions, interrupting the function of two central processes related to attentional control: inhibition and shifting. Inhibition refers to the ability to regulate automatic responses, while shifting refers to the ability to switch attention between tasks. In both cases, anxious individuals show an increase in stimulus-driven attention, meaning that both external, such as threatening task-irrelevant distractors, and internal stimuli, such as worrisome thoughts that are perceived as threatening, can distract them during a task. This distraction is manifested as disrupted inhibition, making it difficult for individuals to demonstrate top-down regulatory control (or goal-driven attention). Additionally, anxiety disrupts shifting, meaning that the impact of the bottom-up process of stimulus-driven attention is increased, resulting in a decreased ability to voluntarily shift attention from one task to another. These disruptions lead to both difficulty in disengaging from a distracting stimulus, such as a threat during a task, and facilitated detection of threat. Difficulty in disengagement from and vigilance to threat are observed in anxiety disorders as well as in typical populations with increased trait anxiety.

According to Bar-Haim et al. (2007), a multidimensional model can be employed to elucidate the mechanisms underlying AB. The model comprises of several stages. First, an incoming stimulus is evaluated by the pre-attentive threat evaluation system (PTES), whereby individuals with anxiety tend to automatically perceive a benign or mildly threatening stimulus as highly threatening. If the stimulus is evaluated as low threatening, the individual continues with their task and ignores the stimulus. However, if the stimulus is deemed highly threatening, the individual's resource allocation system (RAS) causes them to interrupt their current activity, direct their attention towards the threat and become physiologically aroused. Biases arise in the RAS of anxious individuals, who tend to allocate attention even to mild threats.

After initial evaluation, the guided threat evaluation system (GTES) is activated. At this stage, anxious individuals assess the context of the threat, compare it with prior memories and learning and evaluate their coping resources. If GTES evaluates the threat as low, the alert state relaxes, allowing the individual to focus on current goals. However, anxious individuals may still perceive a stimulus as highly threatening even if prior learning or coping skills suggest otherwise. Despite recognizing that their anxiety is irrational, individuals with anxiety may find it difficult to terminate physiological arousal due to deficiencies in the overriding mechanism (RAS), which would have relaxed the alert state when the stimulus was non-threatening. If GTES evaluates the threat as high, a state of high anxiety ensues.

In addition to vigilance to threat, some models suggest the presence of attentional avoidance (Mogg and Bradley 1998; Williams et al. 1988). Williams et al. (1988) proposed that individuals with lower anxiety exhibit attentional avoidance instead of vigilance to threat, but the model does not specify how this is possible and how it is affected by the level of threat value. On the other hand, Mogg and Bradley (1998) acknowledge that AB is a typical process in anxiety but suggest that individuals may exhibit attentional avoidance at lower levels of anxiety or when confronted with a moderately threatening stimulus.

Another dimension of AB addressed in various models is the degree of automaticity. Some models suggest that attentional biases are automatic in nature (Williams et al. 1988), while others propose that they are both automatic and voluntary/strategic (Matthews and Mackintosh 1998; Ohman 1996). For example, the cognitive model of anxiety (Beck and Clark 1997) suggests that biases during the initial evaluation of stimuli are automatic but can be influenced by voluntary or strategic processes. Specifically, the early detection of threat operates outside of conscious awareness and activates a primal threat mode, which aims to minimize threat. This mechanism is comprised of various automatic and strategic processes, including initial appraisal of the stimulus, hypervigilance for threat and negative automatic thoughts, even if it is largely driven by the stimulus itself. Following an initial perception, individuals with anxiety display a schema-driven processing of threat, known as secondary elaboration, which is slow and effortful and involves reappraisal of the stimulus context and coping strategies. Therefore, according to this model, while early attention to threat is largely automatic, the later difficulty in disengagement from threat is strategic in nature.

In contrast, Wells and Matthews (1994) propose a self-regulatory executive function model, which emphasizes the role of top-down processes in attention control and AB. According to this model, individuals are guided towards threat by self-knowledge, voluntary goals and beliefs. AB is seen as a result of a voluntary threat-monitoring strategy, where anxiety involves conscious perception of a stimulus as threatening followed by monitoring of the threat in order to develop a coping plan. The coping plan differs between anxiety disorders and individuals based on personal concerns. AB results from ingrained beliefs that monitoring threat is important.

Focusing on characteristics of SAD, the cognitive-behavioural model of anxiety proposed by Rapee and Heimberg (1997) outlines how social anxiety is maintained, highlighting individuals' fear of negative evaluation and their dependence on positive appraisal from others. During social interactions, socially anxious individuals form a mental image of themselves that incorporates information from long-term memory, internal interoceptive cues and external information. Attentional resources are typically allocated towards self-perceived negative features and external threats, such as audience feedback. At the same time, individuals try to predict the norms or standards they must meet in a given social situation. If the self-image created falls short of these standards, there is a heightened risk of negative evaluation, leading to increased anxiety with associated physiological, cognitive and behavioural symptoms. This, in turn, influences how the individual perceives themselves in the eyes of the audience, perpetuating the cycle of social anxiety.

Similarly, the cognitive model of social phobia proposed by Clark and Wells (1995) posits that social anxiety stems from negative past experiences that lead individuals to believe that they will behave unacceptably and experience negative consequences, such as rejection from others. Thus, individuals present cognitive, somatic, affective and behavioural defensive changes upon entering a social situation. These changes become further signals of danger and maintain or exaggerate anxiety. With regard to attentional processes, this model highlights the importance of self-focused attention and avoidance of eye contact, which can be interpreted as attentional avoidance. Attention is assumed to turn inwards towards heightened physiological sensations and self-evaluative thoughts, interfering with the ability to process social cues and leading to errors in social behaviour. These errors can become interpreted as failures, resulting in new negative learning experiences that perpetuate social anxiety.

Summary Based on the preceding discussion, it appears that current models do not fully converge regarding their assumptions about specific AB that contribute to anxiety and SAD in particular. However, there is a common thread among them, which is the presence of vigilance towards threat, particularly at early stages of processing. On the other hand, elements such as difficulty in disengaging from threat and attentional focus to internal stimuli are more contentious and are only included in some models. For instance, the models of Beck and Clark, Eysenck et al., Bar-Haim et al. and Rapee and Heimberg propose that difficulty in disengaging from threat is a significant factor in anxiety. In contrast, Williams et al. highlight attentional avoidance in trait anxiety, similar to the model proposal by Mogg and Bradley.

Numerous studies support the overall perspective of these models by demonstrating that anxious individuals exhibit threat-related biases, including those with SAD, who tend to pay more attention to socially threatening information, such as signs of disapproval from others, and internal threat stimuli. While there is some evidence for the less common biases proposed by these models, such as difficulty in disengaging from threat and attentional avoidance, further research is necessary to reconcile these models and elucidate the stages of processing during which each type of AB occurs.

Evidence for Attentional Biases in Anxiety

Empirical evidence supports the role of attentional biases in the development and maintenance of anxiety disorders, including SAD, in accord with cognitive models of anxiety (Beard 2011). However, the precise attentional processes underlying AB effects remain unclear, and the most important processes involved in the maintenance of social anxiety are still being described. It has also been noted that AB likely occurs dynamically within individuals, over the duration of the task, rather than at an individual difference level (MacLeod et al. 2019).

Attentional Vigilance Hypervigilance is the 'preference' for the allocation of attention to threatening stimuli (Bögels and Mansell 2004; Cisler and Koster 2010). It received the most consistent and robust support (with a low to medium effect size of $d = .45$, based on meta-analytic findings of 172 studies; Bar-Haim et al. 2007), in both clinical and subclinical samples with anxiety (Mogg and Bradley 2002), even at very brief, pre-conscious presentations of threat stimuli (Mathews and MacLeod 1986; Mogg and Bradley 2002), using a variety of tasks and across anxiety disorders (Cisler and Koster 2010). This conclusion has been challenged, however, by a recent meta-analysis in clinical anxiety and PTSD, including 13 studies and 1005 participants, which found no evidence of AB towards threat (Kruijt et al. 2019). The study used data from only dot-probe task, the reliability of which has been questioned.

Attentional Disengagement According to some theorists, early vigilance to threat, during the first 200 ms of stimulus presence, is normal and adaptive, found in both high and low anxious individuals (Moriya and Tanno 2011). It is the difficulty in disengagement from threat, after the first 200 ms that is characteristic of anxious individuals, and in fact some have suggested that it is the only AB that differentiates anxiety (Amir et al. 2003; Fox et al. 2001). According to Derryberry and Reed (2002), difficulty in disengagement is moderated by individual's differences in attentional control, which is the capacity for effortful regulation of attention, involving focus or shifting, in contrast to less voluntary, automatic, pre-attentive processes (Derryberry & Rothbart, 1988). Trait-anxious individuals high in attentional control could more easily disengage attention from threat at 500 ms than trait-anxious individuals with poor attentional control (Derryberry and Reed 2002). Moriya and Tanno (2011) suggested that socially anxious individuals show difficulty in disengagement after 300 ms of stimulus presentation and that the effect is specific to SAD and not due to comorbid depression or trait anxiety.

Evidence for difficulty in disengagement from threat in SAD have been found using the Posner task (e.g. Amir et al. 2003; McGlade et al. 2020), such that socially anxious individuals were significantly slower to find the invalidly cued targets (when the probe appeared in a different location than the cue) than controls only when the probe followed a social threat word (Amir et al. 2003). The use of other tasks has led to similar conclusions but less consistently. For example, Delchau et al. (2020) found no evidence of difficulty in disengagement with the dot-probe task, whereas the effect was found using eye-tracking by Lazarov et al. (2021). Similarly, Schofield et al. (2012) using eye-tracking during a dot-probe task found that social anxiety was related to AB towards emotional faces and difficulty in disengagement from threatening faces, at later stages of stimulus presentation.

Vigilance-avoidance hypothesis Despite the strong support of hypervigilance effects in anxiety, some studies have found the opposite results, showing attentional avoidance, where attention is directed away from threatening stimuli, especially at later stages of stimulus presentation (Cisler et al. 2009; Cisler and Koster 2010; Mogg et al. 2004), although the exact timeframes remain unclear (Boettcher et al. 2013). For example, Koster et al. (2005) found that trait-anxious individuals present vigilance at 100 ms in comparison with low trait-anxious individuals. However, at 200 ms and 500 ms, they presented a tendency to avoid the threatening stimulus.

In general, at a shorter threat presentation, e.g. 500 ms, trait-anxious individuals (and socially anxious ones; Garner et al. 2006; Mansell et al. 1999; Mühlberger et al. 2008) show vigilance to threat, but at 1500 ms or longer, they typically avoid these stimuli (e.g. Koster et al. 2005, 2006). However, a recent systematic review and meta-analysis using eye-tracking found some evidence for early vigilance (1000 ms) but also attentional avoidance of emotional pictures (either negative or positive) during the same timeframe (Günther et al. 2021).

The vigilance-avoidance hypothesis was proposed to reconcile such findings (Mogg et al. 2004) and suggests that attention is initially and pre-consciously allocated to searching for threat, e.g. a frowning face, and that once the danger is detected it is subsequently avoided. Avoidance during conscious stages of processing may perpetuate anxiety, as it interferes with habituation or reappraisal of the danger as more threatening than it actually is (Bögels and Mansell 2004; Clark and Wells 1995).

Moderating Factors

State Anxiety The inconsistent findings regarding the precise nature of AB in SAD may also be due to methodological features of the different studies, including the manipulation of state anxiety, for example, using public speaking stressors. Although socially anxious people are characterized by trait anxiety, the presence of state anxiety during the experimental task may increase the likelihood that certain AB effects emerge. For example, Garner et al. (2006) and Mühlberger et al. (2008) used eye-tracking with high and low socially anxious individuals who completed the dot-probe task after being informed that they would give a public speech. Socially anxious participants demonstrated initial vigilance to all emotional faces regardless of expression, but they also spent less time looking at the emotional faces compared to low socially anxious individuals, showing evidence of avoidance. Such results suggest that avoidance is especially characteristic of SAD when state stress is present.

Task Type The type of task used to assess AB may also have an influence on results. Common tasks include the visual search task (e.g. Öhman et al. 2001; Rinck et al. 2003), which assesses vigilance to threat, as faster response times to detect a threat among neutral stimuli compared to detecting a neutral stimulus among neutral stimuli. It also measures difficulty in disengagement as slower detection of a neutral stimulus among threatening stimuli compared to detecting a threatening stimulus among neutral stimuli. This is because threatening stimuli have a tendency to capture attention.

The spatial cueing task or Posner task (Fox et al. 2001; Posner 1980) requires participants to focus on a point between two rectangles. One of the rectangles is highlighted, or a threatening stimulus is displayed in it owed by a target stimulus in the position of one of the rectangles. Participants have to identify the rectangle where the target stimulus was shown. Attentional bias is present when individuals respond more quickly to rectangles where a threatening, rather than a neutral stimulus, was previously presented. Difficulty in disengagement is when individuals respond more slowly to invalidly cued responses (the stimulus was not presented after the threatening cue) relative to valid cues (the stimulus is presented after the threatening cue).

The modified Stroop task (Stroop 1935) presents threatening or neutral words in different colours, requiring participants to name the colour of the word while ignoring its meaning. AB is indicated when participants take longer to name the colour of threatening compared to neutral words, as it is assumed that the emotional aspects of the stimulus grasp and maintain attention. However, effects can also be attributed to emotional reactions, cognitive avoidance or mental preoccupation, and these confounding explanations have led to criticism of the emotional Stroop task (Bögels and Mansell 2004).

MacLeod et al. (1986) developed the dot-probe paradigm, the most commonly used task in the field of AB. Its advantages over the Stroop task include simultaneous presentation of the two stimuli, selective attention to one of the stimuli, measurement of AB with reaction time and the ability to measure attentional avoidance (Bögels and Mansell 2004). For SAD, facial expressions are typically used rather than words as stimuli, which is considered a more ecologically valid approach, as faces represent a primary social threat (Öhman 1986).

While several studies have demonstrated the validity of the dot-probe task (e.g. Bar-Haim et al. 2007), other studies have raised concerns about their split-half and test-retest reliability (Schmukle 2005; Staugaard 2010). Recent studies have also reported low reliabilities of it (Price et al. 2014; Waechter et al. 2014; Waechter and Stolz 2015), although larger split-half reliability coefficients were found when clinical samples were used (Bar-Haim et al. 2010). Similarly, relatively good reliabilities were reported by Enock et al. (2014) using a smart-phone delivery of the dot-probe task, but there was disagreement as to the interpretation of these findings (Waechter and Stolz 2015; Rodebaugh et al. 2016).

To overcome these limitations, researchers have suggested using eye-tracking, which provides a direct and continuous measure of visual attention and is ecologically valid as it is not based on individuals' subjective experience (Bögels and Mansell 2004; Chen et al. 2012; Schofield et al. 2012). Eye-tracking can provide four different types of attentional indices, including the proportion and latency of the first fixations, the proportion of fixation frequencies and the proportion of viewing time for the emotional stimuli in comparison to neutral (Calvo and Avero 2005;

Gamble and Rapee 2010; Garner et al. 2006; Hermans et al. 1999). The reliability of eye-tracking indices varies, with the proportion of fixation frequencies and viewing time showing high reliability ($\alpha > .8$) over a 5000 ms duration, while the reliability of the first fixation indices within 1500 ms is relatively low (Waechter et al. 2014). Unfortunately, despite its advantages over the other methods discussed, eye-tracking has not been used extensively due to technical issues and time constraints, but advances in technology are making it more feasible for use in future studies (Jacob and Karn 2003).

Attention Bias Modification Treatment Effectiveness and Mechanisms of Change

An attention bias modification treatment (ABMT) protocol aims at reducing automatic vigilance towards threat, presumed to result in anxiety reduction. The most commonly used task in ABMT is the dot-probe task, where the attention system is trained through implicit learning and repetition (Bar-Haim 2010) to focus more on neutral stimuli by presenting response targets consistently after neutral and not threat stimuli. To date there seem to be mixed results about the effectiveness of ABMT for social anxiety, although meta-analytic findings tend to support its efficacy for anxiety disorders more broadly, and evidence is overall highly promising.

A meta-analysis of 12 randomized controlled trials of ABMT for anxiety (one study with socially anxious, two studies with generalized anxious participants) concluded that this treatment has a medium effect size, which is promising ($d = 0.61$; Hakamata et al. 2010; Linetzky et al. 2015). Specifically, clinician ratings for the intervention group showed improved anxiety with a significant medium effect size ($d = 0.42$). Nonetheless, the effect on self-reported anxiety measures was less promising. Similar results were obtained in a meta-analysis by Price et al. (2016) for anxiety disorders (76% SAD, 13% generalized anxiety and 11% other anxiety disorders) who found that young age (<37 years), receiving training in the laboratory and relying on clinician assessment were significant moderators of treatment effectiveness. Dennison (2018) found that ABMT is efficient for reducing anxiety and indicated that age, method of training (computer vs Internet) and location of training were not significant moderators of treatment effectiveness, in contrast to Price et al. With regard to clinical vs subclinical symptoms, it seems that these groups do not differ for between-group analyses, but a clinical population gives larger effect sizes for within-group analyses. A recent study that compared ABMT vs SSRI and wait-list controls found a significant and equivalent improvement in SAD scores for both active treatments and improvement in attention biases only for the ABMT group (Arad et al. 2023).

There are, however, a small number of studies that did not support the effectiveness of ABMT, but their results may be explainable by methodological limitations. Bunnell et al. (2013) found no differences between the groups with regard to self-report, clinician interview and behavioural measures of social anxiety following ABMT. However, they did not assess pre- and post-intervention AB, and the sample was small. Maoz et al. (2013) examined the efficacy of a subliminal AB intervention on a student sample, finding no improvement on AB or self-reported social anxiety. The negative result may be due to the low baseline AB of the sample and the idiosyncratic task used. Additionally, Neophytou and Panayiotou (2022) in a sample of non-treatment-seeking college students with SAD found no changes in social anxiety after ABMT. Half of the participants presented low baseline AB, and from the remaining almost half presented vigilance and half avoidance. Low AB baseline levels and a non-treatment-seeking population might explain the negative results. It may be that participants with limited attentional biases towards threat do not present with gains in comparison to control groups (Amir et al. 2011), and level of pre-training bias predicts treatment outcome (Aday and Carlson 2017). In support of this conclusion, an fMRI study in combination with the usage of a dot-probe task found that socially anxious individuals with more left amygdala activation at baseline, which is related to vigilance to threat, had greater symptom reduction post-treatment regardless of the training condition (Britton et al. 2014).

Furthermore, it appears that ABMT delivered through the Internet, i.e. without therapist contact (e.g. Boettcher et al. 2012, 2013; Carlbring et al. 2012; Neubauer et al. 2013), showed less effectiveness that when it was delivered in the clinic, perhaps because effectiveness in the context of the clinic was mostly found on clinician-administered measures. It is also possible that participants in the Internet-based intervention who were in the relaxing context of their home were less state-anxious, another potential moderator of effectiveness. Based on a similar rationale, Kuckertz et al. (2014) compared Internet-based AMBT from Carlbring et al. (2012) with Internet-based delivery of ABMT plus activation of state anxiety to Internet-delivered cognitive-behavioural therapy (iCBT). Results showed that Internet ABMT+state anxiety was superior to Internet ABMT-only and the same as iCBT. Higher initial AB was a significant moderator of anxiety reduction.

Despite the overall positive results on the effectiveness of ABMT in reducing anxiety, the precise mechanisms of change remain to be determined. Klumpp and Amir (2010) hypothesized that if ABMT works by training disengagement from threat, then anxiety reduction would only be observed in the attention training away from threat condition. However, if the mechanism of change is improved attentional control, then anxiety reduction should be observed in both training conditions. This study overall supported that ABMT works by improving attentional control, but further research is needed to provide more evidence.

Heeren et al. (2011) investigated the effects of training towards both positive and threat stimuli and found that the group trained towards positive stimuli showed reduced levels of social anxiety. These results suggest that ABMT may be effective by reducing vigilance towards threat or by facilitating disengagement from it through training towards non-threatening stimuli. In contrast, Boettcher et al. (2013) found anxiety reduction in the group that was trained towards threat. While this finding was initially explained by changes in attentional control, it may also be due to the reduction of attentional avoidance through repeated exposure to threat.

Conclusion

Attention biases are a dominant component of many theories of anxiety, including social anxiety, and for the most part, data support the presence of these biases and their role in anxiety maintenance, even though the specific biases that characterize each anxiety disorder need to be further specified. Finding ways to address these biases, through brief computerized interventions, may be an efficient and promising path towards treatment of anxiety disorders that offers multiple benefits, including a limited need of therapists, reduction of drop-out and hesitation to receive therapy, easy accessibility and reduced cost. Although ABMT studies overall show a significant treatment effectiveness, some studies found limited or no effect of this treatment (e.g. Boettcher et al. 2013; Bunnell et al. 2013), which may be attributable to moderating factors or methodological issues that deserve consideration, including the level of attentional biases at baseline and the modality of treatment delivery which it is probably related to the levels of state anxiety present. Most importantly, it is unclear how ABMT works and specifically which attentional processes change after the intervention. Proposed mechanisms of ABMT effectiveness are vigilance to threat and difficulty in disengagement from threat. Moreover, effects of this treatment may be related to exposure towards threatening faces and reductions in attentional avoidance, or increased attention control, a hypothesis that needs to be studied further. The treatment is highly promising, addresses a well-defined target and is easy to subject to rigorous evaluation. For these reasons, further research into ABMT may be an important clinical investment.

References

Aday, J., & Carlson, J. M. (2017). Structural MRI-based measures of neuroplasticity in an extended amygdala network as a target for attention bias modification treatment outcome. *Medical hypotheses*, *109*, 6–16.

Albano, A. M., & DiBartolo, P. M. (2007). *Cognitive–behavioral therapy for social phobia in adolescents, stand up, speak out: therapist guide* (1st edition). Oxford University Press.

American Psychiatric Association: Diagnostic and Statistical Manual of Mental Disorders, Fifth Edition. Arlington, VA, American Psychiatric Association, 2013.

Amir, N., Elias, J., Klumpp, H., & Przeworski, A. (2003). Attentional bias to threat in social phobia: facilitated processing of threat or difficulty disengaging attention from threat?. *Behaviour research and therapy*, *41*(11), 1325–1335.

Amir, N., Taylor, C. T., & Donohue, M. C. (2011). Predictors of response to an attention modification program in generalized social phobia. *Journal of consulting and clinical psychology, 79*, 533–541.

Arad, G., Azriel, O., Pine, D. S., Lazarov, A., Sol, O., Weiser, M., ... & Bar-Haim, Y. (2023). Attention bias modification treatment versus a selective serotonin reuptake inhibitor or waiting list control for social anxiety disorder: a randomized clinical trial. American Journal of Psychiatry, 180(5), 357–366.

Bar-Haim, Y. (2010). Research review: attention bias modification (ABM): a novel treatment for anxiety disorders. *Journal of Child Psychology and Psychiatry*, *51*(8), 859–870.

Bar-Haim, Y., Holoshitz, Y., Eldar, S., Frenkel, T. I., Muller, D., Charney, D. S., Pine, D. S., Fox, N. A., & Wald, I. (2010). Life-threatening danger and suppression of attention bias to threat. *Life, 167*(6).

Bar-Haim, Y., Lamy, D., Pergamin, L., Bakermans-Kranenburg, M. J., & van IJzendoorn, M. H. (2007). Threat-Related Attentional Bias in Anxious and Nonanxious Individuals: A Meta-Analytic Study. *Psychological Bulletin, 133,* 1–24.

Barlow, D. H., & Durand, V. M. (2000). *Ψυχοπαθολογία και παθολογική συμπεριφορά: Μία σύνθετη βιοψυχοκοινωνική προσέγγιση* (1ος τόμος). Εκδόσεις ΕΛΛΗΝ.

Beard, C. (2011). Cognitive bias modification for anxiety: current evidence and future directions. *Expert review of neurotherapeutics, 11,* 299–311.

Beck, A. T., & Clark, D. A. (1997). An information processing model of anxiety: Automatic and strategic processes. *Behaviour research and therapy, 35*(1), 49–58.

Bögels, S. M., & Mansell, W. (2004). Attention processes in the maintenance and treatment of social phobia: hypervigilance, avoidance and self-focused attention. *Clinical psychology review, 24*(7), 827–856.

Britton, J. C., Suway, J. G., Clementi, M. A., Fox, N. A., Pine, D. S., & Bar-Haim, Y. (2014). Neural changes with Attention Bias Modification (ABM) for anxiety: A randomized trial. *Social cognitive and affective neuroscience*, nsu141.

Brown, O., Wells. J. E., & Magnus, M. A. (2006). Twelve–month and lifetime health service use in Te Rau Hinengaro: the New Zealand Mental Health Survey. *Australian and New Zealand Journal of Psychiatry, 40,* 855–864.

Boettcher, J., Berger, T., & Renneberg, B. (2012). Internet-based attention training for social anxiety: a randomized controlled trial. *Cognitive Therapy and Research, 36*(5), 522–536.

Boettcher, J., Leek, L., Matson, L., Holmes, E. A., Browning, M., MacLeod, C., ... & Carlbring, P. (2013). Internet-based attention bias modification for social anxiety: a randomised controlled comparison of training towards negative and training towards positive cues. *PLoS One, 8*(9), e71760.

Bunnell, B. E., Beidel, D. C., & Mesa, F. (2013). A randomized trial of attention training for generalized social phobia: does attention training change social behavior?. *Behavior therapy, 44*(4), 662–673.

Calvo, M. G., & Avero, P. (2005). Time course of attentional bias to emotional scenes in anxiety: Gaze direction and duration. Cognition & Emotion, 19(3), 433–451.

Carlbring, P., Apelstrand, M., Sehlin, H., Amir, N., Rousseau, A., Hofmann, S. G., & Andersson, G. (2012). Internet-delivered attention bias modification training in individuals with social anxiety disorder-a double blind randomized controlled trial. *BMC psychiatry, 12*(1), 66.

Chen, N. T. M., Clarke, P. J. F., MacLeod, C., & Guastella, A. J. (2012) Biased Attentional Processing of Positive Stimuli in Social Anxiety Disorder: An Eye Movement Study. *Cognitive Behaviour Therapy, 41,* 96–107.

Clark, D. M., & Wells, A. (1995). A cognitive model of social phobia. *Social phobia: Diagnosis, assessment, and treatment, 41*(68), 00022–3.

Cisler, J. M., Bacon, A. K., & Williams, N. L. (2009). Phenomenological Characteristics of attentional biases toward threat: a critical review. Cognitive therapy and research, 33, 221–234.

Cisler, J. M., & Koster, E. H. W. (2010). Mechanisms of attentional biases towards threat in anxiety disorders: an integrative review. *Clinical psychology review, 30,* 203–216.

Clarke, P. J. F., MacLeod, C., & Guastella, A. J. (2013). Assessing the role of spatial engagement and disengagement of attention in anxiety-linked attentional bias: a critique of current paradigms and suggestions for future research directions. *Anxiety, Stress, & Coping, 26,* 1–19.

Cuijpers, P., & Schuurmans, J. (2007). Self–help interventions for anxiety disorders: an overview. *Current Psychiatry Reports, 9,* 284–290.

Delchau, H. L., Christensen, B. K., O'Kearney, R., & Goodhew, S. C. (2020). What is top-down about seeing enemies? Social anxiety and attention to threat. *Attention, Perception, & Psychophysics, 82,* 1779–1792.

Dennison, Travis D. (2018). A Meta-Analysis Examining Attention Bias Modification Treatment and the Reduction of Psychological Distress (Doctoral dissertation, Pacific University). Retrieved from: https://commons.pacificu.edu/spp/1297.

Derryberry, D., & Rothbart, M. K. (1988). Arousal, affect, and attention as components of temperament. *Journal of personality and social psychology, 55*(6), 958.

Derryberry, D., & Reed, M. A. (2002). Anxiety-related attentional biases and their regulation by attentional control. *Journal of abnormal psychology, 111*(2), 225.

Dewit, D. J., Ogborne, A., Offord, D. R., & MacDonald, K. M. (1999). Antecedents of the risk of recovery from DSM-IIIR social phobia. *Psychological Medicine, 29,* 569–582.

Enock, P. M., Hofmann, S. G., & McNally, R. J. (2014). Attention bias modification training via smartphone to reduce social anxiety: A randomized, controlled multi-session experiment. *Cognitive therapy and research, 38*(2), 200–216.

Eysenck, M. W., Derakshan, N., Santos, R., & Calvo, M. G. (2007). Anxiety and cognitive performance: attentional control theory. *Emotion, 7*(2), 336.

Fox, E., Russo, R., Bowles, R., & Dutton, K. (2001). Do threatening stimuli draw or hold visual attention in subclinical anxiety? Journal of Experimental Psychology: General, 130, 681−700.

Gamble, A. L., & Rapee, R. M. (2010). The time-course of attention to emotional faces in social phobia. *Journal of behavior therapy and experimental psychiatry, 41*(1), 39–44.

Garner, M., Mogg, K., & Bradley, B. P. (2006). Orienting and maintenance of gaze to facial expressions in social anxiety. *Journal of Abnormal Psychology, 115*(4), 760.

Griffiths, K. M., & Christensen, H. (2007). Internet–based mental health programs: A powerful tool in the rural medical kit. *Australian Journal of Rural Health, 15,* 81–87.

Günther, V., Kropidlowski, A., Schmidt, F. M., Koelkebeck, K., Kersting, A., & Suslow, T. (2021). Attentional processes during emotional face perception in social anxiety disorder: A systematic review and meta-analysis of eye-tracking findings. *Progress in Neuro-Psychopharmacology and Biological Psychiatry, 111,* 110353.

Hakamata, Y., Lissek, S., Bar-Haim, Y., Britton, J. C., Fox, N. A., Leibenluft, E., Monique, E., & Pine, D. S. (2010). Attention bias modification treatment: a meta-analysis toward the establishment of novel treatment for anxiety. *Biological psychiatry, 68*(11), 982–990.

Heeren, A., Lievens, L., & Philippot, P. (2011). How does attention training work in social phobia: disengagement from threat or re-engagement to non-threat?. *Journal of Anxiety Disorders,* 25(8), 1108–1115.

Hermans, D., Vansteenwegen, D., & Eelen, P. (1999). Eye movement registration as a continuous index of attention deployment: data from a group of spider anxious students. Cognition & Emotion, 13(4), 419–434.

Jacob, R. J., & Karn, K. S. (2003). Eye tracking in human-computer interaction and usability research: Ready to deliver the promises. *Mind, 2*(3), 4.

Kessler, R. C., Chiu, W. T., Demler, O., Merikangas, K., & Walters, E. E. (2005). Prevalence, severity, and comorbidity of 12–month DSM–IV disorders in the National Comorbidity Survey Replication. *Archives of General Psychiatry, 62,* 617–627.

Kessler, R. C., Stein, M. B., & Berglund, P. (2014). Social phobia subtypes in the National Comorbidity Survey.

Klumpp, H., & Amir, N. (2010). Preliminary study of attention training to threat and neutral faces on anxious reactivity to a social stressor in social anxiety.*Cognitive Therapy and Research, 34*(3), 263–271.

Koster, E. H., Crombez, G., Verschuere, B., Van Damme, S., & Wiersema, J. R. (2006). Components of attentional bias to threat in high trait anxiety: Facilitated engagement, impaired disengagement, and attentional avoidance. *Behaviour research and therapy, 44*(12), 1757–1771.

Koster, E. H., Verschuere, B., Crombez, G., & Van Damme, S. (2005). Time-course of attention for threatening pictures in high and low trait anxiety. *Behaviour research and therapy, 43*(8), 1087–1098.

Kruijt, A. W., Parsons, S., & Fox, E. (2019). A meta-analysis of bias at baseline in RCTs of attention bias modification: No evidence for dot-probe bias towards threat in clinical anxiety and PTSD. *Journal of abnormal psychology, 128*(6), 563.

Kuckertz, J. M., Gildebrant, E., Liliequist, B., Karlström, P., Väppling, C., Bodlund, O., ... & Carlbring, P. (2014). Moderation and mediation of the effect of attention training in social anxiety disorder. *Behaviour research and therapy, 53,* 30–40.

Lazarov, A., Basel, D., Dolan, S., Dillon, D. G., Pizzagalli, D. A., & Schneier, F. R. (2021). Increased attention allocation to socially threatening faces in social anxiety disorder: A replication study. *Journal of affective disorders*, *290*, 169–177.

Linetzky, M., Pergamin-Hight, L., Pine, D. S., & Bar-Haim, Y. (2015). QUANTITATIVE EVALUATION OF THE CLINICAL EFFICACY OF ATTENTION BIAS MODIFICATION TREATMENT FOR ANXIETY DISORDERS. *Depression and anxiety*, *32*(6), 383–391.

MacLeod, C., Grafton, B., & Notebaert, L. (2019). Anxiety-linked attentional bias: is it reliable?. *Annual review of clinical psychology*, *15*, 529–554.

MacLeod, C., Mathews, A., & Tata, P. (1986). Attentional bias in emotional disorders. *Journal of abnormal psychology*, *95*(1), 15.

Mansell, W., Clark, D. M., Ehlers, A., & Chen, Y. P. (1999). Social anxiety and attention away from emotional faces. *Cognition & Emotion*, *13*(6), 673–690.

Maoz, K., Abend, R., Fox, N. A., Pine, D. S., & Bar-Haim, Y. (2013). Subliminal attention bias modification training in socially anxious individuals. *Frontiers in human neuroscience*, *7*.

Mathews, A., & MacLeod, C. (1986). Discrimination of threat cues without awareness in anxiety states. Journal of abnormal psychology, 95(2), 131.

Matthews, A., & Mackintosh, B. (1998). A cognitive model of selective processing in anxiety. *Cognitive Therapy and Research, 22,* 539–560.

McGlade, A. L., Craske, M. G., & Niles, A. N. (2020). Temporal trends in attention disengagement from social threat as a function of social anxiety. *Journal of Behavior Therapy and Experimental Psychiatry*, *68*, 101529.

Mogg, K., & Bradley, B. P. (1998). A cognitive-motivational analysis of anxiety. *Behaviour Research and Therapy, 36,* 809–848.

Mogg, K., & Bradley, B. P. (2002). Selective orienting of attention to masked threat faces in social anxiety. Behaviour research and therapy, 40(12), 1403–1414.

Mogg, K., Bradley,B., Miles, F., & Dixon, R. (2004). Brief report time course of attentional bias for threat scenes: testing the vigilance-avoidance hypothesis. *Cognition and emotion*, *18*(5), 689–700.

Moriya, J., & Tanno, Y. (2011). The time course of attentional disengagement from angry faces in social anxiety. *Journal of behavior therapy and experimental psychiatry*, *42*(1), 122–128.

Mühlberger, A., Wieser, M. J., & Pauli, P. (2008). Visual attention during virtual social situations depends on social anxiety. *CyberPsychology & Behavior*, *11*(4), 425–430.

Neophytou, K., & Panayiotou, G. (2022). Does attention bias modification reduce anxiety in socially anxious college students? An experimental study of potential moderators and considerations for implementation. *Plos one*, *17*(2), e0264256.

Neubauer, K., von Auer, M., Murray, E., Petermann, F., Helbig-Lang, S., & Gerlach, A. L. (2013). Internet-delivered attention modification training as a treatment for social phobia: a randomized controlled trial. *Behaviour research and therapy*, *51*(2), 87–97.

Öhman, A. (1986). Face the beast and fear the face: Animal and social fears as prototypes for evolutionary analyses of emotion. *Psychophysiology*, *23*(2), 123–145.

Ohman, A. (1996). Preferential preattentive processing of threat in anxiety: Preparedness and attentional biases. In R. M. Rapee (Ed.), Current controversies in the anxiety disorders New York: Guilford Press.

Öhman, A., Flykt, A., & Esteves, F. (2001). Emotion drives attention: Detecting the snake in the grass. Journal of Experimental Psychology: General, 130, 466–478.

Pergamin-Hight, L., Naim, R., Bakermans-Kranenburg, M. J., van IJzendoorn, M. H., & Bar-Haim, Y. (2015). Content specificity of attention bias to threat in anxiety disorders: a meta-analysis. *Clinical psychology review*, *35*, 10–18.

Posner, M. I. (1980). Orienting of attention. Quarterly Journal of Experimental Psychology, 32, 3–25.

Price, R. B., Kuckertz, J. M., Siegle, G. J., Ladouceur, C. D., Silk, J. S., Ryan, N. D., ... & Amir, N. (2014). Empirical Recommendations for Improving the Stability of the Dot-Probe Task in Clinical Research.

Price, R. B., Greven, I. M., Siegle, G. J., Koster, E. H., & De Raedt, R. (2016). A novel attention training paradigm based on operant conditioning of eye gaze: Preliminary findings. Emotion, 16(1), 110.

Rapee, R. M., & Heimberg, R. G. (1997). A cognitive-behavioral model of anxiety in social phobia. *Behaviour research and therapy*, *35*(8), 741–756.

Rinck, M., Becker, E. S., Kellermann, J., & Roth, W. T. (2003). Selective attention in anxiety: Distraction and enhancement in visual search. Depression and Anxiety, 18, 18–28.

Rodebaugh, T. L., Scullin, R. B., Langer, J. K., Dixon, D. J., Huppert, J. D., Bernstein, A., ... & Lenze, E. J. (2016). Unreliability as a threat to understanding psychopathology: The cautionary tale of attentional bias. *Journal of Abnormal Psychology*, *125*(6), 840.

Schneier, F. R., Johnson, J., Horning, C. D., Liebowitz, M. R., & Weissman, M. M. (1992). Social Phobia Comorbidity and Morbidity in an Epidemiologic Sample. *Archives of General Psychiatry, 49*, 282–288.

Schofield, C. A., Johnson, A. L., Inhoff, A. W., & Coles, M. E. (2012). Social anxiety and difficulty disengaging threat: Evidence from eye-tracking. *Cognition & emotion*, *26*(2), 300–311.

Schmukle, S. C. (2005). Unreliability of the dot probe task. *European Journal of Personality: Published for the European Association of Personality Psychology*, *19*(7), 595–605.

Shechner, T., Britton, J. C., Perez-Edgar, K., Bar-Haim, Y., Ernst, M., Fox, N. A., Leibenluft, E., Pine, D. S. (2012). Attention biases, anxiety, and development: Toward or away from threats or rewards? *Depression and Anxiety, 29*, 282–294.

Staugaard, S. R. (2010). Threatening faces and social anxiety: a literature review. *Clinical psychology review*, 30(6), 669–690.

Stein, M. B., & Kean, Y. M. (2000). Disability and Quality of Life in Social Phobia: Epidemiologic Findings. *American Journal of Psychiatry, 157 (10)*, 1606–1613.

Stroop, J. R. (1935). Studies of interference in serial verbal reactions. *Journal of experimental psychology*, *18*(6), 643.

Stuhldreher, N., Leibing, E., Leichsenring, F., Beutel, M. E., Herpertz, S., Hoyer, J., ... & König, H. H. (2014). The costs of social anxiety disorder: The role of symptom severity and comorbidities. *Journal of affective disorders*, *165*, 87–94.

Taylor, C. B., & Luce, K. H. (2003). Computer and internet–based psychotherapy interventions. *Current directions in psychological science, 12*, 18–22.

Titov, N., Andrews, G., Schwencke, G., Drobny, J., & Einstein, D. (2008). Shyness 1: Distance Treatment of Social Phobia over the Internet. *Australian and New Zealand Journal of Psychiatry, 42*, 585–594.

Waechter, S., Nelson, A. L., Wright, C., Hyatt, A., & Oakman, J. (2014). Measuring attentional bias to threat: Reliability of dot probe and eye movement indices. *Cognitive therapy and research*, *38*(3), 313–333.

Waechter, S., & Stolz, J. A. (2015). Trait anxiety, state anxiety, and attentional bias to threat: Assessing the psychometric properties of response time measures. *Cognitive Therapy and Research*, *39*(4), 441–458.

Wells, A., & Matthews, G. (1994). *Attention and emotion: A clinical perspective*. Hillsdale, NJ: Lawrence Erlbaum Associates.

Williams, J. M. G., Watts, F. N., MacLeod, C., & Mathews, A. (1988). *Cognitive psychology and emotional disorders*. John Wiley & Sons.

Wittchen, H. U., Jacobi, F., Rehm, J., Gustavsson, A., Svensson, M., Jönsson, B., ... & Fratiglioni, L. (2011). The size and burden of mental disorders and other disorders of the brain in Europe 2010. *European Neuropsychopharmacology*, *21*(9), 655–679.

Dialogues: Similarities and Differences Between the Psychodynamic Therapy and Cognitive-Behavioural Approaches Regarding Case Conceptualization and Treatment of Anxiety

Georgia Panayiotou and Christos Charis

Psychoanalytic and later psychodynamic traditions (PD) historically preceded behavioural and cognitive-behavioural approaches (CBT). Similarly, several waves of CBT evolved over the years, each one proposing to address the limitations of previous theories and practices. Predictably, the more recent theories were presented as improvements or counter-arguments against the shortcomings of previous traditions, creating an adversarial relationship among proponents of each view. This book discusses various perspectives, within but also outside each of these traditions, based on original reports of experts in each area. The current volume makes no effort to present one view as superior to the other. At the same time, it will make no effort to present an integrative view, as we believe that it is not to the benefit of our patients to promote approaches that have not been put to the test, either empirically or practically, when separate traditions have cumulative evidence to present as to their effectiveness. At a conceptual level, each tradition ought to have the theoretical breadth and depth to encompass most aspects of what the clinician will encounter and that having the need to borrow from other traditions may mark the limits of each perspective. However, what the book does aim for is to present in detail how each tradition conceptualizes and treats anxiety disorders and in doing so to highlight the theoretical constructs and clinical methodologies that may point to similar etiological and maintenance mechanism and to mechanisms of action that bring about positive chance. That is, even when different terminologies, concepts and even aims are presented, the targeted mechanism and produced outcome may share essential similarities. The following sections aim to address these points.

G. Panayiotou
Department of Psychology, Centre for Applied Neuroscience, Nicosia, Cyprus
e-mail: georgiap@ucy.ac.cy

C. Charis (✉)
Private practice for Psychotherapy, Dillenburg, Hessen, Germany
e-mail: christos-charis@outlook.de

C. Charis, G. Panayiotou (eds.), *Anxiety Disorders and Related Conditions*,
https://doi.org/10.1007/978-3-031-56798-8_11

The Psychodynamic Perspective

In this section I (CC) do not limit myself to the anxiety disorders, but I explain some central concepts of psychodynamic psychotherapy that apply to all mental disorders. In doing so, I want to make the basis of the more specific treatment of anxiety disorders more understandable to the reader. Ultimately, the questions here are as follows: (a) how does the psyche function from a psychodynamic point of view or (b) what makes one ill and (c) what works in therapy?

(In the following presentation, I (CC) refer mainly to conflict-related disorders. The description of structural developmental disorders and trauma sequelae would go beyond the scope of this book. Thus, I refer to the relevant literature (e.g. Bateman and Fonagy 2004; Rudolf 2010).)

Central concepts of psychodynamic theory are drive theory and the associated conflicts, affects and defence processes, the unconscious and the significance of experiences with important others (representations) (for details see Benecke 2014):

1. The unconscious in psychoanalysis.

   Freud (1900) argues that the life of the soul is essentially unconscious, and he differentiated different degrees of unconsciousness: processes that are close to consciousness and easily accessible ('preconscious'). These processes can easily enter consciousness by focusing attention. Other mental processes are substantially kept aside. In this context, the term 'dynamic unconscious' was introduced. This expresses the fact that the unconscious contents have a life of their own; they continue to function in order to maintain an inner balance. The 'unconscious mind' is a complex construct in which everything forgotten, repressed and unlived (feelings, thoughts, urges) is kept away from consciousness. It is the result of psychological processing of past experiences (Rudolf 2010; Benecke 2016).
2. Psychoanalytical theory source of drive of motivation and conflict.

   A source of drive (German: 'Triebquelle') is a 'state of arousal in the body' that becomes 'psychically felt' as a desire or need (Freud 1933, p. 530). According to Freud, drives are to be understood as constructs or general principles from which psychological motives emerge, which in turn manifest themselves in the form of desires, needs, fantasies or actions (Benecke 2016). In the meantime, it has become widely accepted that the assumptions of classical psychoanalysis regarding the concept of drives are no longer tenable (Mertens 1994; Benecke 2016). Today, even within psychoanalysis, human motives are essentially seen within an evolutionary biological and evolutionary psychological framework (Benecke 2016). Modern psychoanalytic motivation theory states that the individual has certain basic needs (Benecke 2016):

   (a) Need for secure attachment: a primary object-seeking motivation, seeking love and bonding (Fairbrain 1952; Balint 1966; Bowlby 1969).
   (b) Need for safety: the safety principle is considered a fundamental need of the individual (Sandler 1960) that seeks to control drive impulses that are valued as dangerous.

(c) Need for autonomy and individuation (Erikson 1966; Mentzos 1984).
(d) Need for self-assertion and exploration (Lichtenberg 1991).
(e) Need for sensuality as well as sexual arousal (Lichtenberg 1991).
(f) Need for self-esteem regulation (Kohut 1979).
(g) An important role is attributed to the development of one's own identity (Erikson 1966; Thomä and Kächele 2006).

Freud posited that neuroses are based on psychological forces that are in conflict (Freud 1916–17). More recent theories of psychoanalysis, e.g. OPD 2, also assume unconscious, inner conflicts of an individual. However, these are not necessarily or exclusively drive conflicts. One assumes, as well as traditionally in the analysis, a developmental history: The roots of such conflicts are to be sought in childhood, where external conflicts with nurturers can lead to the 'frowned-upon' desires being unconsciously held (repressed). Since central parts of such a conflict remain unconscious, the conflict cannot be resolved in a healthy way. These conflicts are activated later in life and unfold their pathogenic effect, i.e. the actualisation of the conflict occurs through a triggering situation, often threshold situations (e.g. entry into professional life); the individual gets out of the psychological balance; and intense affects arise, e.g. fear and anger, which contribute to the development of symptoms. To make this clearer, I will give an example here: a patient who, as a child and adolescent, often experiences violent quarrels between his parents and, as a result, is repeatedly afraid for his mother's life because his father, in an alcoholic state, shouts at his mother and sometimes physically harms her, and he learns consequently to be afraid of his anger. He cannot detach himself from his parents against the background of his fears of loss and separation. These relationship experiences lead to the development of pseudo-autonomy (emphasised independence and self-will) in our patient. In this marriage, he has subordinated himself to his wife for a long time and, as he himself reports, put his own autonomy needs on the back burner. When they separate, he suffers panic attacks again. Psychodynamic therapy aims to make the connection between the current stressful experience and old patterns in the patient's life history understandable. The goal is to uncover the patient's unconscious conflict and work through it (working through means working on the conflict repeatedly so that it becomes clear to the patient). The uncovering work on the conflict focuses on affects and works out dysfunctional relationship aspects of the patient together with the patient. By making the patient aware of his dysfunctional relationship design and conflict with the help of therapy today, he can free himself from the burden of the past. In our example, first, the patient becomes aware in therapy that he is panic-stricken by his anger and subsequently suffers panic attacks. With the help of his biography, he can recognise that he has learnt that aggression is dangerous through the frequent and sometimes violent quarrels between his parents. In psychodynamic therapy, it is important to address what has not been experienced and what is longed for or feared. It is also important to deal with real problems of the present and to reorient oneself (a more detailed description of psychodynamic psychotherapy can be found in chapters by Dr. Charis in this book or in more detail in the book of the same name by Rudolf 2010).

3. Representations and transference in psychoanalysis.

   'Representations', a term coined by psychoanalysis, is the consensus today. As a result of interactions with important people from one's own life—real or fantasised interactions—internalised images emerge ('World of representations' Jacobsen 1978). They are formed with the cooperation of defence and regulatory processes. The representations function as a kind of unconscious template, i.e. they are condensations of early affective experiences that are activated in everyday situations. They have a decisive influence on the experience and behaviour of the person concerned. This means they determine the person's perception, interpretation, inner conclusions and expectations and finally also their relational behaviour (Benecke 2016). In other words, one perceives oneself and others from the perspective of representations (self and object representations). These representations are the basis for the so-called transference of psychodynamic therapy.

4. Another important point for research is what works in therapy.

   In psychodynamic psychotherapy, two effective factors have been identified (Benecke 2016; Wöller and Kruse 2018):

   (a) The establishment of a sustainable therapeutic relationship and its use
   (b) The mediation of 'emotional insight' into the patient's unconscious motives, the connections of the symptoms and the patient's experience and actions mainly with the help of interpretations
   (a) A therapeutic relationship takes place on three levels: the real relationship, the transference relationship and the working relationship. The real relationship means the patient's perception of the therapist as a real person. In contrast, the transference relationship: the patient's expectations, hopes and wishes of the therapist based on previous experiences with significant others. The working relationship is dependent on the abilities of both the patient and the therapist (Greenson 2007). A good sustainable therapeutic relationship is an important prerequisite for a successful therapy in all forms of therapy. This is because a patient can engage in therapy all the better if a sustainable working alliance is established. Only then can therapeutic interventions be promising (e.g. Kanfer et al. 2000; Muran and Barber 2010). The influence of the therapeutic relationship on therapy is effective as a moderator and not directly curative (Kazdin 2009). It acts like a good foundation on which the therapeutic interventions take place (Benecke 2016). Each therapist's ability to build a good therapeutic relationship varies from individual to individual (Baldwin et al. 2007). Therefore, suggestions are made in the literature on how to improve the working relationship (Horvarth et al. 2011), and various questionnaires to assess relationship quality have been developed, e.g. Horvath and Greenberg (1989, 'Working Alliance Inventory'); a good working relationship also depends on the therapist's skills (Baldwin et al. 2007). As a result of the relationship offer, i.e. the

therapist's inner attitude and his resulting behaviour, a relationship offer is made to the patient, which in itself has a healing effect. Furthermore, it is ensured that new experiences of the patient in therapy also have a healing effect. This means that the patient has the experience that the therapist does not behave in the same way as his reference persons in his childhood and youth, but in a more loving and caring way (Alexander and French 1946). In this framework, the patient is given the opportunity to have 'corrective experiences' that help change the pathogenic representations stemming from earlier experiences. The patient internalises the care and strategies that the therapist seeks to resolve, conflicts that arise, his handling of impulses and affects and so on (Thomä and Kächele 2006).

(b) The core of psychodynamic interventions is interpretation, which aims to provide emotional insight to the patient. Interpretation requires a lot of tact and a sense for the right moment. An interpretation is most effective when it points to the core relational issue in a way that is understandable to the patient and addresses the conflictual nature of what is happening in the relationship. Examples of interpretations can be found in CC's chapter "Case Study of a 33-Year-Old Patient with a Panic Disorder, an Emetophobia (ICD-10 F 41.0/F 40.2) and a Moderate Depression on the Basis of a Recurrent Depressive Disorder (ICD-10 F 33.1) from Psychodynamic Point of View". Interpretations that are followed by an affect are more likely to have a positive therapeutic effect. They lead to what is called emotional insight (Stigler et al. 2007). Thus, 'insight' is not an intellectual process of understanding contexts. Transference interpretation is done so that the patient recognises that, because of past experiences in important relationships, they have retained fears, expectations, hopes and attitudes beliefs from the past and they direct them towards the therapist today. This shapes or strains the relationship today with significant others (Rudolf 2010). In practice, the patient directs wishes, fantasies and affects to the therapist, which the therapist focuses on in therapy, allowing the patient to become aware of them. In other words, the therapist pays attention to the patient's verbal and non-verbal expressions, asking the question, 'What is the patient trying to tell me with what he is saying right now?' In these expressions, the therapist looks for the patient's fantasies, desires and affects. The therapist's own impulses, fantasies and affects, i.e. the therapist's reactions to the patient, are also taken into account (countertransference analysis). All this reveals the patient's inner world and his conflicts and provides the basis for therapeutic interventions, whereby the patient is patiently invited to deal with his own painful affects (working through) (Milrod et al. 1997; Wöller and Kruse 2018; Benecke 2016). This psychodynamic approach seems to be very well supported based on process outcome research (Benecke 2014).

And here I take the liberty of making a brief supplementary comment to Professor Panayiotou's remarks below regarding the diagnosis in my chapter "Case Study of a 33-Year-Old Patient with a Panic Disorder, an Emetophobia (ICD-10 F 41.0/F 40.2) and a Moderate Depression on the

Basis of a Recurrent Depressive Disorder (ICD-10 F 33.1) from Psychodynamic Point of View". The patient had classic symptoms of panic disorder as described in the diagnostic systems (e.g. DSM-5). In addition, she also had a fear of vomiting ('emetophobia') and strong hypochondriacal fears since childhood. Therefore, the diagnosis of emetophobia was made in addition to the panic disorder on the basis of the present symptoms. In psychodynamic therapy, as I have understood it, it is important to try to find a descriptive diagnosis but more so to try to understand the individual meaning of the symptoms with the patient in order to be able to start therapy regarding these symptoms. However, in therapy we strengthen the patients' ability to introspect to such an extent that they have learnt to pay attention to their 'inner gestures' in the course of the therapy. If they manage to make some progress, they start to recognise connections to their panic attacks, so that the panic attacks no longer cause them so much anxiety. These are the experiences I have had.

To say that what is not measured is disregarded leads to the exclusion of crucial points that contribute to the explanation of symptoms. In my opinion, this is a great loss for practical therapy and also for research. Just because patients are not aware of their feelings does not mean they do not exist. And specifically on the subject of fear of one's own anger, which is repressed against this background, I have seen many patients who had panic attacks out of fear of their own anger, and after we worked on this mental construct of the patient, namely, that anger is not as dangerous as they usually experienced it in their family, e.g. like our patient with her father, this patient was able to allow her anger, as a result of which her panic attacks decreased, completely or partially. And that without psychotropic drugs.

The Cognitive-Behavioural Therapy (CBT) Perspective

Many fundamental CBT theories of anxiety disorders draw from biologically informed and evolutionary views of fear and anxiety (Öhman 1993). Fear and anxiety are conceptualized as basic human emotions that carry an adaptive value. They are closely linked to core motivational systems that initiate defensive responses in the presence of danger, including fight, flight and freeze behaviours, and are therefore necessary for survival (Gray 1991). Fear pertains to imminent danger, while anxiety describes preparation, anticipation and vigilance for dangers anticipated in the future, based on prior learning. For some individuals these responses are exaggerated, sustained or contextually inappropriate and maladaptive. When fear and anxiety occur in the absence of real danger, are disproportionate to the threat or are difficult to control and regulate and cause substantial distress and dysfunction, the person is said to have an anxiety disorder. The causes of these disorders are multifactorial but can in part be attributed to inherited factors, and in part to learning experiences, in accord with a diathesis-stress perspective (Mineka and Zinbarg

2006). Individuals who are at higher risk to develop them often have predispositions such as a propensity for intense, chronic or difficult-to-regulate negative emotions (high neuroticism) and the tendency to be behaviourally inhibited (i.e. show a predominance of withdrawal and avoidance behaviours) and are characterized by high harm avoidance (Papachristou et al. 2018). These temperamental characteristics interact with acquired learning and environmental causes (e.g. traumatic events) to increase the risk for anxiety disorders. Learning that certain things, situations, experiences and emotions are dangerous and to be avoided can come via multiple methods. For example, in addition to transmitting their hereditary temperamental characteristics and genes, the parents of anxious individuals are often themselves anxious and fearful and 'teach' their children vicariously that the world (or particular situations) is dangerous and that avoidant responses should be preferred. Social learning through modelling (Bandura 1962) can take place by observing the fearful responses of others when they are faced with a threatening situation. Classical conditioning processes are also critical in the learning of fear and anxiety responses. Individuals may experience a real traumatic/threatening event and experience an intense surge of fear or a full-blown panic attack (also called a 'true alarm'). This experience can lead to subjective distress and physiological arousal during future encounters with the same or similar situation. Similarly, the individual may experience an unexpected panic attack or intense fear and anxiety in a situation that is not in itself highly threatening, what would be considered a 'false alarm', which also would result in similar fear responses and avoidance in similar situations in the future, through associative learning (Barlow 2000). The association between specific stimuli and anxiety responses is typically operantly reinforced through avoidance or safety behaviours, which prevent the person from experiencing anxiety in the short term (negative reinforcement) but ultimately reinforce the anxiety in the long term (Panayiotou et al. 2014). Additional reinforcement for avoidant, helpless or dependent responses in the presence of feared stimuli or during anxiety episodes can come from what are known as secondary gains (a concept also acknowledged in the psychodynamic tradition). Oftentimes the family and friends of anxious patients will respond to the distress of their loved ones through extra attention, support and care and by facilitating the avoidant behaviours, helping the patient reduce responsibility, stress and effort. These contextual responses can act as additional reinforcers that help maintain anxious and fearful behaviour.

Anxiety disorders represent a classic case where behavioural approaches have been most influential (Emmelkamp 2004). Exposure techniques are a core element of behaviour therapy, cognitive therapies and third-wave approaches like ACT, for all forms of anxiety (but also other disorders where intense emotions or urges are involved, like addictions and eating disorders). Bandelow et al. (2015) found effect sizes of $d = 1.3$ for pre-post exposure therapy improvement for patients with various anxiety disorders. Recent developments in exposure therapy can yield significant effects for, for example, specific phobias, in a single session. Similar, highly effective brief therapies have been designed for other anxiety disorders, e.g., the Bergen program for obsessive compulsive disorder (OCD; Kvale et al. 2018) and somewhat longer panic control treatment for panic disorder (Barlow 1997). Exposure therapy broadly speaking involves the confrontation with the fear/anxiety-eliciting stimulus until the intensity of the response is reduced (Brady and Raines 2009). Exposures are repeated or prolonged, and it is expected that both subjective and physiological fear responses will show reduction both within and between exposure sessions. Exposures can be accomplished in different modalities, for example, in vivo (real-life exposure), in vitro (imaginal exposure) and more recently through virtual reality (VRE). In vivo exposure is known as the most potent version, which sometimes suffers from limitations like the fact that it may re-traumatize the patient if too intense, it may not be easily controlled by the therapist (e.g. the audience's reactions in the treatment of social anxiety) or the situation cannot be easily recreated (exposure to war scenes in post-traumatic stress disorder). For this case, in vitro exposure can be used, while VRE seems to more closely approximate the effects of in vivo treatment (Freitas et al. 2021).

Exposure is typically conducted on the basis of a fear hierarchy, i.e. a collaboratively constructed list of situations that evoke fear and avoidance, which are addressed through exposure in an incremental manner, from less to more intense. Although these are common approaches across anxiety disorders and other conditions, some specific variations are found to be especially suitable for particular disorders, according to some researchers. For example, panic control treatment for panic disorder (with and without agoraphobia) not only includes in vivo exposure for agoraphobic avoidance of situations where panic attacks are anticipated to occur but also includes interoceptive exposure for the panic attacks themselves, where the patient is exposed to the bodily sensations (typically components of the autonomic nervous system response) that trigger fear and set into motion an attack (Barlow 1997). Therefore, the patient is guided through exercises like running in place to increase heart rate, spinning in place to induce dizziness and other activities to induce autonomic-like sensations that the patient fears, in order to produce habituation. In OCD, in addition to response prevention, the patient may be exposed to the content of the disturbing thoughts, for example, by writing them down repeatedly or hearing recordings of them over earphones over and over. In PTSD the emphasis is on gradually filling in the story around the trauma, combating the gaps in memory that are often part of the symptoms and increasing tolerance of the intense associated affect through prolonged exposure (Foa and Rothbaum 1998).

It is typically assumed that extinction is a result of habituation to the prolonged exposure to the threat, without engagement in escape behaviours, also known as safety behaviours. More recently, different sets of processes have been identified as part of extinction, namely, inhibitory learning (Craske et al. 2014). It is assumed that change is a result of new learning, which overrides the strong association between the stimulus and the fear response. Therefore, it is important for the patient to come out of the exposure situation with the knowledge that one's prediction of catastrophic outcomes as a result of contact with the stimulus did not hold and instead one was able to cope and tolerate the distress. Within this framework, it becomes less important that one's fear/anxiety response actually shows a significant decrease during exposure. Aligned with these findings are the claims of cognitive therapies (e.g. Beck 1991), which are a standard part of cognitive-behavioural therapy (CBT), which use behavioural experiments, i.e. deliberate preplanned exposures meant to test the outcomes that the patient predicts, in order to disconfirm cognitive distortions and catastrophizing. The aim again is for the patient to acquire new learning.

Because fear (and erroneous predictions about catastrophic results) may be reinforced if the patient avoids the exposure situation, monitoring safety behaviours (e.g. distraction from the exposure trial) and preventing them from occurring are essential parts of the treatment. In obsessive compulsive disorder, this component is called response prevention, i.e. prohibiting all compulsions from occurring that serve the function of calming anxiety, so that the patient learns that one can tolerate the emotions and the disturbing cognitions or sensations. In social anxiety disorder, self-focused attention and self-directed ruminative thinking form part of avoidance, by turning attention away from the social situation (Aldao et al. 2010). For this reason, attention needs to be monitored, and the patient needs to learn to decrease self-focus in order to be fully present in the social interaction and experience the related discomfort. Because avoidance, escape and safety behaviours can take many forms and shapes, the therapist must be very alert in collaboration with the patient to identify them and reduce them.

Cognitive techniques, in addition to behavioural experiments, include cognitive restructuring, which is the challenging, through Socratic dialogue, of distorted automatic thoughts, specific to a fearful situation, and core beliefs that are stereotypic attitudes that span many different situations. The use of cognitive techniques needs to be considered in terms of cost and benefit, as some patients with anxiety (e.g. in OCD or generalized anxiety) may use the positive restructuring technique as a way to rationalize their fears and experiences and in essence avoid exposure.

CBT Versus Psychodynamic Perspectives in Case Conceptualization and Treatment

To draw comparisons between these two perspectives, we refer to the case presented in chapter "Case Study of a 33-Year-Old Patient with a Panic Disorder, an Emetophobia (ICD-10 F 41.0/F 40.2) and a Moderate Depression on the Basis of a Recurrent Depressive Disorder (ICD-10 F 33.1) from Psychodynamic Point of View" by Dr. Charis. In sum, the patient is a 33-year-old married female with no children, who lives with her older husband, who has a daughter from a previous relationship. The woman is described as having had very close bonds to her family of origin, who were also strictly religious. The patient suffers from panic attacks that apparently started at the age of 17 and occasional depression. The panic attacks started after a stressful period, when the cousins of the patient moved into their home and took over her room, and following a serious rapture of an aneurysm in her father that resulted in him being wheelchair bound. The actual attack took place after the patient observed her cousin vomit in the room. The cousins are described as having had *Salmonella* infection that resulted later in the infection of the patient's father. The patient suffered from various potentially serious illnesses and health problems from an early age and experienced similar problems in her family. The recent precipitant of the recurrence of panic attacks was an episode when the patient herself vomited, and after which the paroxetine dose was reduced. Among the primary therapeutic aims are to reduce panic attacks and discontinue paroxetine treatment that the patient received ever since her first attack.

First of all, at a diagnostic level, some information is unavailable to me as a reader from the brief description provided that would guide DSM-5-based differential diagnosis, such as the frequency and intensity of panic attacks and the severity of other complains, such as the fear of vomiting. It would be important for the clinician in the context of a full history to clarify the details such that alternative diagnostic hypotheses can be evaluated. For example, panic attacks can occur in all forms of anxiety disorders and other conditions (depression) and not just in panic disorder. What is characteristic of panic attacks in panic disorder is that these are experienced as unexpected (out of the blue), and the fear is focused on the bodily symptoms themselves, with catastrophic interpretations of them. The patient typically experiences intense anticipatory anxiety for future unexpected panic attacks and is fearful that they are an indication that the patient is having a heart attack, dying, fainting or losing control. Patients often describe specific autonomic symptoms as being especially disturbing, and often they bring on the rest of the symptoms once they are perceived. Feared and unexpected panic attacks often precipitate the development of agoraphobia (i.e. panic disorder with agoraphobia) where the patient avoids places, experiences, activities and even thoughts that are believed to increase the likelihood of panic occurrence. More information is therefore needed to delineate whether the experienced panic attacks are indeed characteristic of panic disorder or occur exclusively in situations where vomit may be seen or experienced (i.e. emetophobia, an alternative diagnosis suggested by Dr. Charis) or more broadly in situations involving fear of contamination, dirt or even immoral/'dirty' thoughts (i.e. a specific phobia, illness anxiety or OCD). The latter hypothesis can be derived from the family history detailed in chapter "Case Study of a 33-Year-Old Patient with a Panic Disorder, an Emetophobia (ICD-10 F 41.0/F 40.2) and a Moderate Depression on the Basis of a Recurrent Depressive Disorder (ICD-10 F 33.1) from Psychodynamic Point of View" that clearly insinuates the family's strict religious morals, extreme cleanliness behaviours and a punitive, guilt-laden environment that is often characteristic of OCD types of presentations. Also, the patient displays ritualistic hand-washing after her involvement in a motor vehicle accident that triggered emotions of guilt.

Whereas the psychodynamic case conceptualization places a heavy emphasis on interpreting the meaning of the patient's descriptions of her family and relationships, behavioural therapy is focused more on the 'here-and-now', aiming to better understand the precipitants and consequences of current symptoms and maladaptive behaviours. For example, it is common for the onset of panic disorder to occur during a period of increased stress, when autonomic arousal is already at a high baseline. This does not mean that patient descriptions, such as the fact that she is a 'trophy wife' to her husband or that he and her father are the 'rock of the house' are meaningless. With regard to the cognitive component of CBT, these descriptions are important ways of revealing the patient's automatic thoughts and deep-rooted schemas about herself, the world and her future, so that distorted beliefs that shape and sustain her behaviour can be identified (Padesky 1994). Identifying these core beliefs and attempting to make them more consistent with current reality seem to be a common element of the psychodynamic approach described in chapter "Case Study of a 33-Year-Old Patient with a Panic Disorder, an Emetophobia (ICD-10 F 41.0 / F 40.2) and a Moderate Depression on the Basis of a Recurrent Depressive Depression (ICD-10 F 33.1) from Psychodynamic Point of View" and the CBT perspective.

Similarly, the common behaviours between the father and the patient (common symptoms and fears) are recognized as important information from both perspectives. Phobias, anxiety and psychosomatic symptoms, related to intense emotions, primarily of a gastro-intestinal nature, seem to also run in the patient's family and especially her father. From the psychodynamic view, these are interpreted as a sign of poor detachment from the father; in CBT these are seen as indications of potentially shared inherited vulnerabilities and learning of fearful and avoidant responses through modelling and reinforcement. Continuing with further similarities, the conceptualization in chapter "Case Study of a 33-Year-Old Patient with a Panic Disorder, an Emetophobia (ICD-10 F 41.0/F 40.2) and a Moderate Depression on the Basis of a Recurrent Depressive Disorder (ICD-10 F 33.1) from Psychodynamic Point of View" stresses that the patient's 'exploratory behaviour' as a child was reduced, and her dependence on her family members increased because of the many severe health-related issues and stressful home environment (angry paternal outbursts), which resulted in lack of a 'supportive inner ideas of relationships' and poor ability to regulate feelings. CBT would concur that these real threats would easily result in core beliefs that the world is dangerous and that life and somatic integrity can be threatened at any moment by illness. Indeed, both in health anxiety and panic disorder but also in other anxiety conditions, we find a history of family illness. Also, the apparent over-protectiveness of the parents, particularly the father who slept with the patient until the age of 9, a common feature of many anxiety disorders (e.g. generalized anxiety disorder), probably reduced the patient's confidence in her own ability to cope with these challenges and increased her dependence. This continues to date, as her husband apparently takes a similar protective role, which probably reinforces her beliefs about her own abilities and produces secondary gains in relation to her anxieties. Therefore, the patient likely has deficits in adaptive coping skills and emotion regulation and also has not had the opportunity to learn that she can effectively cope with and survive these threats. An inhibitory learning approach to exposure therapy, where the new learning that one can survive these challenges (Craske et al. 2014) is compatible with the necessity to change these perceptions.

A potential difference in the case conceptualizations pertains to the psychodynamic emphasis on the role of repressed anger. The patient is described as angry towards the cousins who moved into the home and also brought infectious diseases, angry against the parents for their rules and for giving her room to the cousins, angry against the mother for making irrational demands and angry against her husband who deprives her of the opportunity to have children. These repressed emotions of fear and anger 'flood' the ego and are presumably expressed through panic attacks. CBT does not typically engage in interpretations that involve constructs that cannot be observed and measured, like repressed emotions. Also, it would be unlikely to conceive of anger as the trigger of an intense fear response (panic), unless one entertains the possibility that anger results in increased physiological arousal, that the patient perceives as threatening due to previous associations with panic, and in turn triggers panic when perceived. This is indeed possible, but overall CBT aims for the principle of parsimony and may not consider the involvement of unobservable emotions as necessary for case conceptualization. To the degree that the patient describes conscious anger towards family members that she has difficulty expressing, the clinician is likely to consider whether the patient lacks assertiveness and emotional expression skills and may engage the patient in therapeutic activities like skills training, role plays and guided practice through homework.

The therapeutic goals of decreasing panic attacks and reducing dependence on medication would be appropriate in both treatment traditions. In CBT reliance on medication could be conceptualized as another safety behaviour. Although SSRIs do have positive effects on anxiety disorders, especially at the acute phase, in the long term, CBT is considered at least equally efficacious. Anxiolytic medications in particular may be counter-indicated as they reduce the intensity of the fear response, making exposure exercises less effective (Otto et al. 2010).

Therapy

Given the conceptualization that the patient has developed deep-rooted beliefs about the degree of dangerousness of the world around her, and her own bodily symptoms, and that she learnt through associative learning that bodily sensations of fear, anxiety and panic (including vomiting) are dangerous and life-threatening, the CBT clinician would proceed with a combination of cognitive and behavioural techniques, depending on the specific diagnosis and symptoms, following detailed assessment and monitoring. In panic disorder treatment, thorough psychoeducation is critical and sometimes enough to bring on significant relief. Once the patient understands the working of the autonomic nervous system during normal fear, the role of anticipatory anxiety and the effects of behaviours like hyper-ventilation and of avoidance and safety behaviours, panic attacks may no longer be experienced as random and unexpected. The patient will come to realize that they are often precipitated by specific thoughts, selective attention to specific sensations and worries and by false associations between situations and bodily experiences and may be able to prevent them through awareness, relaxation exercises and thought restructuring. The knowledge that panic attacks are essentially the same as normal, adaptive fear, but occur at inappropriate times, for specific reasons, and that the body can 'handle them' so that they are extremely unlikely to result in negative consequences like fainting, death or loss of control, is often liberating and hugely comforting. The patient acquires skills to monitor their anxiety and arousal levels, to use relaxation activities, to identify safety behaviours and to tolerate panic symptoms, as something that will come and go without significant consequences. Through exposure exercises, the patient combats agoraphobic avoidance of external situations, and though interoceptive exposure learns to tolerate and control internal physiological symptoms. If additional diagnostic criteria are met, or the symptoms are better explained by a different disorder, then specific modifications to the general treatment will be applied, such as exposure with response prevention for OCD symptoms, behavioural activation for depression and specific exposure exercises for emetophobia. What is less stressed compared to psychodynamic therapy is the interpretation of feelings and fantasies as a way to access inner conflicts, as conflicts, especially unconscious aspects of it, are not considered primary in the case conceptualization. The aim in CBT is to achieve a significant and maintainable change in the context of short treatment (typically 8–15 weekly sessions), to reduce the possibility of dropout and of financial and other burdens. If additional therapeutic goals are identified after the initial primary complaints are addressed, like marital conflict or help with the decision about having a child, additional sessions may be required. However, as the panic/fear of vomiting presentation appears to have played a critical role in this case, reduction of symptoms and improvement in coping, communication and emotion regulation skills may be adequate to address these concerns as well. Nevertheless, given the significant role that the social environment may play in the maintenance of symptoms, in CBT too the effects of therapeutic progress on relationships and vice versa must be carefully monitored. Sometimes, relationships suffer when the patient exits the sick role. At other times, the collaboration of the family is necessary to reduce safety behaviours. In fact, family consultation sessions with the consent of the patient may be necessary in such cases.

In CBT case conceptualization is collaborative (Padesky 2022), and it is important that the patient accepts the theoretical framework of their current symptoms. Also, motivation to engage in the difficult (and frightening) exposure exercises may be needed. The supportive therapeutic relationship is as important to CBT in this direction, as in psychodynamic, or any other form of therapy. In the same way that in chapter "Case Study of a 33-Year-Old Patient with a Panic Disorder, an Emetophobia (ICD-10 F 41.0/F 40.2) and a Moderate Depression on the Basis of a Recurrent Depressive Depression (ICD-10 F 33.1) from Psychodynamic Point of View" the Ithaka poem is presented to showcase the importance of the journey towards the final destination, values clarification exercises and motivational interviewing can be used in CBT. Values clarification helps the patient identify what is important to them, what they want their direction to be in live and why this would make the difficult 'journey' through therapy and the exposure exercises worthwhile. For example, in this case, if it is indeed an important value for the patient to have children and be a good mother, it would make it worthwhile to combat her fear of vomit and contamination to facilitate this ultimately valued life goal.

Concluding Remarks

We hope that the discussion above highlighted the centre tenets of each theoretical approach but also some of the common mechanisms they appear to address. It may also have highlighted their, at points, sharp differences. Anxiety disorders and phobias are common but can cause extreme distress and impact on the quality of life. Psychotherapies are highly effective in addressing them with long-term outcome maintenance and improvement in the quality of life. Irrespective of the tradition, making psychological treatments even more efficacious, accessible to as many patients as possible, reducing dropout and adopting a personalized approach to address the particularities of each person's circumstances, symptom presentation and needs should be the goal of clinical science. The dialogue between different perspectives can be a step in this direction, deepening our understanding of what we do and why we do it.

References

Alexander F. & French T. M. (1946): psychoanalytic therapy: Principles and application. Roland Press. New York.

Aldao, A., Nolen-Hoeksema, S., & Schweizer, S. (2010). Emotion regulation strategies across psychopathology: A meta-analytic review. Clinical Psychology Review, 30, 217–237.

Bandelow, B., Reitt, M., Rover, C., Michaelis, S., Gorlich, Y., Wedekind, D., 2015. Efficacy of treatments for anxiety disorders: a meta-analysis. Int. Clin. Psychopharmacol. 30, 183–192. https://doi.org/10.1097/YIC.0000000000000078.

Bandura, A. (1962). Social learning through imitation.

Baldwin S. A., Wambold B. E. & Imel Z. E., (2007): Untangling in alliance-outcome correlation: Exploring the relative importance of the therapist and patient variability in the alliance. Journal of Consulting Clinical Psychology, 75, 842–852.

Balint M. (1966): Die Urformen der Liebe und die Technik der Psychoanalyse. Klett. Stuttgart.

Barlow, D. H. (2000). Unraveling the mysteries of anxiety and its disorders from the perspective of emotion theory. American psychologist, 55(11), 1247.

Barlow, D. H. (1997). Cognitive-behavioral therapy for panic disorder: current status. Journal of Clinical Psychiatry, 58(2), 32–37.

Bateman A. & Fonagy P. (2004): Psychotherapy for Borderline Personality Disorder. Mentalization. Based Treatment. Oxford University press.

Beck, A. T. (1991). Cognitive therapy: A 30-year retrospective. American psychologist, 46(4), 368.

Benecke C. (2014) Klinische Psychologie und Psychotherapie. Ein integratives Lehrbuch. Kohlhammer. Stuttgart.

Benecke C. (2016) Psychodynamische Therapie und Verhaltenstherapie im Vergleich: zentrale Konzepte und Wirkprinzipien. Vandenhoeck & Ruprecht. Göttingen.

Bowlby J. (1969): Bindung. Eine Analyse der Mutter-Kind-Beziehung. Kinder. München.

Brady, A., & Raines, D. (2009). Dynamic hierarchies: a control system paradigm for exposure therapy. The Cognitive Behaviour Therapist, 2(1), 51–62.

Craske, M. G., Treanor, M., Conway, C. C., Zbozinek, T., & Vervliet, B. (2014). Maximizing exposure therapy: An inhibitory learning approach. Behaviour research and therapy, 58, 10–23.

Emmelkamp, P. M. (2004). Behavior therapy with adults. In Bergin and Garfield's (Eds.) Handbook of psychotherapy and behavior change, 393–446.

Erikson E. H. (1966): Identität und Lebenszyklus. Suhrkamp. Frankfurt am Main.
Fairbrain W. R. (1952): Psychoanalytic studies of the personality. Tavistock/Routledge. London.
Foa, E. B., & Rothbaum, B. O. (1998). Treating the trauma of rape: Cognitive-behavioral therapy for PTSD. Guilford Press.
Freitas, J. R. S., Velosa, V. H. S., Abreu, L. T. N., Jardim, R. L., Santos, J. A. V., Peres, B., & Campos, P. F. (2021). Virtual reality exposure treatment in phobias: a systematic review. Psychiatric Quarterly, 92(4), 1685–1710.
Freud S. (1900): Die Traumdeutung. Band 2/3 in Gesammelte Werke. S. Fischer. Frankfurt am Main.
Freud S. (1916–17): Vorlesungen zur Einführung in die Psychoanalyse. Projekt Gudenberg-De. Edition 16.
Freud S. (1933): Vorlesungen zur Einführung in die Psychoanalyse. Gustav Kiepenheuer. Berlin.
Gray, J. A. (1991). Fear, panic, and anxiety: what's in a name?. Psychological Inquiry, 2(1), 77–78.
Greenson, R. R. (2007) Technik und Praxis der Psychoanalyse. 9 Auflage. Klett – Cotta. Stuttgart.
Horvarth A. O., & Greenberg L. S. (1989): Development and validation of the Working Alliance Inventory. Journal on Counseling Psychology. 36, 223–233.
Horvarth A. O., Del Re A. C., Flückiger C. & Symonds D. (2011): Alliance in individual psychotherapy. Psychotherapy (Chic.) 48, 9–16.
Jacobsen E (1978): Das Selbst und die Welt der Objekte. Suhrkamp. Frankfurt am Main.
Kanfer F. H., Reinecker H., Schmelzer D. (2000): Selbstmanagement-Therapie. Ein Lehrbuch für die Praxis. Springer. Berlin.
Kazdin A. E. (2009): Understanding how and why psychotherapy leads to change. Psychotherapy Research, 19, 418–428.
Kohut H. (1979): Die Heilung des Selbst. Suhrkamp. Frankfurt am Main.
Kvale, G., Hansen, B., Björgvinsson, T., Børtveit, T., Hagen, K., Haseth, S., ... & Öst, L. G. (2018). Successfully treating 90 patients with obsessive compulsive disorder in eight days: the Bergen 4-day treatment. BMC psychiatry, 18, 1–9.
Lichtenberg D (1991): Psychoanalyse und Säuglingsforschung. Springer. Berlin.
Mentzos S. (1984) Neurotische Konfliktverarbeitung. Fischer. Frankfurt am Main.
Mertens W. (1994): Psychoanalyse. Grundlagen, Behandlungstechnik und Anwendung. Kohlhammer. Stuttgart.
Milrod B., Busch F., Cooper A. & Shapiro T. (1997): Manual of Panic Focused Psychodynamic Psychotherapy. American Psychiatric Press. Washington DC.
Mineka, S., & Zinbarg, R. (2006). A contemporary learning theory perspective on the etiology of anxiety disorders: it's not what you thought it was. American psychologist, 61(1), 10.
Muran J. C. & Barber J. P. (2010): The Therapeutic Alliance. An Evidence Based Guide to practice. Guilford Press. New York.
Öhman, A. (1993). Fear and anxiety as emotional phenomena: Clinical phenomenology, evolutionary perspectives, and information-processing mechanisms.
Otto, M. W., McHugh, R. K., & Kantak, K. M. (2010). Combined pharmacotherapy and cognitive-behavioral therapy for anxiety disorders: Medication effects, glucocorticoids, and attenuated treatment outcomes. Clinical Psychology: Science and Practice, 17(2), 91–103. https://doi.org/10.1111/j.1468-2850.2010.01198.x
Padesky, C. A. (1994). Schema change processes in cognitive therapy. Clinical Psychology & Psychotherapy, 1(5), 267–278.
Padesky, C. A. (2022). Collaboration and guided discovery. Cognitive and Behavioral Practice, 29(3), 545–548.
Panayiotou, G., Karekla, M., & Mete, I. (2014). Dispositional coping in individuals with anxiety disorder symptomatology: Avoidance predicts distress. Journal of Contextual Behavioral Science, 3(4), 314–321.
Papachristou, H., Theodorou, M., Neophytou, K., & Panayiotou, G. (2018). Community sample evidence on the relations among behavioural inhibition system, anxiety sensitivity, experien-

tial avoidance, and social anxiety in adolescents. Journal of Contextual Behavioral Science, 8, 36–43.
Rudolf G. (2010): Psychodynamische Therapie. Die Arbeit am Konflikt, Struktur und Trauma. Schattauer. Stuttgart.
Sandler J. (1960): The background of safety. International Review of Psychoanalysis. 41, 352–356.
Stigler M., de Roten Y., Drapeau M., Despland J.-M. (2007): Process research in psychodynamic psychotherapy: a combined measure for accuracy and conflictualiy of interpretations. Schweiz. Arch Neurologie Psychiatrie: 158. 225–232.
Thomä H. und Kächele H. (2006): Lehrbuch der Psychoanalytischen Therapie. Springer. Berlin.
Wöller W. & Kruse J. (2018): Tiefenpsychologisch fundierte Psychotherapie. Basisbuch und Leitfaden. Schattauer. Stuttgart.

Index

C. Charis, G. Panayiotou (eds.), *Anxiety Disorders and Related Conditions*, https://doi.org/10.1007/978-3-031-56798-8

The manufacturer's authorised representative in the EU is Springer Nature Customer Service Centre GmbH, Europaplatz 3, 69115 Heidelberg, Germany. If you have any concerns regarding our products, please contact ProductSafety@springernature.com

Printed and bound by CPI Group (UK) Ltd, Croydon, CR0 4YY
01/10/2026
02225862-0001